Drug Candidates for Allergic Diseases

Drug Candidates for Allergic Diseases

Guest Editor

Luis Manuel Teran

MDPI

Basel • Beijing • Wuhan • Barcelona • Belgrade • Novi Sad • Cluj • Manchester

Guest Editor
Luis Manuel Teran
Department of
Immunogenetics and Allergy
Instituto Nacional de
Enfermedades Respiratorias
Mexico City
Mexico

Editorial Office
MDPI AG
Grosspeteranlage 5
4052 Basel, Switzerland

This is a reprint of the Special Issue, published open access by the journal *Pharmaceuticals* (ISSN 1424-8247), freely accessible at: https://www.mdpi.com/journal/pharmaceuticals/special_issues/allergic_pharmaceutical.

For citation purposes, cite each article independently as indicated on the article page online and as indicated below:

Lastname, A.A.; Lastname, B.B. Article Title. *Journal Name* **Year**, *Volume Number*, Page Range.

ISBN 978-3-7258-6079-1 (Hbk)
ISBN 978-3-7258-6080-7 (PDF)
https://doi.org/10.3390/books978-3-7258-6080-7

Contents

About the Editor

Luis Manuel Teran

Luis Manuel Teran studied medicine at the National Autonomous University of Mexico and undertook his MD in Allergy and Clinical Immunology at the National Institute of Pediatrics, Mexico, and at the University of California, San Diego, USA. His primary interest at the time was the investigation of the effect of allergen challenge on the release of inflammatory mediators in the airways of asthmatic patients. He then went on to pursue a Ph.D. at the University of Southampton, UK. His PhD work focused on establishing the molecular basis that regulates the inflammatory process of this disease, specifically the functions of cytokines and chemokines, including IL-5 and CXCL1, CCL2, CCL3, CCL5, CCL11, CCL24, and CCL26. Numerous drugs were developed to neutralize these inflammatory mediators, with monoclonal antibodies that neutralize IL-5 being the most effective in the treatment of eosinophilic asthma. He was honoured with an award by the National Asthma Campaign, UK, for his outstanding work.

After completing his Ph.D., Prof. Teran received an Alexander von Humboldt Postdoctoral Fellowship award from Germany and worked in the Department of Dermatology at the University of Kiel, Germany. There, he identified several proteins in the supernatant of both lung fibroblasts and airway epithelial cells that exerted either chemotactic (chemokines) or antibiotic activity (defensins). From 2004 to 2012, he was a frequent visitor to the European Molecular Biology Laboratory, supported by the Foundation Alexander von Humboldt. Finally, he established his group at the National Institute of Respiratory Diseases, Mexico.

Preface

This Reprint presents a collection of manuscripts highlighting the impact of novel therapies on allergic diseases including asthma, atopic dermatitis (AD), chronic spontaneous urticaria (CSU), and idiopathic hypereosinophilic syndrome, with featured studies ranging from animal experimental models to human clinical studies. Biologics signify an important breakthrough in allergy management by focusing on specific molecules and pathways related to allergic inflammation, providing a more tailored and effective alternative to traditional therapies. They function by disrupting essential immune responses, including the inhibition of IL-5 and IL-4/IL-13 and TSLP. This collection of manuscripts serves as a helpful resource for researchers, clinicians, and policymakers seeking to advance patient care and enhance outcomes

Luis Manuel Teran
Guest Editor

pharmaceuticals

MDPI

Review

Biologic Therapies for Asthma and Allergic Disease: Past, Present, and Future

Fernando Ramírez-Jiménez , Gandhi Fernando Pavón-Romero, Juancarlos Manuel Velásquez-Rodríguez , Mariana Itzel López-Garza, José Fernando Lazarini-Ruiz, Katia Vanessa Gutiérrez-Quiroz and Luis M. Teran *

Immunogenetics and Allergy Department, Instituto Nacional de Enfermedades Respiratorias Ismael Cosio Villegas, (INER), Mexico City 14080, Mexico
* Correspondence: teranjlm@gmail.com

Abstract: The discovery of the mechanism underlying allergic disease, mouse models of asthma, and bronchoscopy studies provided initial insights into the role of Th2-type cytokines, including interlukin (IL)-4, IL-5 and IL-13, which became the target of monoclonal antibody therapy. Omalizumab, Benralizumab, Mepolizumab, Reslizumab, and Tezepelumab have been approved. These biologicals have been shown to be good alternative therapies to corticosteroids, particularly in severe asthma management, where they can improve the quality of life of many patients. Given the success in asthma, these drugs have been used in other diseases with type 2 inflammation, including chronic rhinosinusitis with nasal polyps (CRSwNP), atopic dermatitis, and chronic urticaria. Like the Th2-type cytokines, chemokines have also been the target of novel monoclonal therapies. However, they have not proved successful to date. In this review, targeted therapy is addressed from its inception to future applications in allergic diseases.

Keywords: asthma; biologic therapies; monoclonal antibodies; cytokines; chemokines

1. Introduction

The discovery of murine T helper 1 (Th1) and T helper 2 (Th2) cell clones has had a high impact on the development of novel therapeutic targets for allergy disease. In 1986 Mossman and Coffman reported that Th1 clones produced interferon (IFN)-y while Th2 clones released IL-4 [1]. Soon after, it was demonstrated that Th2 clones produced IL-5, IL-6, and IL-10 [2]. Th1 clones were involved in helper activity for cell-mediated immunity, while Th2 clones stimulated B-cell development and antibody production. In parallel, the nomenclature of type-2 (T2) cytokines began to be used to describe the immunologic effect of these cytokines [2]. Currently, type-1 cytokines are IFN-y, IL-2, and IL-12 while type-2 cytokines include IL-4, IL-5, IL-6, IL-10, and IL-13. By undertaking bronchoscopy studies, other researchers and we demonstrated that type 2 cytokines are produced in the airways of allergic asthma patients [3–5]. More recently, two specific endotypes, including type 2 high- and low asthma, were described in both allergic and nonallergic eosinophilic asthma, respectively. Allergic asthma involves the production of cytokines such as IL-4, IL-5, and IL-13 produced by the classic Th2 cells, whereas in nonallergic asthma, the airway epithelium release mediators such as thymic stromal lymphopoietin (TSLP) IL-25, and IL-33 upon activation of pollutants or allergens; these cytokines, in turn, activate innate lymphoid cells–type 2 (ILC-2) to release IL-4, IL-5, and IL-13 [6].

The first report of successful therapy with murine monoclonal antibodies in humans was in 1982 in a patient with lymphoma [7], and the first therapeutical murine monoclonal antibody was approved in 1986 for the prevention of kidney transplant rejection. However, it was not until the late 1990s that chimeric monoclonal antibodies were approved and marketed [8]. The development of mAbs has played an important role in the therapy of different disorders, with no exception in the treatment of immune allergic diseases, mainly asthma and skin diseases such as chronic urticaria and atopic dermatitis. Therapeutic mAbs are typically immunoglobulin (Ig) G isotypes; they can be murine (suffix: -omab), chimeric (suffix: -ximab), humanized (suffix: -zumab), or human (suffix -umab) [9].

Asthma has been one of the main objectives in developing mAbs for immunoallergic respiratory diseases; however, the pathophysiology shared between this and other diseases have allowed its use in other conditions, with indications approved by consistent trials. Asthma is a chronic airway disease. It is characterized by variable expiratory airflow limitation and clinically represented by cough, wheezing, shortness of breath, and chest tightness. Asthma is a heterogeneous condition in both children and adults; scientific advances in recent decades have made it possible to understand this heterogeneity, describe disease pathogenesis, and develop new therapeutic strategies, especially in severe diseases [6]. An important molecular mechanism of asthma is type 2 inflammation, which occurs in many but not all patients. The cells involved in type 2 immune response of the airway are Th2 cells, IgE-producing B cells, ILC2s, mast cells, basophils, and eosinophils. This type of inflammation is characterized by the production of interleukin (IL)-4, IL-5, and IL-13, which are produced and released by cells of the adaptive and innate response, such as Th2 and ILC2s, respectively; ILC2 are activated by epithelial damage through the release of TSLP, IL-25, and IL-33 [10].

Soon after the demonstration of the role of Th1 and Th2 cells, a novel family of chemotactic cytokines began to be unraveled, which was named "the chemokines." These cytokines have been subdivided into four subfamilies based on the position of either one or two cysteine residues located near the N-terminus of the protein: CXC, CC, C, and CXXXC. subfamilies that exert their activity through specific chemokine receptors. Among these chemokines, the CCL family attracted [11] the most attention as it exerted potent quimiotactic activity for eosinophils and lymphocytes. Using the endobronchial allergen challenge, we demonstrated that eosinophil-activating CCL chemokines MIP-1α (CCL3), RANTES (CCL5), and MCP-3 (CCL7) were released into the airways of asthmatic patients; levels of these cytokines peaked at 4 h and declined at 24 h [12]. Subsequently, Brown et al. showed that eotaxin-1 (CCL11) also has a similar release; levels of CCL11 peaked at four hours and declined at 24 h after the allergen challenge [13]. Interestingly, our model of asthma using endobronchial challenges demonstrated that IL-5 shows different kinetics of release compared with chemokines [3]. Levels of IL-5 increase gradually in BAL fluid, which peaks 24 h after the challenge, suggesting that IL-5 may maintain lung eosinophilia whereas chemokines may exert biological activity for a shorter time (4-fold lesser length of time). Our IL-5 study was undertaken up to 24 h following an allergen challenge, and it is not known whether IL-5 may be produced locally for a longer period of time.

Chemokines exert their activities by binding chemokine receptors which belong to the G-protein-coupled receptors (GPCRs). These receptors have become one of the most successful therapeutic targets, and they account for approximately one-third of all Food and Drug Administration (FDA)-approved pharmaceutical drugs. Thus, chemokine receptors are promising drug targets in allergy [14]. The chemokine receptor (CCR)3 attracted the most attention since the discovery of chemokines as it is expressed on eosinophils and Th2 lymphocytes and serves as a receptor for CCL5, CCL11, CCL24, and CCL26 [11,15]. Indeed, CCR3-null mice and eotaxin-1 and eotaxin-2 double-knockout mice abolished up to ~99% of allergen-induced airway eosinophilia [15]. Chemokine receptors expressed on Th2 lymphocytes have also been investigated, including CCR4 and CCR8 [14]. CCL17 (TARC) and CCL22 (MDC) are ligands for CCR4, while CCL1 (I-309) binds CCR8, and these three ligands have been associated with asthma [16–18]. The pharmaceutical industry has developed antagonists which also target CCR3, CCR4, and CCR8. For example, GSK developed the molecules GW824575 and GSK2239633, which target CCR3 and CCR4, respectively. However, they did show efficacy in asthma [19]. To date three drugs targeting chemokine receptors have been approved: an anti-CXCR4 antagonist that mobilizes hematopoietic stem cells and is used in oncology (plerixafor), a CCR5 antagonist used for HIV treatment (maraviroc), and a monoclonal-antibody CCR4 antagonist for the treatment of mycosis fungoides or Sézary syndrome (mogamulizumab) [20]. The novel CCR3 antagonist, R321, has been developed, and it is currently under investigation. R321 inhibits G-protein-mediated processes and promotes the endocytosis and degradation of CCR3 [21].

Targeted therapy through mAbs has been focused on mitigating the biological effect of substances produced in type 2 inflammatory response. Here, novel anti-cytokine therapies for asthma and allergy disease are reviewed (Figure 1).

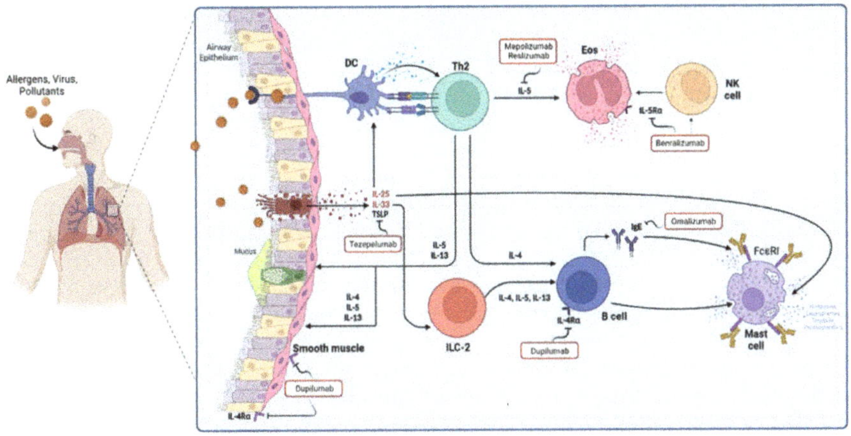

Figure 1. Cells, cytokines, and mediators involved in asthma pathophysiology and the mechanisms of targeted therapy that have been approved in asthma.

2. Omalizumab

Omalizumab (Xolair®, before called rhuMab-E25) is a recombinant humanized monoclonal antibody that binds directly to the Fc portion of the circulating IgE, preventing the activation of mast cells and basophils, and the release of histamine and tryptase, responsible for the clinical symptoms of atopic disease [22,23]. Moreover, by reducing serum-free IgE, Omalizumab downregulates FcεRI expression on mast cells, basophils, dendritic cells, and IgE-CD23 [24]. Omalizumab was first tested in vitro models as well as animal models [25,26]. At the end of the 20th century, the first randomized, double-blind, placebo-controlled clinical trials were carried out in the United States. They showed that Omalizumab decreased corticosteroid consumption compared to placebo. However, statistically significant results were not obtained [27].

Omalizumab for asthma and allergic rhinitis. The first double-blind placebo-controlled randomized clinical trial in asthma was published in 1997. The response to Omalizumab treatment was evaluated in a group of patients diagnosed with mild asthma who had at least one allergic sensitivity (mainly dust mites, cat epithelium, and grasses). A weekly dose of 0.5 mg/kg was administered as a 5-min intravenous infusion for 9 weeks. The main result was the decrease in serum IgE levels within the first doses, as well as the decrease in symptoms (shortness of breath, chest tightness, wheezing, cough, and sputum) in relation to the allergen challenge. However, no difference was shown in lung function tests compared to the control group [28]. In that same year, the first study was carried out to evaluate the effectiveness in the management of allergic rhinitis; 240 patients from 7 different centers in the United States were included, all of them with allergic sensitivity to ragweed. They were divided into five groups with different doses and routes of administration over 12 weeks period. Weekly doses were administered in the first 2 weeks and then biweekly, the safety of this treatment was demonstrated in this trial, and no difference was found in pharmacokinetics properties when administered intravenously or subcutaneously [29]. However, these studies did not show significant differences in control of asthma or rhinitis symptoms compared to control groups. It was until 1999 that the first trial was published in moderate and severe asthma, in patients aged between 11 to 50 years., who required management with inhaled and systemic corticosteroids and in whom allergic sensitivity to at least 2 aeroallergens was proven; the effectiveness of Omalizumab treatment was evaluated in a period of 20 weeks administering a dosage schedule during the first week: on days 0 (half dose), 4 (half dose) and 7 (full dose) with additional biweekly doses, using 2 different treatment schemes: high dose (5.8 mcg/kilogram/ng of Ig/mL) or low dose (2.5 mc/kilogram/ng of IgE/mL), it was reported a 40% difference in symptoms in the low-dose group ($p = 0.005$) and 42% in the high-dose group ($p = 0.008$) compared to control group, also the need for systemic corticosteroids was reduced by 50% and 65% in high-dose group ($p = 0.045$) and low-dose group ($p = 0.11$), respectively; Moreover, a single dose of Omalizumab rapidly reduced serum free IgE serum concentrations by more than 95% [27].

The first trial conducted in Europe (Sweden, Finland, and Norway) was published in 2000. In this study, 251 patients diagnosed with allergic rhinitis sensitive to birch pollen were divided into two treatment groups. In the first one, patients with serum IgE levels less than 150 IU/mL received 300 mg of subcutaneous Omalizumab at weeks 0 and 4 while the second group with serum IgE levels above 150 IU/mL also received 300 mg of subcutaneous Omalizumab over 6 weeks period a (weeks 0, 3 and 6). The safety of this treatment was demonstrated, as well as a decrease in the need for treatment of antihistamine rescue. Moreover, patients having Omalizumab showed a statistically significant difference in symptoms as well as in the quality of life compared to the control group [30]. Similarly, asthmatic children (334 children aged 6 and 12 years) treated with omalizumab significantly reduced the use of a daily dose of inhaled corticosteroids (ICS), and the withdrawal of this medication was greater in those with Omalizumab compared with placebo (55% vs. 39%, respectively; $p = 0.004$) [21]. Serum IgE levels ranged from 30 to 1300 IU/mL; however, following treatment, levels of this immunoglobulin decreased by 95–99% on average [31]. Omalizumab dose was given at 0.016 mg/kg/IgE [IU/mL] per 4 weeks.

The first systematic review by the Cochrane collaboration was published in 2004, which included the results of 8 studies and 2037 patients with a diagnosis of moderate to severe asthma, where a decrease in the need for systemic corticosteroid uses by 50% (OR 2.44, 95% CI 1.93–3.08). Likewise, a lower probability of presenting asthma exacerbation was demonstrated in patients treated with omalizumab (OR 0.47, 95% CI 0.37–0.6) [32].

Omalizumab in other diseases. Omalizumab has proved useful in chronic urticaria. The first series of 3 patients diagnosed with chronic urticaria, with variable levels of serum IgE, who did not improve with conventional treatment, was published in 2007. Chronic spontaneous urticaria (CSU) is defined as the development of wheals, angioedema, or both that last for at least 6 weeks. 50% of these patients have an autoimmune background with either an anti-IgE or anti-IgE receptor triggering the release of histamine; Theoretically, the mechanism by which patients with chronic urticaria can benefit from Omalizumab is due to the decrease in the expression of specific receptors for IgE, so anti-IgE and anti-IgE receptor antibodies cannot trigger their function [33]. The first meta-analysis of randomized clinical trials comparing using omalizumab versus placebo in the management of chronic urticaria showed that patients treated with omalizumab had remission rates, defined as a UAS (urticaria activity score 7) of 0, up to 36% after treatment with doses of 300 mg subcutaneous every 4 weeks for 24 weeks. Likewise, it was shown that there is a safety profile similar to that found in a placebo. (RR, 6.55; 95% CI, 4.17–10.28; $p < 0.00001$) [34]. In the most recent systematic review, it is shown that using omalizumab at a dose of 300 mg every 4 weeks is related to an improvement in quality of life, evaluated by the result obtained by the chronic urticaria quality of life questionnaire. (Mean difference −4.03; 95% CI −5.56 to −2.25) [35].

The administration of omalizumab before the start of allergen-specific immunotherapy in patients with allergic asthma, in whom symptoms persisted after administering optimal doses of inhaled steroid, showed a decrease in allergic reactions induced by allergen-specific immunotherapy, compared with placebo (13.5% vs. 26.2; $p = 0.017$; 95% CI 2.91–22.56%);

Likewise, using Omalizumab increased the rate of patients who reached maintenance dose (87.3% vs. 72.1%, respectively; $p = 0.004$) [36].

Doses and eligibility criteria (Figure 2). The safety and efficacy of Omalizumab have been evaluated, and it has been approved for use in individuals over 6 years of age with a diagnosis of moderate to severe allergic asthma and in whom allergic sensitivity has been demonstrated by an objective method: these patients did not achieve control of their symptoms after management with high-dose of inhaled corticosteroids (ICS) and serum IgE levels between 30–700 IU/mL (in patients older than 12 years) or between 30–1300 IU/mL (in patients 6 to 11 years old) [37]. According to the guidelines published by the global initiative for asthma, the eligibility criteria for this type of therapy in asthma are allergic sensitization (determined by skin prick test or by specific IgE), total serum IgE, and weight within the dose range, and asthma exacerbations during the past year. Likewise, the predictors of good response are serum eosinophils > 260/μL, fraction exhaled nitric oxide (FeNo) > 20 ppb, allergen-driven symptoms, and childhood-onset asthma [38]. The dose of Omalizumab is determined by the serum levels of IgE before biological treatment as well as the weight of each patient, calculated based on 0.016 mg/kg per IU of IgE, with doses for patients older than 12 years between 150–375 mg, subcutaneously every 2–4 weeks, and between 75 and 375 mg every 2 to 4 weeks in patients between 6 and 12 years of age [39].

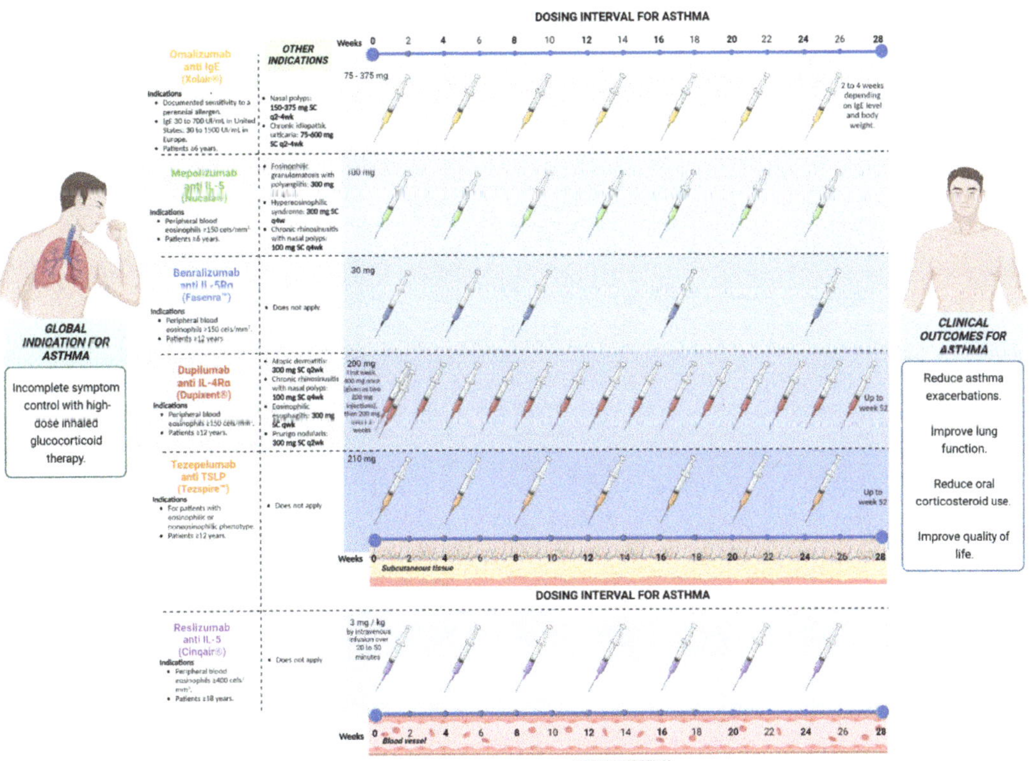

Figure 2. Doses and eligibility criteria of targeted therapy that has been approved for asthma.

3. Mepolizumab

Mepolizumab (Nucala® before called SB-240563) is an N-glycosylated IgG1 (k) antibody that binds to human IL-5 preventing its interaction with the α chain of the IL-5 receptor complex expressed on the cell surface of eosinophils. This cytokine is responsible for the growth, differentiation, activation, recruitment, and survival of eosinophils [40].

Mepolizumab in asthma. The phase 2 trials of Mepolizumab were conducted in early 2002 as a potential treatment for asthma and atopic dermatitis [41]. While in 2000, Leckie et al. demonstrated that a single intravenous infusion of Mepolizumab in patients with allergic asthma reduced the number of circulating blood eosinophils, with suppression maintained over 16 weeks, with no significant effect on the late asthmatic response to allergen challenge or on airway hyperresponsiveness to inhaled histamine [42]. Subsequently, it was demonstrated that Mepolizumab suppresses eosinophils in blood and sputum but did not affect T-cell activation [43]. A significant reduction in bronchial and bone marrow eosinophil counts was seen in patients with mild atopic asthma after three doses of Mepolizumab IV. Additional changes seen in this study include a significant reduction in tenascin thickness, luminal density, procollagen III density, and bronchial mucosal eosinophils expressing Transforming growth factor-beta 1 (TGF-β1) mRNA [44–46].

In 2007, Flood-Page et al. reported the use of three doses of Mepolizumab in subjects with moderate to severe asthma with persistent symptoms despite treatment with ICS reaching a 50% reduction in the exacerbation rates but without significance [47]. It was until 2009 that Haldar et al. associated Mepolizumab with significantly fewer exacerbations of refractory eosinophilic asthma (RR: 0.57; 95% CI, 0.32–0.92; $p = 0.02$) and increased asthma-related quality of life in these patients (mean 0.35%; 95% CI, 0.08–0.52; $p = 0.02$), by suppressing eosinophilic airway inflammation, suggested a causal link with the exacerbations. Nevertheless, there was no significant difference in lung function, asthma symptoms, and FeNO [48]. Nair et al. demonstrated a significant reduction in prednisone use without a clinical exacerbation and a decrease in eosinophil number [49]. In DREAM (Dose Ranging Efficacy and Safety with Mepolizumab) study in severe asthma reported that the use of anti-IL-5 represented an important treatment option in patients with severe eosinophilic asthma [50]. Ortega et al. performed a cluster analysis to identify distinctive characteristics within subgroups of patients included in the DREAM trial. Higher decrease in exacerbations was observed in the patients treated with Mepolizumab and elevated eosinophils. The low airway reversibility was associated with a reduction in exacerbations by 53% in the non-obese compared with obese patients [51]. The route of administration was suggested to influence the response to Mepolizumab. The double-blind study, Mepolizumab as adjunctive therapy in patients with severe asthma (MENSA), demonstrated a reduction by 47% of the exacerbations rate in intravenous administration and by 53% in patients receiving subcutaneous SC, both being significantly ($p < 0.001$) [52]. In another study, Ortega et al. demonstrated that Mepolizumab produced a clinical reduction in the exacerbation rate and an improvement in asthma control and quality of life (measured by SGRQ) in patients with severe eosinophilic asthma who had at least two exacerbations in the previous year and had a baseline blood eosinophil threshold of a minimum of 150 cells/mm^3 [53]. In a randomized, double-blind, placebo-controlled, parallel-group, multicenter, phase 3b trial (MUSCA), Mepolizumab was associated with an important improvement in health-related quality of life, asthma control, lung function, and asthma symptoms [54]. Mepolizumab demonstrated comparable efficacy with Benralizumab, reducing the exacerbations and improving pre-bronchodilator forced expiratory volume in 1 s (FEV$_1$) [55].

In 2018, Henriksen et al., in a systematic review and meta-analysis, reported a significant clinical improvement in exacerbation rate and oral corticosteroids (OCS) reduction with Mepolizumab and Reslizumab equally, besides improvement in FEV$_1$, asthma control and asthma-related quality of life, with no differences between both drugs in efficacy and safety measures [56]. Kelly E. et al. described that the exacerbation events in Mepolizumab treatment were less severe in terms of symptoms and less responsive to prednisolone, associated with a lower induced sputum eosinophil count compared with placebo [57]. In a multicenter, open-label, long-term safety study (COLUMBIA), patients who participated in the DREAM study with severe asthma reported injection-site reactions and headaches [58]. In 2019 Carpagnano et al. reported the efficacy of Mepolizumab in patients with severe uncontrolled asthma and diagnosed bronchiectasis, suggesting that the presence of these could be a criterion to identify an emerging phenotype of severe eosinophil asthma [59].

Claude S. et al. showed the ability of Mepolizumab to improve small airway function, associated with clinical control of the disease [60].

Mepolizumab in other diseases. Mepolizumab function by blocking IL-5 and makes it a candidate to treat various eosinophil-associated disorders. Most investigated are CRSwNP, eosinophilic esophagitis, hypereosinophilic syndrome (HES), eosinophilic granulomatosis with polyangiitis, allergic bronchopulmonary aspergillosis and eosinophilic chronic obstructive pulmonary disease. In 2004, a study demonstrated that anti-IL5 appeared to be safe in 4 patients with manifestations of hypereosinophilic syndromes, suggesting that Mepolizumab may exhibit a steroid-sparing effect in the disease [61]. Consistent with this observation, Roufosse et al. demonstrated that 750 mg of once a month of Mepolizumab produced satisfactory results in HES patients [62]. In phase 3, a randomized, placebo-controlled trial, it was further demonstrated a 50% reduction in HES symptoms during 32 weeks of treatment compared with a placebo [63]. Interestingly, patients treated with 750 mg of Mepolizumab monthly who were receiving topical corticosteroid therapy and had severe, recurrent bilateral nasal polyps showed a significant improvement in efficacy outcomes after 9 weeks of treatment compared with placebo-treated patients [64]. Cavaliere et al. presented a case report associated with an improvement in olfactory capacity after 4 months of treatment [65]. About eosinophilic esophagitis (EoE) is an eosinophilic inflammation of the esophagus. The first trial with Mepolizumab treatment was in 2010, with a significant reduction in esophageal eosinophilia after 4 weeks of Mepolizumab treatment; also reduced the expression of TGF-β1 and tenascin C (TN-C) in the esophageal epithelium after 13 weeks of treatment [66]. However, a systematic review and network meta-analysis that compared the efficacy of six pharmacologic treatments, budesonide suspension, and couscous, fluticasone, esomeprazole, prednisone, Mepolizumab, and placebo, found viscous budesonide, to be the most effective therapy for EoE [67].

Doses and eligibility criteria (Figure 2). According to Global Strategy for Asthma Management and Prevention (GINA) 2022, the doses approved for patients with 12 years and older are 100 mg SC every 4 weeks, and for patients with 6 to 11 years, a dose of 40 mg SC every 4 weeks, both with a minimum of 4 months of treatment. The eligibility criteria vary but usually include the number of severe exacerbations in the last year and blood eosinophils (>150 or >300/m) with a different cut point for patients with OCS. Potential predictors of good response the higher blood eosinophils, higher number of severe exacerbations in previous years, adult-onset asthma, nasal polyposis, maintenance of OCSs at baseline, and low lung function ($FEV_1 < 65\%$ predicted in one study) [38].

4. Reslizumab

Reslizumab (Cinqair®, before SCH55700) is an IgG4/k humanized monoclonal antibody composed of the complementarity-determining regions of a murine antibody to human IL-5. It neutralizes circulating IL-5 by preventing its binding to eosinophils [68].

Reslizumab for asthma. Pre-clinical trials showed that reslizumab inhibited both pulmonary eosinophilia and airway hyperresponsiveness [69]. The first clinical trial was developed in 2003 that showed a decreased blood eosinophils dose-dependently, with a single dose of 1.0 mg/kg—the decrease remained significant up to day 30; a trend toward improvement in baseline FEV_1 was observed too, but no significant changes occurred in other clinical indices of disease activity [69]. In 2011, Castro et al. conducted the first controlled clinical trial in which they identified a phenotype of patients with asthma who benefited from anti–IL-5 therapy. They documented a reduction in eosinophils, and an improved level of asthma control and airway function, particularly in patients with higher ACQ scores and nasal polyps [70].

The same group undertook two clinical trials in phase 3 and reported a significant frequency reduction in asthma exacerbations in patients with asthma and blood counts of eosinophil > 400 cells/μL that receive intravenous Reslizumab (3.0 mg/kg) every 4 weeks for 1 year (RR, 0.50; 95% CI: 0.37–0.67) and (RR, 0.41; 95% CI: 0.28–0.59) in each study (both $p < 0.0001$) compared with those receiving placebo, these studies could show significant changes in FEV_1, Asthma Quality of Life Questionnaire (AQLQ), Asthma Control Questionnaire-7 (ACQ-7), Asthma Symptom Utility Index (ASUI) scores, and blood eosinophil count at 16 and 52 weeks of treatment [71]. One year later, Corren et al. reported the results of another randomized, double-blind, placebo-controlled, phase 3 trial in the United States. They conducted the study in a population with asthma unselected for baseline blood eosinophil counts to determine the impact of baseline eosinophil level on efficacy. It confirmed the benefit lung function of intravenous Reslizumab (3.0 mg/kg) every 4 weeks only in patients with asthma and blood eosinophil counts >400 cells/mL; the subgroup with eosinophils > 400 cells/mL, the treatment with Reslizumab was associated with a significant increase in FEV_1 (0.270 + 0.1320 L, p: 0.0436) compared to the subgroup with eosinophils < 400 (0.033 + 0.0539 L, p: 0.5422), this trial didn't report a significant difference in ACQ-7 and SABA use in both subgroups [72]. An open-label extension study of these phase III trials was reported in 2017. Long-term efficacy and safety were evaluated in moderate-to-severe eosinophilic asthma. Patients received Reslizumab 3.0 mg/kg intravenously every 4 weeks for up to 24 months, patients that previously received placebo were enrolled to receive Reslizumab, FEV_1, and ACQ score had a significant change at 4 and 16 weeks of treatment. However, blood eosinophil counts appeared to be returning to baseline after Reslizumab discontinuation. The most common adverse effect reported was worsening asthma (29%), nasopharyngitis (14%), and respiratory tract infections (10%). There were two drug hypersensitivity reactions reported and two events of drug eruption reported; all were related to other allergen exposure and did not result in discontinuation of Reslizumab, and only 2% discontinued treatment because of adverse events [73].

Doses and eligibility criteria (Figure 2). Reslizumab is indicated in patients aged >18 years with severe eosinophilic asthma uncontrolled dose approved is 3 mg/kg by intravenous infusion every 4 weeks; potential predictors of good response are the same as those recommended for Mepolizumab and Benralizumab [38].

5. Benralizumab

Benralizumab (FasenraTM before called MEDI-563) is a humanized fucosylated Mab recombinant immunoglobulin IgG1K isotype, which binds to the IL-5 with high affinity to the domain 1 of the α-chain of the IL-5 receptor [74,75]. A fucosylation of the oligosaccharide of IgG1 results in an up to 50 times higher affinity to Fcg receptor (FcgR) expressed on natural killer cells, macrophages, and neutrophils [76]. Fucosylation of the Benralizumab enhances the interaction more than 1000 times. Therefore, it can increase the functions of antibody-dependent cell-mediated cytotoxicity [75]. These characteristics may result in a complete depletion of eosinophils in the airway lumen without degranulation of eosinophils [77].

Benralizumab in asthma. It was first described in knockout mice in 2009 by Koike et al., as a strong hIL-5Ralpha neutralizing mAb hIL-5Ralpha that blocks the binding of the IL-5 ligand to its receptor [74]. Evidence for its role in asthma derived from a study showing patients that mild atopic asthmatics giving a single dose from 0.03 mg/kg to 3 mg/kg depleted circulating eosinophils at 24 h, and the effect persisted for at least 2 to 3 months [78]. Laviolette et al. conducted another phase 1 study. It was a multicentered, randomized, double-blinded, and placebo-controlled study from 2008 to 2011 in asthmatics that had a sputum eosinophil count $\geq$2.5%. In this study, there was a reduction in 100% of eosinophils in both sputum and blood in the group of asthmatic patients treated with Benralizumab (1 mg/kg single IV or SC) per day 28 [79].

In a separate study, benralizumab was applied at three different doses (2 mg, 20, and 100 mg) to patients with eosinophilic asthma who were using medium-dose or high-dose inhaled corticosteroids and long-acting β agonists. Interestingly, those patients with benralizumab doses of 20 mg and 100 mg showed lower exacerbations than the placebo group proving its usefulness in adults with uncontrolled eosinophilic asthma [80]. Similar outcomes were presented by Nowak et al., who reported a 49% reduction in exacerbations and hospitalizations rates [81]. The first phase 3a studies, SIROCCO AND CALIMA, showed that Benralizumab given as a 30 mg dose for 4 to 8 weeks for 48 weeks (the first three doses were given every 4 weeks) resulted in improved lung function and fewer exacerbations rates in the 8-week cohort [82,83]. In this phase 3, studies researchers concluded that the effects seemed to be better in patients with blood eosinophilia >300 cells/µL [77]. In contrast, low to medium doses of ICS or low dosage and LABA did not improve significantly in subjects with- or without eosinophilia [73). The first phase 3a studies, SIROCCO AND CALIMA, showed that Benralizumab given as a 30 mg dose every 4 to 8 weeks for 48 weeks (the first three doses were given every 4 weeks) resulted in improved lung function and fewer exacerbations rates in the 8-week cohort [82,83]. These phase 3 studies observed that the therapeutic effects seemed to be better in patients with blood eosinophilia >300 cells/µL [77]. Belralizumab also plays an important role in reducing the use of corticosteroids (OCS). Indeed [73–76], the phase 3a study called ZONDA showed that Benralizumab at 30 mg dose given every 4 to 8 weeks reduced the use of OCS by 75% as compared with a reduction in 25% in the OCS doses in the placebo group [84]. As an add, Blecker and Nair found an improvement in the quality of life assessed with the Asthma Quality of Life Questionnaire for 12 years and older (AQLQ(S) + 12 scores; 0.30, 0.10–0.50; $p = 0.0036$), (95% CI, 0.14 to 0.76 $p = 0.004$) [82–84].

The US Food and Drug Administration (FDA)'s approved Benralizumab in 2017 for the add-on maintenance treatment of patients with severe asthma aged 12 years and older and with an eosinophilic phenotype [77,85]. In 2019, Liu et al. published a meta-analysis about the adverse events of Benralizumab in moderate to severe eosinophilic asthma considering previous studies which described the risk of headache (RR 1.42, 95% CI 1.07–1.87) and pyrexia (RR 2.26, 95% CI 1.32–3.87) was higher in the Benralizumab group. However, there was a reduced risk of serious adverse effects and decreased moderately to severe asthma symptoms [86]. In 2019, the GRECO study reported that Benralizumab was safe for patients who were under treatment administered by themselves or a caregiver at home. Despite this, it was recommended that the first three doses should be applied by the physician's office or with supervision. Only 1.7% of autoinjector administrations were unsuccessful during 28 weeks of treatment (98.3% successful administration; 95% CI: 91.41–99.05) [87]. BORA trial was a 2-year follow-up of the patients enrolled in the SIROCCO and CALIMA studies. It reported no new consequences of long-term eosinophil depletion. The exacerbation rate was (0.48; 95% CI 0.42 to 0.56) and (0.46; 95% CI 0.39 to 0.53) for the 4 and 8 weeks groups, respectively [88]; following the same trend, Korn et al. published in 2021 a 5 year follow up of 345 subjects who were in the SIROCCO, CALIMA, and ZONDA trials, this integrated analysis reported that the adverse events and serious adverse events were stable over the 5 years and did not increase with higher Benralizumab exposure [89].

Benralizumab in other diseases. In recent years, Benralizumab has been used to treat other diseases, such as chronic obstructive pulmonary disease (COPD), and to date, three-phase trials have investigated the impact of Benralizumab on COPD exacerbation rates. Unfortunately, there is no evidence that this treatment can ameliorate exacerbation outcomes for most patients with COPD [90]. In contrast, 30% of patients with polyps treated with Benralizumab no longer required surgery at week 25. Moreover, there was a significant improvement in nasal polyposis severity, visual analog scale score, and endoscopic nasal polyp score [83]. There is not enough evidence that supports Benralizumab as a treatment in patients with no response to antihistamines with chronic spontaneous urticaria. The role of Benralizumab was studied in a small group of patients ($n = 12$) suffering from chronic spontaneous urticaria who were unresponsive to second-generation H1-antihistamines in a 24-week, single-blind study. At the completion of the treatment, symptoms decreased by −15.7 points in the urticaria activity score during a 7-day interval (95% CI, −6.6 to −24.8; $p < 0.001$); only nine patients completed the study, five patients had a very good response, two patients had only a partial response, the rest of the patients showed no improvement. However, a trial in a larger patient population is required [91].

Doses and eligibility criteria (Figure 2). The FDA has approved Benralizumab for the add-on maintenance treatment of patients with severe asthma aged 12 years and older and with an eosinophilic phenotype. It is not indicated for the treatment of any other eosinophilic conditions, including acute bronchospasm relief or status asthmaticus [75]. Step 5 of the GINA main report is established to add-on anti-interleukin/5R treatment (subcutaneous Benralizumab for ages ≥12 years) with severe eosinophilic asthma that is uncontrolled in Step 4 [38]. The recommended dose is 30 mg, administered once every 4 weeks for the first three doses and then once every 8 weeks thereafter by subcutaneous injection into the upper arm, thigh, or abdomen.

6. Dupilumab

Dupilumab (Dupixent® previously called REGN668) is a recombinant IgG4 monoclonal antibody against the IL-4/IL-13 alpha receptor, avoiding the subsequent activation of type-2 inflammation pathways [92,93]. Dupilumab also reduced the expression of genes involved in type 2 inflammation (IL13, IL31, CCL17, CCL18, and CCL26), epidermal hyperplasia (keratin 16 and MKi67), T cells, dendritic cells (ICOS, CD11c, and CTLA4), and TH17/TH22 activity (IL17A, IL-22, and S100As) and concurrently increased expression of epidermal differentiation, barrier, and lipid metabolism genes (filaggrin, loricrin, claudins, and ELOVL3). Additionally, this biological agent suppressed type 2 CCL17, CCL18, periostin, and total and allergen-specific IgE. [94].

Dupilumab in asthma. Several clinical trials have evaluated the efficacy of the anti-IL-4 receptor in asthma at different doses and times (EXPEDITION, P2b, QUEST, VENTURE, and TRANSVERSE). Most clinically evaluated tests include changes in lung function (FEV1), the score of specific quality life questionnaires (ACQ-5 and AQLQ), and/or levels in biomarkers (serum eosinophils and IgE levels) [95]. 200–300 mg of Dupilumab every 2 to 4 weeks were used in most clinical trials [95]. For example, the LIBERTY study evaluated the administration of 200 and 300 mg of Dupilumab applied every 15 days for one year; both dosages reduced the annualized rate of asthma exacerbation and improved around 300 mL of the FEV_1 at week 12 when were compared with the placebo group; these results were maintained even when stratified by eosinophil levels. Likewise, asthma control was better with Dupilumab from the second week, an effect that persisted throughout the entire study [96].

Dupilumab has also been evaluated in 6 to 11 children in a multicenter study with severe asthma. Doses of 100 mg were given if the patient weighed less than 30 kg and 200 mg if heavier, every two weeks for 52 weeks); Dupilumab reduced asthma exacerbations at one year, improved 10% the pre-bronchodilator FEV_1, and reduced inflammatory biomarkers such as Thymus and activation-regulated chemokine (TARC), FENO, and total IgE compared to the placebo group. In addition, patients with anti-IL-4 therapy improved asthma control at 24 weeks. Regarding safety in this group, approximately 10% of patients developed viral upper respiratory tract infections, which was the main adverse reaction [97].

Dupilumab in other diseases. Dupilumab has also been used in moderate-to-severe atopic dermatitis. The SOLO1 and SOLO2 studies enrolled adults from the USA, Europe, and Asia with moderate-to-severe atopic dermatitis whose disease was inadequately controlled by topical steroids. They applied 300 mg of Dupilumab weekly or every two weeks for 16 weeks, and the therapeutic targets were compared versus the placebo group. Both groups showed a reduction in clinical symptoms at 16 weeks, as the extension and severity of atopic eczema by EASI score decreased the pruritus around 3 points of peak score, being these changes notorious from week 2. Patients also reported improvements in pruritus, sleep, symptoms of anxiety or depression, and quality of life. The placebo group had more need for rescue therapy for control of symptoms. Reactions at the injection site and conjunctivitis were more frequent in the Dupilumab groups than in the placebo [98]. Similar results were reported in the LIBERTY AD CHRONOS trial (NCT02260986). This analysis compared dupilumab (300 mg every 2 weeks for 1 year) plus topical steroid versus topical steroid alone. The Dupilumab group had a lower annualized flare rate (78% reduction in annual flare-ups) than the topical steroid group suggesting that Dupilumab can be used as therapy in adults with moderate to severe AD by providing continuous, long-term disease control [99]. To investigate mechanisms mediating the effects of Dupilumab, a transcriptomics analysis of skin biopsies was carried out in atopic dermatitis patients administered 200 mg weakly. Interestingly, Dupilumab significantly reduced the expression of genes associated with Th 2 inflammation (IL13, CCL17, CCL18, CCL26, and IL31), epidermal hyperplasia (keratin 16 and MKi67), T cells, and dendritic cells while increased expression of epidermal differentiation, barrier, and lipid metabolism genes (filaggrin, loricrin, claudins, and ELOVL3). Dupilumab also reduced cellular infiltrates, including CD31 T cells. The changes in gene expression were observed at 4 weeks and even higher at week 16. In contrast, there was no comparable modulation in placebo-treated patients [94].

Patients suffering from CRSwNP require recurring systemic corticosteroid and sinus surgery repeatedly. Two multinational, multicentre, randomized, double-blind, placebo-controlled studies, the LIBERTY NP SINUS-24 and the LIBERTY NP SINUS-52, assessed Dupilumab in adults with severe CRSwNP [93,94]. Dupilumab was given at 200 mg every two weeks for 24 and 52 weeks, diminished nasal congestion and nasal polyp score from week 4 and still improved at week 24. Other clinical and radiographic targets also showed improvement as the Lund MacKay score, or SNOT-22 score [100]. Similar findings have been reported in a study using 300 mg of Dupilumab weekly. There were improved clinical-radiographic outcomes after 16 weeks of treatment in comparison to the placebo. Decreased Th2 inflammation biomarkers were also observed in both nasal secretions and nasal tissue [101].

In the surgical scenario, Dupilumab demonstrated significant improvements in disease signs and symptoms and reduced need for both sinonasal surgery and the use of systemic corticosteroid compared to placebo in patients with severe nasal polyposis, regardless of the use of SCS in the previous 2 years, or previous sinonasal surgery [102]. These findings support the use of adding Dupilumab in patients with severe CRwNP with asthma [103].

The contraindications for the use of Dulipumab include another chronic lung disease, pregnancy, breastfeeding, active parasitic infection, HIV infection or immunosuppression condition, and eosinophils count >1500 cell/mm^3 [104].

Doses and eligibility criteria (Figure 2). Dulipumab is approved in the USA and Europe for treating moderate-to-severe asthma, CRSwNP, and atopic dermatitis [92]. For its prescription in asthma, patients must have ICS at medium or high doses in addition to OCS [104] According to GINA, patients with severe eosinophilic/type 2 asthma are eligible when they have a history of exacerbations in the last year and blood eosinophils > 150 and <1500 cells/µL or FeNO > 25 ppb or taking maintenance oral corticoids. Children 6–11 require a weight-dependent dose and frequency by subcutaneous injection for age >12 years, 200 or 300 mg by subcutaneous injection every 2 weeks for patients with OCSs-dependent severe asthma or concomitant moderate/severe atopic dermatitis, 300 mg by subcutaneous injection every 2 weeks. Patients with chronic rhinosinusitis with polyps should be considered due to the benefits (reduced size of nasal polyps, improved nasal symptoms, and reduced need for OCSs or surgery).

7. Tezepelumab

Tezepelumab (TezspireTM before called AMG157/MEDI9929) is a human anti-TSLP monoclonal immunoglobulin G2λ that binds human TSLP and prevents its interaction with receptor complex. TSLP is an epithelial-cell–derived cytokine that is produced in response to proinflammatory stimuli and drives allergic inflammatory responses through its activity on innate immune cells, including dendritic cells, mast cells, and CD34+ progenitor cells [105,106].

Tezepelumab in asthma. A proof-of-concept, randomized, double-blind, placebo-controlled study demonstrated that Tezepelumab attenuated the early- and late asthmatic responses to allergen challenges in mild allergic asthma patients. In this study, 700 mg of Tezepelumab was given in three monthly doses or placebo intravenously, and allergen challenges were carried out on days 42 and 84 to evaluate the late asthmatic response, as measured 3 to 7 h after the allergen challenge. Indeed, Tezepelumab prevented allergen-induced bronchoconstriction by 34.0% and 45.9% on days 42 and 84, respectively, as determined by the FEV_1 measurements in asthmatics compared with the normal group. In addition, levels of blood- and sputum eosinophils decreased before and after the allergen challenge and in the fraction of exhaled nitric oxide [106].

Additional studies have evaluated the therapeutic effects of Tezepelumab. Corren et al. conducted the phase 2b study PATHWAY, a randomized, placebo-controlled, dose-ranging trial with subcutaneous Tezepelumab in adults with moderate to severe, uncontrolled asthma and a history of exacerbations during the year, and they randomized patients for received low dose (70 mg every 4 weeks), medium dose (210 mg every 4 weeks) or high dose (280 mg every 2 weeks) or of placebo every 2 weeks over 52 weeks. Prebronchodilator FEV_1 was higher in all Tezepelumab groups than in the placebo group; In addition, a reduction in annualized rate of asthma exacerbations was reported: 62% (90% CI: 42–75), 71% (90% CI: 54–82), and 66% (90% CI: 47–79), in low, medium, or high dose Tezepelumab groups, respectively, when was compared to placebo ($p < 0.001$) [107]. A post hoc analysis of data from the PATHWAY phase 2b study reported that treatment with Tezepelumab resulted in clinically meaningful improvements in asthma control; the proportion of ACQ-6 responders (reduction in >0.5 in ACQ-6 total score) and of AQLQ(S)+ 2 responders (increase in overall AQLQ(S) + 12 scores of >0.5), 82% and 77% of tezepelumab-treated patients, respectively, were higher at week 50 compared with 70% and 64% of placebo-treated patients, respectively [108].

Two phase 3, multicentre, randomized, double-blind, placebo-controlled, parallel-group studies were conducted to evaluate the efficacy and safety (NAVIGATOR and SOURCE) of Tezepelumab treatment in patients with severe asthma. NAVIGATOR trial was made in adults and adolescents with uncontrolled asthma with medium- or high-dose inhaled glucocorticoids and at least additional asthma controller medication with or without oral glucocorticoids. Patients received 210 mg of Tezepelumab or placebo subcutaneously every 4 weeks for 52 weeks. Consistent with what has been reported, a reduction in the annualized rate of asthma exacerbations was showed: 0.93 (95% CI: 0.80–1.07) in Tezepelumab-treated patients vs. 2.10 (95% CI: 1.84–2.39) in placebo-treated patients (rate ratio, 0.44; 95% CI, 0.37 to 0.53; $p < 0.001$); in addition, prebronchodilator FEV_1 and ACQ-6, AQLQ + 12, and ASD scores were better in Tezepelumab group [109].

The SOURCE trial was conducted in adults with oral corticoid-dependent asthma to evaluate the effect of Tezepelumab 210 mg administered subcutaneously every 4 weeks on oral corticoid dose reduction; eligible patients must have been receiving a stable dose of 7.5–30 mg prednisone for >1 month. Authors did not observe a significant improvement in OCS dose reduction with Tezepelumab versus placebo in the overall population at week 48; however, when the analysis was performed on subgroups categorized by blood eosinophil counts, Tezepelumab increased the cumulative odds of achieving a category of greater percentage reduction (although not significantly) in daily maintenance oral corticoids (OR, 2.58; 95% CI: 1.16–5.75 and OR, 3.49; 95% CI: 1.16–10.49) in patients with $\geq$150 cells/µL or $\geq$300 cells/µL, respectively, compared with placebo [110].

DESTINATION is an ongoing Phase 3 randomized, double-blind, placebo-controlled trial to assess the long-term safety and tolerability of Tezepelumab over 104 weeks that it is ongoing. The study population comprised patients who completed the 52- and 48-week NAVIGATOR and SOURCE studies, respectively [111].

PATH-HOME is a phase 3, multicenter, randomized, open-label, parallel-group study that enrolled adults and adolescents with severe, uncontrolled asthma to assess the functionality and performance of an accessorized pre-filled syringe (APFS) and an autoinjector (AI) for the administration of Tezepelumab in the clinic and at home. Both devices were effectively employed. Tezepelumab administered via APFS was successful by 91.7% of the participants and via AI by 92.4%. After 24 weeks of treatment, improvements in ACQ-6 score were recorded in 81.1% and 76.2% of the patients in the APFS and AI groups, respectively. Nasopharyngitis was reported as the most common adverse effect (9.3%).

Injection-site reactions occurred in 5.7% (AI) and 0% (AFPS) of the patients [112]. Taken together, these results from phase 2/3 trials suggest that blocking the upstream alarmin TSLP with tezepelumab results in clinically meaningful improvements in asthma control in patients with T2-high asthma concerning exacerbations.

Tezepelumab and another indication. ALLEVIAD is a phase 2a, randomized, double-blind, placebo-controlled study that assesses the effect of subcutaneous Tezepelumab 280 mg or placebo every 2 weeks, plus class 3 topical corticosteroids in severe atopic dermatitis. The primary endpoint was the response rate for a >50% reduction in the Eczema Area and Severity Index (EASI50) at week 12. The treatment difference was not statistically significant (OR, 1.97; 95% IC: 0.90–4.33; $p = 0.091$). However, there was a numerically greater percentage of tezepelumab-treated patients who achieved EASI50 (64.7%) versus placebo-treated (48.2%) [105].

Doses and eligibility criteria (Figure 2). According to the GINA report 2022, the dose approved for Tezepelumab is 210 mg subcutaneously every 4 weeks for patients aged > 12 years with severe asthma. Greater benefits (reduction in severe exacerbations) should be considered in patients with high blood eosinophil or high FeNO. There are no recommendations of benefit in patients with severe asthma who have no evidence of Type 2 inflammation [38]. A systematic review of the EAACI guidelines on the use of biologicals in severe asthma in 2020 evaluated Benralizumab, Dupilumab, Mepolizumab, Omalizumab, and Reslizumab and mentioned a high reduction in severe asthma exacerbations as add-on therapy for patients with severe uncontrolled eosinophilic asthma. Regarding the reduction in the daily dose of OCS, only Benralizumab, Dupilumab, and Mepolizumab showed a reduction compared with the standard of care [113].

8. New Monoclonal Antibodies in Asthma and Other Diseases with Type 2 Inflammation

Itepekimab: IL-33 induces the response of the Th2 adaptive immunity through a complex including the binding of ST2 protein, which is in the membrane of mast cells, basophils, eosinophils, T cells, dendritic cells, ILC2 and NK cells [114]. In vivo trials demonstrated that IL-33 stimulates Th2 cytokine expression, with increased eosinophils levels due to an increase in IL-5 expression and IgE synthesis by IL-4 stimulation, identifying that IL-33 induces gene expression of IL-13 in all tissues, expression of both IL-4 and IL-5 was higher in thymus, spleen, liver, and lung [115]. Itepekimab is a human IgG4P monoclonal antibody against interleukin-33. According to the current nomenclature, it has the infix *-ki-* to refer to its target class (cytokine). In a phase 2 trial, 296 patients with moderate-to-severe asthma were randomly assigned to receive: Itepekimab monotherapy (300 mg subcutaneous), Itepekimab plus Dupilumab (300 mg subcutaneous of each one), Dupilumab monotherapy (300 mg subcutaneous) or placebo every 2 weeks for 12 weeks. Two efficiency endpoints were analyzed, the primary being loss of asthma control; 22% of patients have a loss of asthma control in the Itepikimab group, 27% in the combination group, 19% in the Dupilumab group, and 41% in the placebo group. The OR were calculated comparing each group versus placebo: Itepekimab monotherapy, 0.42 (95% CI, 0.20 to 0.88; $p = 0.02$); combination therapy, 0.52 (95% CI, 0.26 to 1.06; $p = 0.07$); and dupilumab monotherapy, 0.33 (95% CI, 0.15 to 0.70; p value not reported). The secondary endpoint was the change in the prebronchodilator FEV_1 from baseline to week 12. An increase in this was reported in the groups with monotherapy (Itepekimab or Dupilumab) but not in the combination group when compared to placebo [116].

Brodalumab. IL-25 (IL-17E) is produced by bronchial subepithelial mucosa cells, such as basophils, eosinophils, and mast cells, up-regulated their receptors on basophils, inhibiting their apoptosis and promoting their degranulation [117,118]. It has been demonstrated ex vivo that IL-25 is associated with angiogenesis through its effects on the proliferation of endothelial cells and the expression of vascular endothelial growth factor and with airway remodeling, maybe because fibroblasts and smooths muscle cells also express IL-25R, both factors contributing to asthma severity [119]. IL-25 binds to its receptor composed of

IL-17RA and IL-17RB for signal transduction, IL-17RA being the key component used by IL-25. IL-17 family cytokines (IL-17A-17F) play an essential role in various diseases such as autoimmune disorders, of which IL-25 exacerbates allergic inflammation by promoting the production of type 2 cytokines. Brodalumab (AMG 827) is a human anti-IL-17AR immunoglobulin G2 (IgG2) monoclonal antibody that binds to human IL-17RA, blocking IL-25, IL-17A, and IL-17F. In 2013 phase 2a, a randomized, double-blind, placebo-controlled, dose-ranging study evaluated the efficacy and safety of the anti-IL-17 in patients with inadequately controlled moderate to severe asthma, not statistically significant in clinical efficacy on ACQ were observed, neither in lung function nor asthma symptoms [120]. Consequently, further studies are required.

Tralokinumab and lebrokizumab. IL-13 is produced by Th2 cells, this cytokine is responsible for eosinophils proliferation and macrophage activation and induces globet cell hyperplasia, which increases the production of mucus [121]. Tralokinumab and Lebrokizumab are anti-human IL-13 monoclonal antibodies developed for the treatment of severe, uncontrolled asthma [122,123]. Phase 1 studies have shown that intratracheal administration of human IL-13 specifically inhibited IL-13-induced eosinophil recruitment to the lung and suggested the potential for both anti-inflammatory and possible airway remodeling effects [124,125]. Phase II studies also supported the finding that there was an improvement in FEV_1 but didn´t show any improvement in quality of life or reduced asthma exacerbation [126,127], but phase 3 studies didn't show any statistical significance in any of these variables [128–130].

Lirentelimab. It is a monoclonal antibody targeting a sialic acid-binding Ig-like lectin 8, an inhibitory receptor that is a receptor expressed on eosinophils and mast cells. In a phase 2 study, Lirentelimab improved symptoms in adults suffering either eosinophilic gastritis or resistant chronic spontaneous and inducible urticaria [131,132].

9. Conclusions

Over the last few years, biologicals have been used successfully for the treatment of allergic diseases. They can be effective in reducing the severity and frequency of allergic reactions and may be recommended for individuals who have not responded to other types of treatment. The most successful biologic therapies are those that target cytokines regulating the Th2 response. Surprisingly, targeting chemokines that are involved in the allergic response has not been successful. It has been proposed that the redundancy of the chemokine system and insufficient blockade of the receptors in different cell types may be the cause of the failure to develop an efficient anti-chemokine therapy in allergic diseases. In addition, the demonstration that chemokines are released for a shorter period compared with Th2 cytokines such as IL-5 limits their biological effect at the allergic site. Currently, there are novel biologicals under development. The development of novel monoclonal antibodies targeting the type 2 inflammation pathway increases the potential for success in further improving the treatment of allergic diseases and other conditions related to this type of inflammation.

Author Contributions: Conceptualization, F.R.-J. and L.M.T.; methodology, F.R.-J. and L.M.T.; software, G.F.P.-R.; validation, L.M.T.; F.R.-J. and G.F.P.-R.; formal analysis, F.R.-J.; investigation, F.R.-J.; G.F.P.-R.; J.M.V.-R.; M.I.L.-G.; J.F.L.-R.; K.V.G.-Q. and L.M.T.; resources, L.M.T.; data curation, not-applied; writing—original draft preparation, F.R.-J.; G.F.P.-R.; J.M.V.-R.; M.I.L.-G.; J.F.L.-R.; K.V.G.-Q. and L.M.T.; writing—review and editing, F.R.-J.; G.F.P.-R. and L.M.T.; visualization, F.R.-J.; and L.M.T.; supervision, F.R.-J.; and L.M.T.; project administration, L.M.T.; funding acquisition, L.M.T. All authors have read and agreed to the published version of the manuscript.

Funding: This research received no external funding.

Institutional Review Board Statement: Not applicable.

Informed Consent Statement: Not applicable.

Data Availability Statement: Not applicable.

Conflicts of Interest: Authors whose names appear at the beginning of the document do not have affiliations or participation in any organization or entity. There is no financial, personal, or professional interest in any of the topics of study of this manuscript.

References

1. Mosmann, T.R.; Cherwinski, H.; Bond, M.W.; Giedlin, M.A.; Coffman, R.L. Two types of murine helper T cell clone. I. Definition according to profiles of lymphokine activities and secreted proteins. *J. Immunol.* **1986**, *136*, 2348–2357. [CrossRef]
2. Mosmann, T.R.; Coffman, R.L. Heterogeneity of Cytokine Secretion Patterns and Functions of Helper T Cells. *Adv. Immunol.* **1989**, *46*, 111–147.
3. Teran, L.M.; Carroll, M.P.; Shute, J.K.; Holgate, S.T. Interleukin 5 release into asthmatic airways 4 and 24 hours after endobronchial allergen challenge: Its relationship with eosinophil recruitment. *Cytokine* **1999**, *11*, 518–522. [CrossRef]
4. Bentley, A.M.; Hamid, Q.; Robinson, D.S.; Schotman, E.; Meng, Q.; Assoufi, B.; Kay, A.B.; Durham, S.R. Prednisolone Treatment in Asthma: Reduction in the Numbers of Eosinophils, T Cells, Tryptase-only Positive Mast Cells, and Modulation of IL-4, IL-5, and Interferon-gamma Cytokine Gene Expression within the Bronchial Mucosa. *Am. J. Respir. Crit. Care Med.* **1996**, *153*, 551–556. [CrossRef]
5. Bodey, K.J.; Semper, A.E.; Redington, A.E.; Madden, J.; Teran, L.M.; Holgate, S.T.; Frew, A.J. Cytokine profiles of BAL T cells and T-cell clones obtained from human asthmatic airways after local allergen challenge. *Allergy* **1999**, *54*, 1083–1093. [CrossRef]
6. Papi, A.; Brightling, C.; Pedersen, S.E.; Reddel, H.K. Asthma. *Lancet* **2018**, *391*, 783–800. [CrossRef]
7. Miller, R.A.; Maloney, D.G.; Warnke, R.; Levy, R. Treatment of B-Cell Lymphoma with Monoclonal Anti-Idiotype Antibody. *N. Engl. J. Med.* **1982**, *306*, 517–522. [CrossRef] [PubMed]
8. Ecker, D.M.; Jones, S.D.; Levine, H.L. The Therapeutic Monoclonal Antibody Market. In *MAbs*; Taylor & Francis: Milton, UK, 2015; Volume 7, pp. 9–14.
9. Buss, N.A.; Henderson, S.J.; McFarlane, M.; Shenton, J.M.; de Haan, L. Monoclonal antibody therapeutics: History and future. *Curr. Opin. Pharmacol.* **2012**, *12*, 615–622. [CrossRef] [PubMed]
10. Fahy, J.v. Type 2 inflammation in asthma—Present in most, absent in many. *Nat. Rev. Immunol.* **2015**, *15*, 57–65. [CrossRef] [PubMed]
11. Teran, L.M. CCL Chemokines and asthma. *Immunol. Today* **2000**, *21*, 235–242. [CrossRef] [PubMed]
12. Holgate, S.T.; Bodey, K.S.; Janezic, A.; Frew, A.J.; Kaplan, A.P.; Teran, L.M. Release of RANTES, MIP-1α, and MCP-1 into asthmatic airways following endobronchial allergen challenge. *Am. J. Respir. Crit. Care Med.* **1997**, *156*, 1377–1383. [CrossRef] [PubMed]
13. Brown, J.R.; Kleimberg, J.; Marini, M.; Sun, G.; Bellini, A.; Mattoli, S. Kinetics of eotaxin expression and its relationship to eosinophil accumulation and activation in bronchial biopsies and bronchoalveolar lavage (BAL) of asthmatic patients after allergen inhalation. *Clin. Exp. Immunol.* **1998**, *114*, 137–146. [CrossRef] [PubMed]
14. Castan, L.; Magnan, A.; Bouchaud, G. Chemokine receptors in allergic diseases. *Allergy* **2017**, *72*, 682–690. [CrossRef]
15. Fulkerson, P.C.; Fischetti, C.A.; McBride, M.L.; Hassman, L.M.; Hogan, S.P.; Rothenberg, M.E. A central regulatory role for eosinophils and the eotaxin/CCR3 axis in chronic experimental allergic airway inflammation. *Proc. Natl. Acad. Sci. USA* **2006**, *103*, 16418–16423. [CrossRef]
16. Lezcano-Meza, D.; Negrete-Garcia, M.C.; Dante-Escobedo, M.; Teran, L.M. The monocyte-derived chemokine is released in the bronchoalveolar lavage fluid of steady-state asthmatics. *Allergy* **2003**, *58*, 1125–1130. [CrossRef]
17. Sandoval-López, G.; Teran, L.M. TARC: Novel mediator of allergic inflammation. *Clin. Exp. Allergy* **2001**, *31*, 1809–1812. [CrossRef]
18. Montes-Vizuet, R.; Vega-Miranda, A.; Valencia-Maqueda, E.; Negrete-García, M.C.; Velásquez, J.R.; Teran, L.M. CC chemokine ligand 1 is released into the airways of atopic asthmatics. *Eur. Respir. J.* **2006**, *28*, 59–67. [CrossRef]
19. Solari, R.; Pease, J.E.; Begg, M. Chemokine receptors as therapeutic targets: Why aren't there more drugs? *Eur. J. Pharmacol.* **2015**, *746*, 363–367. [CrossRef] [PubMed]
20. Miao, M.; de Clercq, E.; Li, G. Clinical significance of chemokine receptor antagonists. *Expert Opin. Drug Metab. Toxicol.* **2020**, *16*, 11–30. [CrossRef]
21. Grozdanovic, M.; Laffey, K.G.; Abdelkarim, H.; Hitchinson, B.; Harijith, A.; Moon, H.-G.; Park, G.Y.; Rousslang, L.K.; Masterson, J.C.; Furuta, G.T.; et al. Novel peptide nanoparticle–biased antagonist of CCR3 blocks eosinophil recruitment and airway hyperresponsiveness. *J. Allergy Clin. Immunol.* **2019**, *143*, 669–680.e12. [CrossRef]
22. Pennington, L.F.; Tarchevskaya, S.; Brigger, D.; Sathiyamoorthy, K.; Graham, M.T.; Nadeau, K.C.; Eggel, A.; Jardetzky, T.S. Structural basis of omalizumab therapy and omalizumab-mediated IgE exchange. *Nat. Commun.* **2016**, *7*, 11610. [CrossRef]
23. Kawakami, T.; Blank, U. From IgE to Omalizumab. *J. Immunol.* **2016**, *197*, 4187–4192. [CrossRef]
24. Nagata, Y.; Suzuki, R. FcεRI: A Master Regulator of Mast Cell Functions. *Cells* **2022**, *11*, 622. [CrossRef]
25. Shields, R.L.; Whether, W.R.; Zioncheck, K.; O'Connell, L.; Fendly, B.; Presta, L.G.; Thomas, D.; Saban, R.; Jardieu, P. Inhibition of Allergic Reactions with Antibodies to IgE. *Int. Arch. Allergy Immunol.* **1995**, *107*, 308–312. [CrossRef]
26. Coleman, J.W.; Helm, B.A.; Stanworth, D.R.; Gould, H.J. Inhibition of mast cell sensitization in vitro by a human immunoglobulin ε-chain fragment synthesized in Escherichia coli. *Eur. J Immunol.* **1985**, *15*, 966–999. [CrossRef] [PubMed]
27. Milgrom, H.; Fick, R.B., Jr.; Su, J.Q.; Reimann, J.D.; Bush, R.K.; Watrous, M.L.; Metzger, W.J. Treatment of Allergic Asthma with Monoclonal Anti-IgE Antibody. *N. Engl. J. Med.* **1999**, *341*, 1966–1973. [CrossRef]

28. Fahy J v Fleming, H.E.; Wong, H.H.; Liu, J.T.; Su, J.Q.; Reimann, J.; Fick, R.B., Jr.; Boushey, H.A. The effect of an anti-IgE monoclonal antibody on the early- and late-phase responses to allergen inhalation in asthmatic subjects. *Am. J. Respir. Crit. Care Med.* **1997**, *155*, 1828–1834. [CrossRef] [PubMed]
29. Casale, T.B.; Bernstein, I.; Busse, W.W.; LaForce, C.F.; Tinkelman, D.G.; Stoltz, R.R.; Dockhorn, R.J.; Reimann, J.; Su, J.Q.; Jr., Fick, R.B. Use of an anti-IgE humanized monoclonal antibody in ragweed-induced allergic rhinitis. *J. Allergy Clin. Immunol.* **1997**, *100*, 110–121. [CrossRef]
30. Ädelroth, E.; Rak, S.; Haahtela, T.; Aasand, G.; Rosenhall, L.; Zetterstrom, O.; Byrne, A.; Champain, K.; Thirlwell, J.; Della Cioppa, G.; et al. Recombinant humanized mAb-E25, an anti-IgE mAb, in birch pollen–induced seasonal allergic rhinitis. *J. Allergy Clin. Immunol.* **2000**, *106*, 253–259. [CrossRef]
31. Milgrom, H.; Berger, W.; Nayak, A.; Gupta, N.; Pollard, S.; McAlary, M.; Taylor, A.F.; Rohane, P. Treatment of Childhood Asthma With Anti-Immunoglobulin E Antibody (Omalizumab). *Pediatrics* **2001**, *108*, e36. [CrossRef] [PubMed]
32. Walker, S.; Monteil, M.; Phelan, K.; Lasserson, T.; Walters, E. Anti-IgE for Chronic Asthma in Adults and Children. In *Cochrane Database of Systematic Reviews*; Walker, S., Ed.; John Wiley & Sons, Ltd: Chichester, UK, 2004.
33. Spector, S.L.; Tan, R.A. Effect of omalizumab on patients with chronic urticaria. *Ann. Allergy Asthma Immunol.* **2007**, *99*, 190–193. [CrossRef]
34. Zhao, Z.-T.; Ji, C.-M.; Yu, W.-J.; Meng, L.; Hawro, T.; Wei, J.-F.; Maurer, M. Omalizumab for the treatment of chronic spontaneous urticaria: A meta-analysis of randomized clinical trials. *J. Allergy Clin. Immunol.* **2016**, *137*, 1742–1750.e4. [CrossRef] [PubMed]
35. Agache, I.; Rocha, C.; Pereira, A.; Song, Y.; Alonso-Coello, P.; Solà, I.; Beltran, J.; Posso, M.; Akdis, C.; Akdis, M.; et al. Efficacy and safety of treatment with omalizumab for chronic spontaneous urticaria: A systematic review for the EAACI Biologicals Guidelines. *Allergy* **2021**, *76*, 59–70. [CrossRef]
36. Massanari, M.; Nelson, H.; Casale, T.; Busse, W.; Kianifard, F.; Geba, G.P.; Zeldin, R.K. Effect of pretreatment with omalizumab on the tolerability of specific immunotherapy in allergic asthma. *J. Allergy Clin. Immunol.* **2010**, *125*, 383–389. [CrossRef] [PubMed]
37. Krings, J.G.; McGregor, M.C.; Bacharier, L.B.; Castro, M. Biologics for Severe Asthma: Treatment-Specific Effects Are Important in Choosing a Specific Agent. *J. Allergy Clin. Immunol. Pract.* **2019**, *7*, 1379–1392. [CrossRef]
38. Global Initiative for Asthma. *Global Strategy for Asthma Management and Prevention*; GINA: Fontana, WI, USA, 2002. Available online: https://ginasthma.org/ (accessed on 15 November 2022).
39. McGregor, M.C.; Krings, J.G.; Nair, P.; Castro, M. Role of Biologics in Asthma. *Am. J. Respir. Crit. Care Med.* **2019**, *199*, 433–445. [CrossRef]
40. Hart, T.K.; Cook, R.M.; Zia-Amirhosseini, P.; Minthorn, E.; Sellers, T.S.; Maleeff, B.E.; Eustis, S.; Schwartz, L.W.; Tsui, P.; Appelbaum, E.R.; et al. Preclinical efficacy and safety of mepolizumab (SB-240563), a humanized monoclonal antibody to IL-5, in cynomolgus monkeys. *J. Allergy Clin. Immunol.* **2001**, *108*, 250–257. [CrossRef]
41. Golab, J.; Stoklosa, T. Technology evaluation: SB-485232, GlaxoSmithKline. *Curr. Opin. Mol. Ther.* **2005**, *7*, 85–93. [PubMed]
42. Leckie, M.J.; Brinke, A.; Khan, J.; Diamant, Z.; Connor, B.J.O.; Walls, C.M.; Mathur, A.; Cowley, H.; Chung, K.; Djukanovic, R.; et al. Early reports Effects of an interleukin-5 blocking monoclonal antibody on eosinophils, airway hyper-responsiveness, and the late asthmatic response. *Lancet* **2000**, *356*, 2144–2148. [CrossRef] [PubMed]
43. Büttner, C.; Lun, A.; Splettstoesser, T.; Kunkel, G.; Renz, H. Monoclonal anti-interleukin-5 treatment suppresses eosinophil but not T-cell functions. *Eur. Respir. J.* **2003**, *21*, 799–803. [CrossRef]
44. Flood-page, P.T.; Menzies-gow, A.N.; Kay, A.B.; Robinson, D.S.; Cells, B.M. Eosinophil' s Role Remains Uncertain as Anti–Interleukin-5 only Partially Depletes Numbers in Asthmatic Airway. *Am. J. Respir. Crit. Care Med.* **2002**, *167*, 199–204. [CrossRef]
45. Menzies-Gow, A.; Flood-Page, P.; Sehmi, R.; Burman, J.; Hamid, Q.; Robinson, D.S.; Kay, A.; Denburg, J. Anti—IL-5 (mepolizumab) therapy induces bone marrow eosinophil maturational arrest and decreases eosinophil progenitors in the bronchial mucosa of atopic asthmatics. *J. Allergy Clin. Immunol.* **2003**, *5*, 714–719. [CrossRef]
46. Flood-Page, P.; Menzies-Gow, A.; Phipps, S.; Ying, S.; Wangoo, A.; Ludwig, M.S.; Barnes, N.; Robinson, D.; Kay, A.B. Anti-IL-5 treatment reduces deposition of ECM proteins in the bronchial subepithelial basement membrane of mild atopic asthmatics. *J. Clin. Investig.* **2003**, *112*, 1029–1036. [CrossRef] [PubMed]
47. Flood-Page, P.; Swenson, C.; Faiferman, I.; Matthews, J.; Williams, M.; Brannick, L.; Robinson, D.; Wenzel, S.; Busse, W.; Hansel, T.T.; et al. A Study to Evaluate Safety and Efficacy of Mepolizumab in Patients with Moderate Persistent Asthma. *Am. J. Respir. Crit. Care Med.* **2007**, *176*, 1062–1071. [CrossRef] [PubMed]
48. Haldar, P.; Brightling, C.E.; Hargadon, B.; Gupta, S.; Monteiro, W.; Sousa, A.; Marshall, R.P.; Bradding, P.; Green, R.H.; Wardlaw, A.J.; et al. Mepolizumab and Exacerbations of Refractory Eosinophilic Asthma. *N. Engl. J. Med.* **2009**, *360*, 973–984. [CrossRef]
49. Dasgupta, A.; Kjarsgaard, M.; Capaldi, D.; Radford, K.; Aleman, F.; Boylan, C.; Altman, L.C.; Wight, T.N.; Parraga, G.; O'Byrne, P.M.; et al. A pilot randomised clinical trial of mepolizumab in COPD with eosinophilic bronchitis. *Eur. Respir. J.* **2017**, *49*, 1602486. [CrossRef]
50. Pavord, I.D.; Korn, S.; Howarth, P.; Bleecker, E.R.; Buhl, R.; Keene, O.N.; Ortega, H.; Chanez, P. Mepolizumab for severe eosinophilic asthma (DREAM): A multicentre, double-blind, placebo-controlled trial. *Lancet* **2012**, *380*, 651–659. [CrossRef] [PubMed]
51. Analysis, C. Cluster Analysis and Characterization of Response to Mepolizumab. A Step Closer to Personalized Medicine for Patients with Severe Asthma. *Ann. Am. Thorac. Soc.* **2014**, *11*, 1011–1017.

52. Ortega, H.G.; Liu, M.C.; Pavord, I.D.; Brusselle, G.G.; Fitzgerald, J.M.; Chetta, A.; Humbert, M.; Katz, L.E.; Keene, O.N.; Yancey, S.W.; et al. Mepolizumab Treatment in Patients with Severe Eosinophilic Asthma. *N. Engl. J. Med.* **2014**, *371*, 1198–1207. [CrossRef]
53. Ortega, H.G.; Yancey, S.W.; Mayer, B.; Gunsoy, N.B.; Keene, O.N.; Bleecker, E.R.; Brightling, C.; Pavord, I. Severe eosinophilic asthma treated with mepolizumab stratifi ed by baseline eosinophil thresholds: A secondary analysis of the DREAM and MENSA studies. *Lancet Respir.* **2016**, *2600*, 1–8.
54. Chupp, G.L.; Bradford, E.S.; Albers, F.C.; Bratton, D.J.; Wang-Jairaj, J.; Nelsen, L.M.; Trevor, J.L.; Magnan, A.; Brinke, A.T. Efficacy of mepolizumab add-on therapy on health-related quality of life and markers of asthma control in severe eosinophilic asthma (MUSCA): A randomised, double-blind, placebo-controlled, parallel-group, multicentre, phase 3b trial. *Lancet Respir. Med.* **2017**, *5*, 390–400. [CrossRef]
55. Bourdin, A.; Husereau, D.; Molinari, N.; Golam, S.; Siddiqui, M.K.; Lindner, L.; Xu, X. Matching-adjusted indirect comparison of benralizumab versus interleukin-5 inhibitors for the treatment of severe asthma: A systematic review. *Eur. Respir. J.* **2018**, *52*, 1801393. [CrossRef]
56. Henriksen, D.P.; Bodtger, U.; Sidenius, K.; Maltbaek, N.; Pedersen, L.; Madsen, H.; Madsen, L.K.; Chawes, B.L. Efficacy, adverse events, and inter-drug comparison of mepolizumab and reslizumab anti-IL-5 treatments of severe asthma—A systematic review and meta-analysis. *Eur. Clin. Respir. J.* **2018**, *5*, 1536097. [CrossRef] [PubMed]
57. Shrimanker, R.; Pavord, I.D.; Yancey, S.; Heaney, L.G.; Green, R.H.; Bradding, P.; Hargadon, B.; Brightling, C.E.; Wardlaw, A.J.; Haldar, P. Exacerbations of severe asthma in patients treated with mepolizumab. *Eur. Respir. J.* **2018**, *52*, 1801127. [CrossRef] [PubMed]
58. Khatri, S.; Moore, W.; Gibson, P.G.; Leigh, R.; Bourdin, A.; Maspero, J.; Barros, M.; Buhl, R.; Howarth, P.; Albers, F.C.; et al. Assessment of the long-term safety of mepolizumab and durability of clinical response in patients with severe eosinophilic asthma. *J. Allergy Clin. Immunol.* **2019**, *143*, 1742–1751.e7. [CrossRef]
59. Scioscia, G.; Curradi, G.; Foschino, M.P. Severe uncontrolled asthma with bronchiectasis: A pilot study of an emerging phenotype that responds to mepolizumab. *J. Asthma Allergy* **2019**, *12*, 83–90.
60. Farah, C.S.; Badal, T.; Reed, N.; Rogers, P.G.; King, G.G.; Thamrin, C.; Peters, M.J.; Seccombe, L.M. Mepolizumab improves small airway function in severe eosinophilic asthma. *Respir Med.* **2019**, *148*, 49–53. [CrossRef]
61. Garrett, J.K.; Jameson, S.C.; Thomson, B.; Collins, M.H.; E Wagoner, L.; Freese, D.K.; A Beck, L.; A Boyce, J.; Filipovich, A.H.; Villanueva, J.M. Anti-interleukin-5 (mepolizumab) therapy for hypereosinophilic syndromes. *J. Allergy Clin. Immunol.* **2004**, *113*, 115–119. [CrossRef]
62. Roufosse, F.E.; Kahn, J.-E.; Gleich, G.J.; Schwartz, L.B.; Singh, A.D.; Rosenwasser, L.J.; Denburg, J.A.; Ring, J.; Rothenberg, M.E.; Sheikh, J.; et al. Long-term safety of mepolizumab for the treatment of hypereosinophilic syndromes. *J. Allergy Clin. Immunol.* **2012**, *131*, 461–467.e5. [CrossRef]
63. Roufosse, F.; Kahn, J.-E.; Rothenberg, M.E.; Wardlaw, A.J.; Klion, A.D.; Kirby, S.Y.; Gilson, M.J.; Bentley, J.H.; Bradford, E.S.; Yancey, S.W.; et al. Efficacy and safety of mepolizumab in hypereosinophilic syndrome: A phase III, randomized, placebo-controlled trial. *J. Allergy Clin. Immunol.* **2020**, *146*, 1397–1405. [CrossRef] [PubMed]
64. Bachert, C.; Sousa, A.R.; Lund, V.J.; Scadding, G.K.; Gevaert, P.; Nasser, S.; Durham, S.R.; Cornet, M.E.; Kariyawasam, H.H.; Gilbert, J.; et al. Reduced need for surgery in severe nasal polyposis with mepolizumab: Randomized trial. *J. Allergy Clin. Immunol.* **2017**, *140*, 1024–1031.e14. [CrossRef]
65. Cavaliere, C.; Incorvaia, C.; Frati, F.; Messineo, D.; Ciotti, M.; Greco, A.; De Vincentiis, M.; Masieri, S. Recovery of smell sense loss by mepolizumab in a patient allergic to Dermatophagoides and affected by chronic rhinosinusitis with nasal polyps. *Clin. Mol. Allergy* **2019**, *17*, 1–4. [CrossRef] [PubMed]
66. Straumann, A.; Conus, S.; Grzonka, P.; Kita, H.; Kephart, G.; Bussmann, C.; Beglinger, C.; Smith, D.; Patel, J.; Byrne, M.; et al. Anti-interleukin-5 antibody treatment (mepolizumab) in active eosinophilic oesophagitis: A randomised, placebo-controlled, double-blind trial. *Gut* **2010**, *59*, 21–30. [CrossRef]
67. Tomizawa, Y.; Melek, J.; Komaki, Y. Efficacy of Pharmacologic Therapy for Eosinophilic Esophagitis. *J. Clin. Gastroenterol.* **2018**, *52*, 596–606. [CrossRef] [PubMed]
68. Egan, R.W.; Athwal, D.; Bodmer, M.W.; Carter, J.M.; Chapman, R.W.; Choua, C.-C.; Coxa, M.A.; Emtage, S.J.; Fernandez, X.; Genatt, N.; et al. Effect of Sch 55700, a Humanized Monoclonal Antibody to Human Interleukin-5, on Eosinophilic Responses and Bronchial Hyperreactivity. *Arzneimittelforschung* **1999**, *49*, 779–790. [CrossRef]
69. Kips, J.C.; O'Connor, B.J.; Langley, S.J.; Woodcock, A.; Kerstjens, H.A.M.; Postma, D.S.; Danzig, M.; Cuss, F.; Pauwels, R.A. Effect of SCH55700, a Humanized Anti-Human Interleukin-5 Antibody, in Severe Persistent Asthma. *Am. J. Respir. Crit. Care Med.* **2003**, *167*, 1655–1659. [CrossRef]
70. Castro, M.; Mathur, S.; Hargreave, F.; Boulet, L.-P.; Xie, F.; Young, J.; Wilkins, H.J.; Henkel, T.; Nair, P. Reslizumab for Poorly Controlled, Eosinophilic Asthma. *Am. J. Respir. Crit. Care Med.* **2011**, *184*, 1125–1132. [CrossRef]
71. Castro, M.; Zangrilli, J.E.; Wechsler, M.E.; Bateman, E.D.; Brusselle, G.G.; Bardin, P.; Murphy, K.; Maspero, J.F.; O'Brien, C.; Korn, S. Reslizumab for inadequately controlled asthma with elevated blood eosinophil counts: Results from two multicentre, parallel, double-blind, randomised, placebo-controlled, phase 3 trials. *Lancet Respir. Med.* **2015**, *3*, 355–366. [CrossRef] [PubMed]
72. Corren, J.; Weinstein, S.; Janka, L.; Zangrilli, J.; Garin, M. Phase 3 Study of Reslizumab in Patients with Poorly Controlled Asthma. *Chest* **2016**, *150*, 799–810. [CrossRef]

73. Murphy, K.; Jacobs, J.; Bjermer, L.; Fahrenholz, J.M.; Shalit, Y.; Garin, M.; Zangrilli, J.; Castro, M. Long-term Safety and Efficacy of Reslizumab in Patients with Eosinophilic Asthma. *J. Allergy Clin. Immunol. Pract.* **2017**, *5*, 1572–1581.e3. [CrossRef] [PubMed]
74. Koike, M.; Nakamura, K.; Furuya, A.; Iida, A.; Anazawa, H.; Takatsu, K.; Hanai, N. Establishment of humanized anti-interleukin-5 receptor alpha chain monoclonal antibodies having a potent neutralizing activity. *Hum. Antibodies* **2009**, *18*, 17–27. [CrossRef] [PubMed]
75. Kolbeck, R.; Kozhich, A.; Koike, M.; Peng, L.; Andersson, C.K.; Damschroder, M.M.; Reed, J.; Woods, R.; Dall, W.; Stephens, G.; et al. MEDI-563, a humanized anti–IL-5 receptor α mAb with enhanced antibody-dependent cell-mediated cytotoxicity function. *J. Allergy Clin. Immunol.* **2010**, *125*, 1344–1353.e2. [CrossRef] [PubMed]
76. Shields, R.L.; Lai, J.; Keck, R.; O'Connell, L.Y.; Hong, K.; Meng, Y.G.; Weikert, S.; Presta, L.G. Lack of fucose on human IgG1 N-linked oligosaccharide improves binding to human Fcgamma RIII and antibody-dependent cellular toxicity. *J. Biol. Chem.* **2002**, *277*, 26733–26740. [CrossRef] [PubMed]
77. Maselli, D.J.; Rogers, L.; Peters, J.I. Benralizumab, an add-on treatment for severe eosinophilic asthma: Evaluation of exacerbations, emergency department visits, lung function, and oral corticosteroid use. *Ther. Clin. Risk Manag.* **2018**, *14*, 2059–2068. [CrossRef]
78. Busse, W.W.; Katial, R.; Gossage, D.; Sari, S.; Wang, B.; Kolbeck, R.; Coyle, A.J.; Koike, M.; Spitalny, G.L.; Kiener, P.A.; et al. Safety profile, pharmacokinetics, and biologic activity of MEDI-563, an anti-IL-5 receptor alpha antibody, in a phase I study of subjects with mild asthma. *J. Allergy Clin. Immunol.* **2010**, *125*, 1237–1244.e2. [CrossRef]
79. Laviolette, M.; Gossage, D.L.; Gauvreau, G.; Leigh, R.; Olivenstein, R.; Katial, R.; Busse, W.W.; Wenzel, S.; Wu, Y.; Datta, V.; et al. Effects of benralizumab on airway eosinophils in asthmatic patients with sputum eosinophilia. *Allergy Clin. Immunol.* **2013**, *132*, 1086–1096.e5. [CrossRef]
80. Castro, M.; Wenzel, S.E.; Bleecker, E.R.; Pizzichini, E.; Kuna, P.; Busse, W.W.; Gossage, D.L.; Ward, C.K.; Wu, Y.; Wang, B.; et al. Benralizumab, an anti-interleukin 5 receptor α monoclonal antibody, versus placebo for uncontrolled eosinophilic asthma: A phase 2b randomised dose-ranging study. *Lancet Respir. Med.* **2014**, *2*, 879–890. [CrossRef] [PubMed]
81. Nowak, R.M.; Parker, J.M.; Silverman, R.A.; Rowe, B.H.; Smithline, H.; Khan, F.; Fiening, J.; Kim, K.; Molfino, N.A. A randomized trial of benralizumab, an antiinterleukin 5 receptor α monoclonal antibody, after acute asthma. *Am. J. Emerg. Med.* **2015**, *33*, 14–20. [CrossRef] [PubMed]
82. Bleecker, E.R.; FitzGerald, J.M.; Chanez, P.; Papi, A.; Weinstein, S.F.; Barker, P.; Sproule, S.; Gilmartin, G.; Aurivillius, M.; Werkström, V.; et al. Efficacy and safety of benralizumab for patients with severe asthma uncontrolled with high-dosage inhaled corticosteroids and long-acting β2-agonists (SIROCCO): A randomised, multicentre, placebo-controlled phase 3 trial. *Lancet* **2016**, *388*, 2115–2127. [CrossRef] [PubMed]
83. FitzGerald, J.M.; Bleecker, E.R.; Nair, P.; Korn, S.; Ohta, K.; Lommatzsch, M.; Ferguson, G.T.; Busse, W.; Barker, P.; Sproule, S.; et al. Benralizumab, an anti-interleukin-5 receptor α monoclonal antibody, as add-on treatment for patients with severe, uncontrolled, eosinophilic asthma (CALIMA): A randomised, double-blind, placebo-controlled phase 3 trial. *Lancet* **2016**, *388*, 2128–2141. [CrossRef]
84. Nair, P.; Wenzel, S.; Rabe, K.F.; Bourdin, A.; Lugogo, N.L.; Kuna, P.; Barker, P.; Sproule, S.; Ponnarambil, S.; Goldman, M. Oral Glucocorticoid–Sparing Effect of Benralizumab in Severe Asthma. *N. Engl. J. Med.* **2017**, *376*, 2448–2458. [CrossRef]
85. AstraZeneca. Fasenra^{TM} (benralizumab). Prescribing Information. Available online: www.azpicentral.com/fasenra/fasenra_pi.pdf (accessed on 10 November 2022).
86. Liu, W.; Ma, X.; Zhou, W. Adverse events of benralizumab in moderate to severe eosinophilic asthma. *Medicine* **2019**, *98*, e15868. [CrossRef]
87. Ferguson, G.T.; Cole, J.; Aurivillius, M.; Roussel, P.; Barker, P.; Martin, U.J. Single-Use Autoinjector Functionality and Reliability for At-Home Administration af Benralizumab for Patients with Severe Asthma: GRECO Trial Results. *J. Asthma Allergy* **2019**, *12*, 363–373. [CrossRef] [PubMed]
88. Busse, W.W.; Bleecker, E.R.; FitzGerald, J.M.; Ferguson, G.T.; Barker, P.; Sproule, S.; Olsson, R.; Martin, U.J.; Goldman, M.; Yañez, A.; et al. Long-term safety and efficacy of benralizumab in patients with severe, uncontrolled asthma: 1-year results from the BORA phase 3 extension trial. *Lancet Respir. Med.* **2019**, *7*, 46–59. [CrossRef]
89. Korn, S.; Bourdin, A.; Chupp, G.; Cosio, B.G.; Arbetter, D.; Shah, M.; Gil, E.G. Integrated Safety and Efficacy Among Patients Receiving Benralizumab for Up to 5 Years. *J. Allergy Clin. Immunol. Pract.* **2021**, *9*, 4381–4392.e4. [CrossRef] [PubMed]
90. Criner, G.J.; Celli, B.R.; Brightling, C.E.; Agusti, A.; Papi, A.; Singh, D.; Sin, D.D.; Vogelmeier, C.F.; Sciurba, F.C.; Bafadhel, M.; et al. Benralizumab for the Prevention of COPD Exacerbations. *N. Engl. J. Med.* **2019**, *381*, 1023–1034. [CrossRef]
91. Bernstein, J.A.; Singh, U.; Rao, M.B.; Berendts, K.; Zhang, X.; Mutasim, D. Benralizumab for Chronic Spontaneous Urticaria. *N. Engl. J. Med.* **2020**, *383*, 1389–1391. [CrossRef] [PubMed]
92. Zhang, L.; Gao, Y.; Li, M.; Xu, C.; Davis, J.D.; Kanamaluru, V.; Lu, Q. Population pharmacokinetic analysis of dupilumab in adult and adolescent patients with asthma. *CPT Pharmacometrics Syst. Pharmacol.* **2021**, *10*, 941–952. [CrossRef]
93. Matsunaga, K.; Katoh, N.; Fujieda, S.; Izuhara, K.; Oishi, K. Dupilumab: Basic aspects and applications to allergic diseases. *Allergol. Int.* **2020**, *69*, 187–196. [CrossRef]
94. Guttman-Yassky, E.; Bissonnette, R.; Ungar, B.; Suárez-Fariñas, M.; Ardeleanu, M.; Esaki, H.; Suprun, M.; Estrada, Y.; Xu, H.; Peng, X.; et al. Dupilumab progressively improves systemic and cutaneous abnormalities in patients with atopic dermatitis. *J. Allergy Clin. Immunol.* **2019**, *143*, 155–172. [CrossRef]

95. Corren, J.; Castro, M.; Chanez, P.; Fabbri, L.; Joish, V.N.; Amin, N.; Graham, N.M.; Mastey, V.; Abbé, A.; Taniou, C.; et al. Dupilumab improves symptoms, quality of life, and productivity in uncontrolled persistent asthma. *Ann. Allergy Asthma Immunol.* **2018**, *122*, 41–49.e2. [CrossRef]
96. Castro, M.; Corren, J.; Pavord, I.D.; Maspero, J.; Wenzel, S.; Rabe, K.F.; Busse, W.W.; Ford, L.; Sher, L.; Fitzgerald, J.M.; et al. Dupilumab Efficacy and Safety in Moderate-to-Severe Uncontrolled Asthma. *N. Engl. J. Med.* **2018**, *378*, 2486–2496. [CrossRef] [PubMed]
97. Bacharier, L.B.; Maspero, J.F.; Katelaris, C.H.; Fiocchi, A.G.; Gagnon, R.; de Mir, I.; Jain, N.; Sher, L.D.; Mao, X.; Liu, D.; et al. Dupilumab in Children with Uncontrolled Moderate-to-Severe Asthma. *N. Engl. J. Med.* **2021**, *385*, 2230–2240. [CrossRef]
98. Simpson, E.L.; Akinlade, B.; Ardeleanu, M. Two Phase 3 Trials of Dupilumab versus Placebo in Atopic Dermatitis. *N. Engl. J. Med.* **2016**, *375*, 2335–2348. [CrossRef] [PubMed]
99. Merola, J.F.; Sidbury, R.; Wollenberg, A.; Chen, Z.; Zhang, A.; Shumel, B.; Rossi, A.B. Dupilumab prevents flares in adults with moderate to severe atopic dermatitis in a 52-week randomized controlled phase 3 trial. *J. Am. Acad. Dermatol.* **2021**, *84*, 495–497. [CrossRef]
100. Bachert, C.; Han, J.K.; Desrosiers, M.; Hellings, P.W.; Amin, N.; E Lee, S.; Mullol, J.; Greos, L.S.; Bosso, J.V.; Laidlaw, T.M.; et al. Efficacy and safety of dupilumab in patients with severe chronic rhinosinusitis with nasal polyps (LIBERTY NP SINUS-24 and LIBERTY NP SINUS-52): Results from two multicentre, randomised, double-blind, placebo-controlled, parallel-group phase 3 trials. *Lancet* **2019**, *394*, 1638–1650. [CrossRef]
101. Jonstam, K.; Swanson, B.N.; Mannent, L.P.; Cardell, L.; Tian, N.; Wang, Y.; Zhang, D.; Fan, C.; Holtappels, G.; Hamilton, J.D.; et al. Dupilumab reduces local type 2 pro-inflammatory biomarkers in chronic rhinosinusitis with nasal polyposis. *Allergy* **2018**, *74*, 743–752. [CrossRef]
102. Desrosiers, M.; Mannent, L.; Amin, N.; Canonica, G.; Hellings, P.; Gevaert, P.; Mullol, J.; Lee, S.; Fujieda, S.; Han, J.; et al. Dupilumab reduces systemic corticosteroid use sinonasal surgery rate in, C.R.S.w.N.P. *Rhinology* **2021**, *59*, 301–311.
103. Laidlaw, T.M.; Bachert, C.; Amin, N.; Desrosiers, M.; Hellings, P.W.; Mullol, J.; Maspero, J.F.; Gevaert, P.; Zhang, M.; Mao, X.; et al. Dupilumab improves upper and lower airway disease control in chronic rhinosinusitis with nasal polyps and asthma. *Ann. Allergy Asthma Immunol.* **2021**, *126*, 584–592.e1. [CrossRef]
104. E Wechsler, M.; Ford, L.B.; Maspero, J.F.; Pavord, I.D.; Papi, A.; Bourdin, A.; Watz, H.; Castro, M.; Nenasheva, N.M.; Tohda, Y.; et al. Long-term safety and efficacy of dupilumab in patients with moderate-to-severe asthma (TRAVERSE): An open-label extension study. *Lancet Respir. Med.* **2021**, *10*, 11–25. [CrossRef]
105. Simpson, E.L.; Parnes, J.R.; She, D.; Crouch, S.; Rees, W.; Mo, M.; van der Merwe, R. Tezepelumab, an anti–thymic stromal lymphopoietin monoclonal antibody, in the treatment of moderate to severe atopic dermatitis: A randomized phase 2a clinical trial. *J. Am. Acad. Dermatol.* **2019**, *80*, 1013–1021. [CrossRef] [PubMed]
106. Gauvreau, G.M.; O'Byrne, P.M.; Boulet, L.-P.; Wang, Y.; Cockcroft, D.; Bigler, J.; FitzGerald, J.M.; Boedigheimer, M.; Davis, B.E.; Dias, C.; et al. Effects of an Anti-TSLP Antibody on Allergen-Induced Asthmatic Responses. *N. Engl. J. Med.* **2014**, *370*, 2102–2110. [CrossRef]
107. Corren, J.; Parnes, J.R.; Wang, L.; Mo, M.; Roseti, S.L.; Griffiths, J.M.; van der Merwe, R. Tezepelumab in Adults with Uncontrolled Asthma. *N. Engl. J. Med.* **2017**, *377*, 936–946. [CrossRef]
108. Corren, J.; Gil, E.G.; Griffiths, J.M.; Parnes, J.R.; van der Merwe, R.; Sałapa, K.; O'Quinn, S. Tezepelumab improves patient-reported outcomes in patients with severe uncontrolled asthma in, P.A.T.H.W.A.Y. *Ann. Allergy Asthma Immunol.* **2020**, *126*, 187–193. [CrossRef] [PubMed]
109. Menzies-Gow, A.; Corren, J.; Bourdin, A.; Chupp, G.; Israel, E.; Wechsler, M.E.; Brightling, C.E.; Griffiths, J.; Hellqvist, Å.; Bowen, K.; et al. Tezepelumab in Adults and Adolescents with Severe, Uncontrolled Asthma. *N. Engl. J. Med.* **2021**, *384*, 1800–1809. [CrossRef] [PubMed]
110. E Wechsler, M.; Menzies-Gow, A.; E Brightling, C.; Kuna, P.; Korn, S.; Welte, T.; Griffiths, J.M.; Sałapa, K.; Hellqvist, Å.; Almqvist, G.; et al. Evaluation of the oral corticosteroid-sparing effect of tezepelumab in adults with oral corticosteroid-dependent asthma (SOURCE): A randomised, placebo-controlled, phase 3 study. *Lancet Respir. Med.* **2022**, *10*, 650–660. [CrossRef]
111. Menzies-Gow, A.; Ponnarambil, S.; Downie, J.; Bowen, K.; Hellqvist; Colice, G. DESTINATION: A phase 3, multicentre, randomized, double-blind, placebo-controlled, parallel-group trial to evaluate the long-term safety and tolerability of tezepelumab in adults and adolescents with severe, uncontrolled asthma. *Respir. Res.* **2020**, *21*, 1–10. [CrossRef]
112. Alpizar, S.; Megally, A.; Chen, C.; Raj, A.; Downie, J.; Colice, G. Functionality and Performance of an Accessorized Pre-Filled Syringe and an Autoinjector for At-Home Administration of Tezepelumab in Patients with Severe, Uncontrolled Asthma. *J. Asthma Allergy* **2021**, *14*, 381–392. [CrossRef]
113. Agache, I.; Beltran, J.; Akdis, C.; Akdis, M.; Canelo-aybar, C.; Walter, G.; Casale, T.; Chivato, T.; Corren, J.; Del Giacco, S.; et al. Efficacy and safety of treatment with biologicals (benralizumab, dupilumab, mepolizumab, omalizumab and reslizumab) for severe eosinophilic asthma. A systematic review for the EAACI Guidelines—Recommendations on the use of biologicals in severe asthma. *Allergy* **2020**, *75*, 1023–1042. [CrossRef]
114. Préfontaine, D.; Nadigel, J.; Chouiali, F.; Audusseau, S.; Semlali, A.; Chakir, J.; Martin, J.G.; Hamid, Q. Increased IL-33 expression by epithelial cells in bronchial asthma. *J. Allergy Clin. Immunol.* **2010**, *125*, 752–754. [CrossRef]

115. Schmitz, J.; Owyang, A.; Oldham, E.; Song, Y.; Murphy, E.; McClanahan, T.K.; Zurawski, G.; Moshrefi, M.; Qin, J.; Li, X.; et al. IL-33, an interleukin-1-like cytokine that signals via the IL-1 receptor-related protein ST2 and induces T helper type 2-associated cytokines. *Immunity* **2005**, *23*, 479–490. [CrossRef] [PubMed]
116. Wechsler, M.E.; Ruddy, M.K.; Pavord, I.D.; Israel, E.; Rabe, K.F.; Ford, L.B.; Maspero, J.F.; Abdulai, R.M.; Hu, C.-C.; Martincova, R.; et al. Efficacy and Safety of Itepekimab in Patients with Moderate-to-Severe Asthma. *N. Engl. J. Med.* **2021**, *385*, 1656–1668. [CrossRef]
117. Corrigan, C.J.; Wang, W.; Meng, Q.; Fang, C.; Eid, G.; Caballero, M.R.; Lv, Z.; An, Y.; Wang, Y.-H.; Liu, Y.-J.; et al. Allergen-induced expression of IL-25 and IL-25 receptor in atopic asthmatic airways and late-phase cutaneous responses. *J. Allergy Clin. Immunol.* **2011**, *128*, 116–124. [CrossRef]
118. Salter, B.M.; Oliveria, J.P.; Nusca, G.; Smith, S.; Tworek, D.; Mitchell, P.; Watson, R.M.; Sehmi, R.; Gauvreau, G.M. IL-25 and IL-33 induce Type 2 inflammation in basophils from subjects with allergic asthma. *Respir. Res.* **2016**, *17*, 1–13. [CrossRef]
119. Corrigan, C.J.; Wang, W.; Meng, Q.; Fang, C.; Wu, H.; Reay, V.; Lv, Z.; Fan, Y.; An, Y.; Wang, Y.-H.; et al. T-helper cell type 2 (Th2) memory T cell-potentiating cytokine IL-25 has the potential to promote angiogenesis in asthma. *Proc. Natl. Acad. Sci. USA* **2011**, *108*, 1579–1584. [CrossRef] [PubMed]
120. Busse, W.W.; Holgate, S.; Kerwin, E.; Chon, Y.; Feng, J.Y.; Lin, J.; Lin, S.-L. Randomized, double-blind, placebo-controlled study of brodalumab, a human anti-IL-17 receptor monoclonal antibody, in moderate to severe asthma. *Am. J. Respir. Crit. Care Med.* **2013**, *188*, 1294–1302. [CrossRef] [PubMed]
121. Zhu, Z.; Homer, R.J.; Wang, Z.; Chen, Q.; Geba, G.P.; Wang, J.; Zhang, Y.; Elias, J.A. Pulmonary expression of interleukin-13 causes inflammation, mucus hypersecretion, subepithelial fibrosis, physiologic abnormalities, and eotaxin production. *J. Clin. Investig.* **1999**, *103*, 779–788. [CrossRef] [PubMed]
122. May, R.; Monk, P.; Cohen, E.; Manuel, D.; Dempsey, F.; Davis, N.; Dodd, A.; Corkill, D.; Woods, J.; Joberty-Candotti, C.; et al. Preclinical development of CAT-354, an IL-13 neutralizing antibody, for the treatment of severe uncontrolled asthma. *Br. J. Pharmacol.* **2011**, *166*, 177–193. [CrossRef] [PubMed]
123. Corren, J.; Lemanske, R.F.; Hanania, N.A.; Korenblat, P.E.; Parsey, M.V.; Arron, J.R.; Harris, J.M.; Scheerens, H.; Wu, L.C.; Su, Z.; et al. Lebrikizumab Treatment in Adults with Asthma. *N. Engl. J. Med.* **2011**, *365*, 1088–1098. [CrossRef]
124. Blanchard, C.; Mishra, A.; Saito-Akei, H.; Monk, P.; Anderson, I.; Rothenberg, M.E. Inhibition of human interleukin-13-induced respiratory and oesophageal inflammation by anti-human-interleukin-13 antibody (CAT-354). *Clin. Exp. Allergy* **2005**, *35*, 1096–1103. [CrossRef] [PubMed]
125. Maselli, D.J.; Keyt, H.; Rogers, L. Profile of lebrikizumab and its potential in the treatment of asthma. *J. Asthma Allergy* **2015**, *8*, 87–92. [CrossRef] [PubMed]
126. A Hanania, N.; Noonan, M.; Corren, J.; Korenblat, P.; Zheng, Y.; Fischer, S.K.; Cheu, M.; Putnam, W.S.; Murray, E.; Scheerens, H.; et al. Lebrikizumab in moderate-to-severe asthma: Pooled data from two randomised placebo-controlled studies. *Thorax* **2015**, *70*, 748–756. [CrossRef]
127. Piper, E.; Brightling, C.; Niven, R.; Oh, C.; Faggioni, R.; Poon, K.; She, D.; Kell, C.; May, R.; Geba, G.P.; et al. A phase II placebo-controlled study of tralokinumab in moderate-to-severe asthma. *Eur. Respir. J.* **2012**, *41*, 330–338. [CrossRef]
128. Busse, W.W.; Brusselle, G.G.; Korn, S.; Kuna, P.; Magnan, A.; Cohen, D.; Bowen, K.; Piechowiak, T.; Wang, M.M.; Colice, G. Tralokinumab did not demonstrate oral corticosteroid-sparing effects in severe asthma. *Eur. Respir. J.* **2019**, *53*, 1800948. [CrossRef]
129. A Hanania, N.; Korenblat, P.; Chapman, K.R.; Bateman, E.D.; Kopecky, P.; Paggiaro, P.; Yokoyama, A.; Olsson, J.; Gray, S.; Holweg, C.T.J.; et al. Efficacy and safety of lebrikizumab in patients with uncontrolled asthma (LAVOLTA I and LAVOLTA II): Replicate, phase 3, randomised, double-blind, placebo-controlled trials. *Lancet Respir. Med.* **2016**, *4*, 781–796. [CrossRef] [PubMed]
130. A Panettieri, R.; Sjöbring, U.; Péterffy, A.; Wessman, P.; Bowen, K.; Piper, E.; Colice, G.; E Brightling, C. Tralokinumab for severe, uncontrolled asthma (STRATOS 1 and STRATOS 2): Two randomised, double-blind, placebo-controlled, phase 3 clinical trials. *Lancet Respir. Med.* **2018**, *6*, 511–525. [CrossRef]
131. Altrichter, S.; Staubach, P.; Pasha, M.; Singh, B.; Chang, A.T.; Bernstein, J.A.; Rasmussen, H.S.; Siebenhaar, F.; Maurer, M. An open-label, proof-of-concept study of lirentelimab for antihistamine-resistant chronic spontaneous and inducible urticaria. *J. Allergy Clin. Immunol.* **2021**, *149*, 1683–1690.e7. [CrossRef] [PubMed]
132. Dellon, E.S.; Gonsalves, N.; Rothenberg, M.E.; Hirano, I.; Chehade, M.; Peterson, K.A.; Falk, G.W.; Murray, J.A.; Gehman, L.T.; Chang, A.T.; et al. Determination of Biopsy Yield That Optimally Detects Eosinophilic Gastritis and/or Duodenitis in a Randomized Trial of Lirentelimab. *Clin. Gastroenterol. Hepatol.* **2021**, *20*, 535–545.e15. [CrossRef] [PubMed]

pharmaceuticals

MDPI

Article

Sustained Effectiveness of Upadacitinib in Moderate-to-Severe Atopic Dermatitis: A 48-Week Real-World Study

Teppei Hagino [1,*], Risa Hamada [2], Mai Yoshida [2], Hidehisa Saeki [2], Eita Fujimoto [3] and Naoko Kanda [1]

1 Department of Dermatology, Nippon Medical School Chiba Hokusoh Hospital, Inzai 270-1694, Japan
2 Department of Dermatology, Nippon Medical School, Tokyo 113-8602, Japan; h-risa@nms.ac.jp (R.H.); m-mai@nms.ac.jp (M.Y.); h-saeki@nms.ac.jp (H.S.)
3 Fujimoto Dermatology Clinic, Funabashi 274-0063, Japan; doctor@fujimoto-derma.com
* Correspondence: teppei-hagino@nms.ac.jp; Tel.: +81-476-99-1111

Abstract: Clinical trials and real-world studies have shown the effectiveness of upadacitinib for treating rash and pruritus in patients with atopic dermatitis (AD). This study aimed to determine whether the early reduction in rash or pruritus at week 12 of upadacitinib treatment could be maintained at later treatment stages. This retrospective study involved 227 and 73 patients with moderate-to-severe AD treated with 15 and 30 mg upadacitinib daily, respectively. The eczema area and severity index (EASI) scores, peak pruritus numerical rating scale (PP-NRS), and investigator's global assessment (IGA) were analyzed. At week 12, patients were divided into achievers and non-achievers of EASI 75, 90, 100, absolute EASI $\leq$ 2, IGA0/1, PP-NRS4, or absolute PP-NRS $\leq$ 1. Achievement rates for each endpoint were assessed at later time points (weeks 24, 36, and 48) in both groups. Week 12 achievers largely maintained their endpoint achievements until week 48, regardless of dosage (15 mg or 30 mg). Week 12 non-achievers saw an increasing achievement rate of EASI 75 until week 48. The initial reduction in rash and pruritus at week 12 persisted until week 48 with upadacitinib treatment, suggesting potential benefits for patients requiring prolonged treatment despite not achieving EASI 75 at week 12.

Keywords: atopic dermatitis; upadacitinib; Janus kinase; long-term; real-world

1. Introduction

Atopic dermatitis (AD) is a chronic inflammatory skin disease characterized by a type 2-skewed immune response, pruritus, and impairment of the skin barrier [1,2]. Previous studies have shown that the development of AD is related to specific cytokines, such as interleukin (IL)-4, IL-5, IL-13, IL-22, IL-31, and thymic stromal lymphopoietin, which intracellularly signal via the Janus kinase (JAK)/signal transducer and activator of transcription pathways [3]. The Janus kinase inhibitors upadacitinib, baricitinib, and abrocitinib have been approved as systemic treatments for AD. Clinical trials and real-world studies have shown the efficacy and safety of upadacitinib for moderate-to-severe AD [4–11]. A post hoc analysis of the Phase III JADE COMPARE trial showed that patients who achieved $\geq$4-point improvement on the peak pruritus numerical rating scale (PP-NRS) at week 2 of abrocitinib treatment achieved higher rates of the eczema area and severity index (EASI) 75, 90, and investigator's global assessment (IGA) 0/1 at week 12 compared to non-achievers [12]. Patients who achieved absolute PP-NRS $\leq$ 1 at week 2 attained a higher rate of EASI 100 at weeks 12 and 24 compared to non-achievers [13]. In the BREEZE-AD3 study, patients with AD receiving baricitinib who achieved IGA $\leq$ 2 at week 16 maintained high rates of EASI 75 and IGA 0/1 until week 68 [14]. These results suggest that early improvement in pruritus or rash may predict strong therapeutic outcomes in the later stages of treatment with baricitinib and abrocitinib. However, it remains unclear whether the early reduction in rash or pruritus is sustained at later stages of upadacitinib treatment.

This study aimed to investigate whether the early improvement in rash or pruritus at week 12 could be maintained until week 48 of upadacitinib treatment in real-world clinical practice. We also investigated whether patients with an insufficient response to upadacitinib at week 12 could achieve greater therapeutic effects at later stages of treatment.

2. Results

2.1. Demographic and Baseline Characteristics

Of the 300 patients with AD in this study, 227 and 73 were treated with 15 mg and 30 mg of upadacitinib daily, respectively. The baseline demographics of patients in the two treatment groups are presented in Table 1. The proportion of pretreatment with dupilumab and baricitinib (4 mg) was higher in the 30 mg group than in the 15 mg group, indicating more refractory symptoms of AD in the former group. Baseline EASI, IGA, and PP-NRS scores were lower in the 30 mg group than in the 15 mg group, which may reflect the effects of systemic pretreatments in the former group. The number of week 12 achievers and non-achievers of individual endpoints was longitudinally assessed throughout the 48 weeks of treatment (Tables 2 and 3). Table 2 presents the longitudinal analysis of achievement rates for EASI 75, EASI 90, and EASI 100 responses, while Table 3 shows the outcomes for EASI $\leq$ 2, IGA 0/1, PP-NRS 4, and PP-NRS $\leq$ 1.

Table 1. Baseline demographics and disease characteristics of patients with atopic dermatitis treated with upadacitinib.

	Total Population (*n* = 300)	15 mg (*n* = 227)	30 mg (*n* = 73)	*p* (15 mg versus 30 mg)
Male sex, *n* (%)	216 (72.0)	162 (71.4)	54 (74.0)	0.765
Age (years) [a]	37.0 [18.0–51.0]	35.5 [16.0–51.0]	40.0 [31–48]	0.327
Body mass index (kg/m^2) [a]	22.7 [15.6–25.9]	22.2 [20.1–25.0]	23.6 [21.5–27.2]	0.0133 *
Disease duration (years) [a]	30.0 [15.0–44.0]	28.0 [13.0–44.0]	33 [22–43]	0.114
Presence of allergic conjunctivitis	46 (15.3)	34 (15.0)	12 (16.4)	0.852
Presence of allergic rhinitis	99 (33)	70 (30.8)	29 (39.7)	0.198
Presence of bronchial asthma	94 (31.3)	65 (28.6)	29 (39.7)	0.0829
		Pretreatment, *n* (%)		
Previous dupilumab	24 (8.0)	12 (5.3)	12 (16.4)	<0.01 **
Previous upadacitinib (15 mg)	32 (10.7)	NA	32 (43.8)	NA
Previous baricitinib (4 mg)	33 (11.0)	6 (2.6)	27 (37.0)	<0.01 **
		Clinical indices		
EASI [a]	20.3 [14.4–30.0]	23.8 [17.2–32.0]	12.5 [8.5–19.4]	<0.01 **
IGA, *n* (%)				
Mild (score of 2)	51 (17.0)	23 (10.1)	28 (38.4)	<0.01 **
Moderate (score of 3)	153 (51.0)	120 (52.9)	33 (45.2)	
Severe (score of 4)	96 (32.0)	84 (37.0)	12 (16.4)	
PP-NRS [a]	8.0 [6.0–9.0]	8 [7–9.5]	6 [3–8.0]	<0.01 **

[a] Data provided as the median [interquartile range]. * Statistically significant at $p < 0.05$, ** $p < 0.01$ by Fisher's exact test or Mann–Whitney U test. EASI, eczema area and severity index; IGA, investigator's global assessment; PP-NRS, peak pruritus numerical rating scale; NA, not applicable.

Table 2. The number of week 12 achievers and non-achievers of EASI 75, 90, and 100 throughout 48 weeks of upadacitinib treatment.

Outcome	Time Point	Week 12 Achievers in 15 mg Group (%)	Week 12 Achievers in 30 mg Group (%)	*p*	Week 12 Non-Achievers in 15 mg Group (%)	Week 12 Non-Achievers in 30 mg Group (%)	*p*
EASI 75	Week 12	129/182 (70.9)	45/64 (70.3)	0.351	53/182 (29.1)	19/64 (29.7)	1
	Week 24	107/145 (73.8)	34/54 (63)	0.173	38/145 (26.2)	20/54 (37)	0.515
	Week 36	72/99 (72.7)	32/44 (72.7)	0.247	27/99 (27.2)	12/44 (31.8)	0.0606
	Week 48	51/74 (68.9)	26/36 66.7)	0.139	23/74 (31.1)	10/36 (27.8)	0.0606
EASI 90	Week 12	69/182 (37.9)	19/64 (29.7)	1	113/182 (62.1)	45/64 (70.3)	0.289
	Week 24	56/145 (38.6)	23/54 (42.6)	1	89/145 (6.1)	31/54 (57.4)	0.153
	Week 36	40/99 (40.4)	20/44 (45.5)	0.143	59/99 (59.6)	24/44 (54.5)	0.463
	Week 48	25/74 (33.8)	18/36 (50)	0.703	49/74 (66.2)	18/36 (50)	0.0942
EASI 100	Week 12	26/182 (14.4)	6/64 (9.4)	1	156/182 (85.7)	58/64 (90.6)	0.274
	Week 24	22/145 (15.2)	4/54 (7.4)	0.161	123/145 (84.8)	50/54 (92.6)	0.182
	Week 36	11/99 (11.1)	6/44 (13.6)	1	88/99 (88.9)	38/44 (86.4)	0.344
	Week 48	7/74 (9.5)	1/36 (2.8)	1	67/74 (90.5)	35/36 (97.2)	0.086

EASI, eczema area and severity index.

Table 3. The number of week 12 achievers and non-achievers of EASI $\leq$ 2, IGA 0/1, PP-NRS 4, and PP NRS $\leq$ 1 throughout 48 weeks of upadacitinib treatment.

Outcome	Time Point	Week 12 Achievers in 15 mg Group (%)	Week 12 Achievers in 30 mg Group (%)	*p*	Week 12 Non-Achievers in 15 mg Group (%)	Week 12 Non-Achievers in 30 mg Group (%)	*p*
EASI $\leq$ 2	Week 12	75/186 (40.3)	29/64 (45.3)	1	111/186 (59.7)	35/64 (54.7)	0.245
	Week 24	59/149 (40.7)	27/54 (50)	0.778	90/149 (60.4)	27/54 (50)	0.171
	Week 36	34/100 (34)	23/44 (52.3)	0.488	66/100 (66)	21/44 (47.7)	0.173
	Week 48	49/75 (65.3)	21/37 (56.8)	1	26/75 (34.7)	16/37 (43.2)	0.268
IGA 0/1	Week 12	48/175 (27.4)	19/63 (30.2)	1	127/175 (72.6)	44/63 (69.8)	0.262
	Week 24	43/139 (30.9)	22/53 (41.5)	0.36	96/139 (69.1)	31/53 (58.5)	0.248
	Week 36	27/99 (27.3)	18/44 (40.9)	0.432	72/99 (72.7)	26/44 (59.1)	0.275
	Week 48	21/75 (28)	21/36 (58.3)	1	54/75 (72)	15/36 (41.7)	0.38
PP-NRS 4	Week 12	121/168 (72)	29/48 (60.4)	0.199	47/168 (28)	19/48 (39.6)	1
	Week 24	97/129 (75.2)	24/41 (58.5)	0.0347 *	32/129 (24.8)	17/41 (41.5)	0.506
	Week 36	71/95 (74.7)	19/35 (54.3)	0.0471 *	24/95 (40.7)	16/35 (45.7)	0.444
	Week 48	56/73 (76.7)	16/29 (55.2)	0.0401 *	17/73 (23.3)	13/29 (44.8)	0.199
PP-NRS $\leq$ 1	Week 12	76/179 (42.5)	30/62 (48.4)	1	103/179 (57.5)	32/62 (51.6)	0.425
	Week 24	48/134 (35.8)	19/52 (36.5)	0.611	86/134 (64.2)	33/52 (6.4)	0.25
	Week 36	34/99 (34.3)	21/46 (45.7)	0.593	65/99 (65.7)	25/46 (54.3)	0.474
	Week 48	23/75 (30.7)	16/35 (45.7)	0.392	52/75 (69.3)	19/35 (54.3)	0.294

EASI, eczema area and severity index; IGA, investigator's global assessment; PP-NRS, peak pruritus numerical rating scale. * Statistically significant at $p < 0.05$ by Fisher's exact test.

2.2. The Transition of Achievement Rates of EASI 75 at the Later Stages of Upadacitinib Treatment

The achievement rate for EASI 75 in week 12 achievers was mostly maintained in both the 15 mg and 30 mg groups (Figure 1a): 82.7%, 79.7%, and 80.6% in the 15 mg group and 76.9%, 79.4%, and 85.2% in the 30 mg group at weeks 24, 36, and 48, respectively.

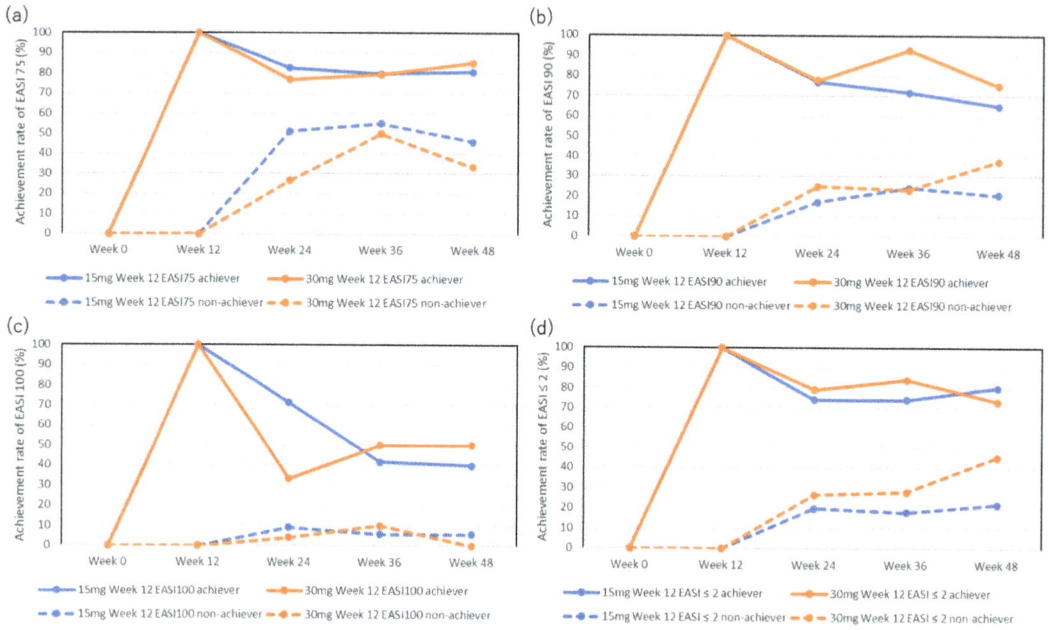

Figure 1. Achievement rates for EASI 75 (**a**), EASI 90 (**b**), EASI 100 (**c**), and absolute EASI $\leq$ 2 (**d**) in week 12 achievers or non-achievers during treatment with upadacitinib (15 mg or 30 mg daily).

The achievement rate for EASI 75 in week 12 non-achievers increased at later stages: 51.2%, 55.2%, and 46.2% in the 15 mg group and 26.7%, 50%, and 33.3% in the 30 mg group at weeks 24, 36, and 48, respectively, although there were no statistically significant differences in the achievement rates compared to week 12 (0%).

2.3. The Transition of Achievement Rates of EASI 90 at the Later Stages of Upadacitinib Treatment

The achievement rates for EASI 90 in week 12 achievers in the 15 mg group slightly decreased at the later stages, although this was not statistically significant compared to week 12 (100%): 76.9%, 71.9%, and 65% at weeks 24, 36, and 48, respectively (Figure 1b). The achievement rate for EASI 90 in week 12 achievers in the 30 mg group was mostly maintained: 77.8%, 92.9%, and 75% at weeks 24, 36, and 48, respectively.

The achievement rate for EASI 90 in week 12 non-achievers in the 15 mg group slightly increased during the later stages, although this was not statistically significant compared to week 12 (0%): 17.2%, 24.2%, and 20.8% at weeks 24, 36, and 48, respectively. The achievement rate for EASI 90 in week 12 non-achievers in the 30 mg group also slightly increased during the later stages without statistically significant differences compared to week 12 (0%): 25%, 23.3%, and 37.5% at weeks 24, 36, and 48, respectively.

2.4. The Transition of Achievement Rates of EASI 100 at the Later Stages of Upadacitinib Treatment

The achievement rates for EASI 100 in week 12 achievers decreased during the later stages of treatment in both the 15 mg and 30 mg groups, although without statistically significant differences compared to week 12 (100%): 71.4%, 41.7%, and 40% in the 15 mg group, and 33.3%, 50%, and 50% in the 30 mg group at weeks 24, 36, and 48, respectively (Figure 1c).

The achievement rate of EASI 100 in week 12 non-achievers was low and did not significantly increase during the later stages: 9.2%, 5.8%, and 5.9% in the 15 mg group and 4.2%, 10%, and 0% in the 30 mg group at weeks 24, 36, and 48, respectively.

2.5. The Transition of Achievement Rates of EASI ≤ 2 at the Later Stages of Upadacitinib Treatment

The achievement rates for EASI ≤ 2 in week 12 achievers were mostly maintained during the later stages in both groups (Figure 1d): 74.1%, 74.1%, and 80% in the 15 mg group and 79.2%, 84.2%, and 73.3% in the 30 mg group at weeks 24, 36, and 48, respectively.

The achievement rates for EASI ≤ 2 in week 12 non-achievers in the 15 mg group slightly increased during the later stages, although this was not statistically significant compared to week 12 (0%): 20%, 18.1%, and 22% at weeks 24, 36, and 48, respectively. The achievement rate for absolute EASI ≤ 2 in week 12 non-achievers in the 30 mg group increased, although this was not statistically significant, compared to week 12 (0%): 26.7%, 28%, and 45.5% at weeks 24, 36, and 48, respectively.

2.6. The Transition of Achievement Rates of IGA 0/1 at Later Stage of Upadacitinib Treatment

The achievement rates for IGA0/1 in week 12 achievers in the 15 mg group slightly decreased at later stages, although without statistically significant differences compared to week 12 (100%): 62.5%, 68.2%, and 75% at weeks 24, 36, and 48, respectively (Figure 2). The achievement rates for IGA0/1 in week 12 achievers in the 30 mg group were mostly maintained: 76.5%, 85.7%, and 83.3% at weeks 24, 36, and 48, respectively.

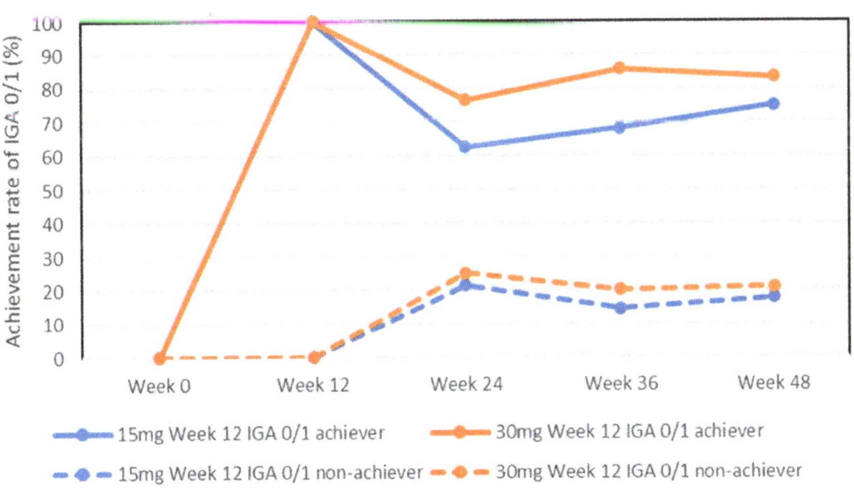

Figure 2. Achievement rates for IGA 0/1 in week 12 achievers or non-achievers during treatment with upadacitinib (15 mg and 30 mg daily).

The achievement rates for IGA0/1 in week 12 non-achievers in both the 15 mg and 30 mg groups slightly increased at later stages, although without statistically significant differences compared to week 12 (0%): 21.5%, 14.5%, and 17.7% in the 15 mg group, and 25%, 20%, and 20.8% in the 30 mg group at weeks 24, 36, and 48, respectively.

2.7. The Transition of Achievement Rates of PP-NRS 4 at the Later Stages of Upadacitinib Treatment

The achievement rates for PP-NRS 4 in week 12 achievers in the 15 mg group were mostly maintained during the later stages: 92.4%, 89.7%, and 90% at weeks 24, 36, and 48, respectively (Figure 3a). The achievement rates for PP-NRS 4 in week 12 achievers in the 30 mg group slightly decreased at the later stages, although this was not statistically significant compared with week 12 (100%): 80.8%, 73.9%, and 71.4% at weeks 24, 36, and 48, respectively. The achievement rates for PP-NRS 4 were significantly higher in week 12 achievers in the 15 mg group than those in the 30 mg group at weeks 24, 36, and 48.

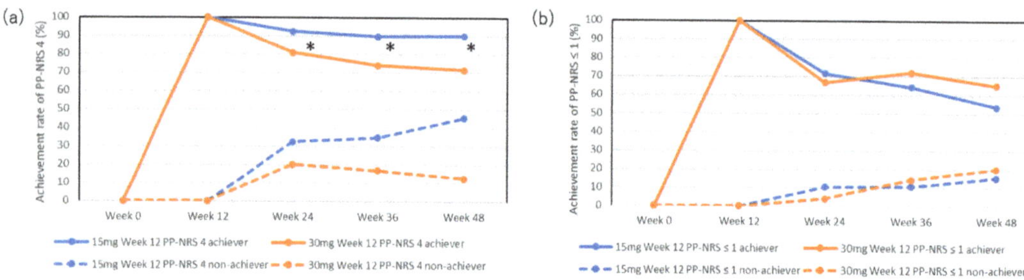

Figure 3. Achievement rates for PP-NRS 4 (**a**) or PP-NRS $\leq$ 1 (**b**) in week 12 achievers or non-achievers during treatment with upadacitinib (15 mg or 30 mg daily). * $p < 0.05$, week 12 achievers of PP-NRS 4 in the 15 mg group versus those in the 30 mg group, analyzed using Fisher's exact test.

The achievement rates for PP-NRS 4 in week 12 non-achievers in the 15 mg group increased during the later stages, although this was not statistically significant compared with week 12 (0%): 32.4%, 34.6%, and 45.4% at weeks 24, 36, and 48, respectively. The achievement rates for week 12 non-achievers in the 30 mg group slightly increased during the later stages, although this was not statistically significant compared to week 12 (0%): 20%, 16.7%, and 12.5%.

2.8. The Transition of Achievement Rates of Absolute PP-NRS $\leq$ 1 at the Later Stages of Upadacitinib Treatment

The achievement rates for PP-NRS $\leq$ 1 in week 12 achievers in both the 15 mg and 30 mg groups decreased during the later stages, although this was not statistically significant compared to week 12 (100%): 71.4%, 64.3%, and 53.6% in the 15 mg group and 66.7%, 72%, and 65% in the 30 mg group at weeks 24, 36, and 48, respectively (Figure 3b).

The achievement rates for PP-NRS $\leq$ 1 in week 12 non-achievers in both the 15 mg and 30 mg groups were low and did not significantly increase during the later stages: 10.3%, 10.7%, and 15.2% in the 15 mg group, and 4%, 14.3%, and 20% in the 30 mg group at weeks 24, 36, and 48, respectively.

2.9. Adjusted Transition of Achievement Rates of Clinical Indexes at the Later Stages of Upadacitinib (30 mg) Treatment

Including patients previously treated with upadacitinib (15 mg) could potentially show unclear results due to the lack of response to upadacitinib (30 mg) treatment. Therefore, an analysis was conducted after excluding patients who had been treated with upadacitinib (15 mg) from the upadacitinib 30 mg group. New figures were created for the achievement rates of EASI 75, EASI 90, EASI 100, and EASI $\leq$ 2 (Supplemental Figure S1a–d), the achievement rate of IGA 0/1 (Supplemental Figure S2), and PP-NRS $\leq$ 1, PP-NRS 4 (Supplemental Figure S3a,b), similar to existing ones. Essentially, the results for the upadacitinib 30 mg group, after excluding patients with a history of upadacitinib (15 mg) treatment, showed almost similar outcomes, suggesting that prior treatment with upadacitinib (15 mg) might not have influenced the results.

3. Discussion

In this study, the achievement rates for EASI 75, 90, EASI $\leq$ 2, IGA0/1, PP-NRS 4, or PP-NRS $\leq$ 1 in week 12 achievers were consistent until week 48 of upadacitinib treatment. Although the achievement rate for EASI 100 in week 12 achievers decreased at later stages, the differences in frequency compared to week 12 were not statistically significant, possibly because of the decrease in the number of patients in later phases. Consistent with this study, a previous clinical trial of the JAK 1/2 inhibitor baricitinib reported long-term maintenance of therapeutic effects in early responders/partial responders who achieved IGA $\leq$ 2 at week 16 [14]. Specifically, in the baricitinib (4 mg) treatment group, the early responders/partial responders maintained the achievement rate of validated IGA-AD 0/1: 45.7% or 47.1% at week 16 or 68, respectively, although that of EASI 75 slightly decreased from 70% at week 16 to 55.7% at week 68. Similarly, in the baricitinib 2 mg treatment group, early responders/partial responders maintained achievement rates of validated IGA-AD 0/1 (46.3% or 59.3%) and EASI 75 (74.1% or 81.5%) at weeks 16 or 68, respectively. The results of that study indicated the long-term maintenance of early responses to JAK inhibitors in the treatment of AD.

Our previous real-world study showed that the achievement of IGA 0/1 at week 12 may be predicted by lower baseline EASI and higher age in the 15 mg upadacitinib treatment group and by lower immunoglobulin E and LDH in the 30 mg treatment group [15]. This indicates that patients with the above background may achieve IGA0/1 at week 12 and maintain a good response in the later stages of upadacitinib treatment at the respective doses.

In this study, the achievement rates of EASI 75 in week 12 non-achievers in both the upadacitinib 15 mg and 30 mg groups increased at later stages of treatment until week 48, although the differences were not statistically significant compared with week 12. These results indicate that slow responders may exist latently among early non responders to upadacitinib treatment. Relating to our findings, a post hoc analysis of the dupilumab open-label extension study [16] revealed that patients who did not achieve EASI 75 or IGA 0/1 at week 16 in SOLO 1 or 2 studies had high achievement rates at week 100: 91% for EASI 75 and 45% (biweekly treatment) or 49% (monthly treatment) for IGA 0/1. In our present study, the reason why some non-achievers of EASI 75 at week 12 benefited from prolonged treatment with upadacitinib remains unknown. However, it may be related to the patient's phenotypes/endotypes, genetic factors, or medication adherence levels. Our current findings indicate that some early non-responders at week 12 may benefit from continued upadacitinib treatment, implying a need for a longer evaluation period to fully assess the responsiveness to upadacitinib. Although determining the assessment time point is challenging, our results suggest that monitoring effects for up to a year might be reasonable. Patients who achieved EASI 75 at a later stage without early response may exhibit higher baseline EASI scores and younger age in the 15 mg treatment group or higher baseline IgE and LDH in the 30 mg treatment group, as analogized from our previous real-world data [15]. Alternatively, slow responders may mainly present with lichenification, whose response to upadacitinib is delayed compared to the other clinical signs, excoriation, erythema, or edema/papulation [11].

In this study, we observed that week 12 non-achievers of EASI 100, IGA 0/1, or PP-NRS $\leq$ 1 did not show a trend towards increased achievement rates of these endpoints at later stages of treatment until week 48. Achieving these endpoints suggests a complete or near-complete resolution of rash or pruritus, indicating that the potential to attain these stringent endpoints might be limited to early responders by week 12.

It is a very critical issue to choose between the continuation of upadacitinib treatment or switching to another treatment for patients who did not achieve EASI 75 at week 12. Because nearly half of the patients may potentially achieve EASI 75 in the later phase of treatment, physicians may continue treatment. However, this continuation may have a psychological impact on patients with AD, subjecting them to a potential insufficient response for a prolonged period. Identifying predictive factors for long-term effectiveness or slow responders could aid in choosing appropriate treatments for early non-responders by week 12.

Week 12 non-achievers of PP-NRS 4 in the 15 mg group showed higher achievement rates of PP-NRS 4 at the late stage compared to the 30 mg group, although the difference was not statistically significant (Figure 3a). This is possible because patients in the 15 mg group had higher baseline PP-NRS values and might have more room to reduce their PP-NRS than those in the 30 mg group (Table 1). Furthermore, the maintenance rate of PP-NRS 4 in week 12 achievers was significantly higher in the 15 mg group than in the 30 mg group (Figure 3a). These results were rather unexpected and may be because of bias owing to the much smaller number of week 12 achievers in the 30 mg group than that in the 15 mg group (Table 2) and/or because week 12 achievers in the 15 mg group may have a higher potential to sustain the response to upadacitinib on pruritus compared to those in the 30 mg group. The results indicate that the therapeutic effects of upadacitinib on pruritus may not consistently align with those on rash and may not always be dose-dependent.

Reports on the long-term effectiveness and safety of upadacitinib in managing AD in real-world clinical studies are increasing, illustrating the sustained therapeutic potential of the drug. This is highlighted in studies from Italy, such as those by Chiricozzi A et al. 2023 and Gargiulo et al. 2023, as well as the systematic review by Ibba L et al. [17] and others [8,10,18–20]. Chiricozzi A et al. detailed the outcomes for 146 patients with moderate-to-severe AD, most of whom (87.0%) received upadacitinib as monotherapy [8]. With 80.8% of these patients on a daily dose of 30 mg, significant clinical improvements were observed at week 16, and achievement rates of EASI 75, EASI 90, and EASI 100 were 78.2%, 47.6%, and 28.2%, respectively, at 16 weeks. At week 48, the achievement rates of EASI 75, EASI 90, and EASI 100 reached 87.6%, 69.1%, and 44.3%, respectively. The study underscored the consistent effectiveness of upadacitinib throughout the observation period. Gargiulo L et al.'s retrospective analysis of 71 patients demonstrated high achievement rates of IGA 0/1 (90.9%), EASI 75 (87.9%), EASI 90 (75.8%), and EASI 100 (57.6%) after one year, with significant symptom relief reported [10]. The effectiveness of upadacitinib was robust, regardless of previous dupilumab exposure, and the study reported no serious AEs. Ibba L et al.'s systematic review further confirms the long-term effectiveness and safety of upadacitinib for severe AD in real-world studies [17]. Through these comparative analyses, the vital role of upadacitinib in the AD treatment landscape is reinforced, endorsing its application as a primary treatment option for achieving long-term disease control.

This study had some limitations. First, the observation period of 48 weeks may be insufficient to fully assess the long-term effectiveness of upadacitinib treatment for AD. Future studies with longer treatment durations are necessary to provide a more comprehensive understanding of the long-term effects of this drug. Second, there was an imbalance in the number of patients between the upadacitinib 15 mg and 30 mg groups, indicating the need for further investigation with a more balanced proportion of participants. Thirdly, this study predicts the maintenance of effectiveness at week 48 based on the classification of subjects into achievers and non-achievers of various clinical indexes at week 12. While we identified baseline patient characteristics that reflect short-term effectiveness in our previous studies with upadacitinib (15 mg and 30 mg) at week 12, future research should focus on identifying baseline characteristics that could predict long-term effectiveness based on the clinical indexes evaluated in this study (achievement rate of EASI 75, 90, 100, IGA 0/1, EASI $\leq$ 2).

4. Materials and Methods

4.1. Study Design and Data Collection

This retrospective study was conducted from August 2021 to November 2023 and involved 300 Japanese patients (aged $\geq$ 12 years) with moderate to severe AD. These patients, diagnosed with AD based on the Japanese Guidelines for Atopic Dermatitis 2021, were identified as having moderate to severe AD with EASI $\geq$ 16 or head-and-neck EASI $\geq$ 2.4. All patients received daily oral upadacitinib (15 mg or 30 mg) combined with moderate to strong topical corticosteroids twice daily. Before upadacitinib treatment, data were collected on the patient's age, sex, body mass index, disease duration, history of bronchial asthma, allergic conjunctivitis, allergic rhinitis, and previous treatment with dupilumab, upadacitinib (15 mg), or baricitinib (4 mg). This study was conducted in accordance with the Declaration of Helsinki (2004) and approved by the Ethics Committee of Nippon Medical School Chiba Hokusoh Hospital. Written informed consent was obtained from all the patients.

4.2. Outcomes of Effectiveness

The EASI, PP-NRS, and IGA scores were analyzed before and after updacitinib treatment. At week 12, patients were divided into achievers and non-achievers of EASI 75, 90, or 100 (at least a 75%, 90%, or 100% reduction from baseline EASI, respectively), absolute EASI $\leq$ 2, IGA 0/1 (IGA scores of 0 (clear) or 1 (almost clear)), PP-NRS4 (PP-NRS reduction $\geq$ 4 points among patients with baseline PP-NRS $\geq$ 4-point), or absolute PP-NRS $\leq$ 1 (Table 2). The achievement rate of each endpoint was analyzed at later time points (weeks 24, 36, and 48) in week 12 achievers and non-achievers.

4.3. Statistical Analysis

Results were expressed as medians and interquartile ranges for nonparametrically distributed variables. Differences in frequencies were assessed using Fisher's exact test. Differences between the two groups were analyzed using the Mann–Whitney U test for variables with a nonparametric distribution. Statistical significance was set at $p < 0.05$. In cases of missing data, the affected patients were excluded from the analysis to ensure data integrity and accuracy. All statistical analyses were conducted using EZR software (version 1.55) (Saitama Medical Center, Jichi Medical University).

5. Conclusions

The reduction in rash and pruritus achieved at week 12 was maintained until week 48 of upadacitinib treatment. The achievement rate for EASI 75 in week 12 non-achievers increased until week 48 of treatment at both the 15 mg and 30 mg doses. These results indicate that a subset of non-achievers of EASI 75 at week 12 may benefit from prolonged treatment.

Supplementary Materials: The following supporting information can be downloaded at: https://www.mdpi.com/article/10.3390/ph17040519/s1, Supplemental Figure S1: Achievement rates for EASI 75 (a), EASI 90 (b), EASI 100 (c), and absolute EASI $\leq$ 2 (d) in week 12 achievers or non-achievers during treatment with upadacitinib 15 mg or 30 mg daily, excluding patients with a history of treatment with upadacitinib 15 mg. Supplemental Figure S2: Achievement rates for IGA 0/1 in week 12 achievers or non-achievers during treatment with upadacitinib 15 mg and 30 mg daily, excluding patients with a history of treatment with upadacitinib 15 mg. Supplemental Figure S3: Achievement rates for PP-NRS 4 (a) or PP-NRS $\leq$ 1 (b) in week 12 achievers or non-achievers during treatment with upadacitinib (15 mg or 30 mg daily), excluding patients with a history of treatment with upadacitinib 15 mg.

Author Contributions: All the authors contributed significantly to the manuscript and agree with its content. Conceptualization, T.H.; manuscript organization, T.H.; formal analysis, M.Y. and R.H.; supervision, N.K.; writing—review and editing, H.S. and E.F. All authors have read and agreed to the published version of the manuscript.

Funding: This research received no external funding.

Institutional Review Board Statement: This study was conducted according to the guidelines of the Declaration of Helsinki and approved by the Ethics Committee of Nippon Medical School Chiba Hokusoh Hospital (protocol codes: H-2022-945; approved 10 February 2022).

Informed Consent Statement: Informed consent was obtained from all subjects involved in the study.

Data Availability Statement: Data are contained within the article and Supplementary Materials.

Conflicts of Interest: H.S. received lecture fees and research costs from AbbVie. T.H. and N.K. received lecture fees from AbbVie. The remaining authors declare that the research was conducted in the absence of any commercial or financial relationships that could be construed as a potential conflict of interest.

References

1. Honda, T.; Kabashima, K. Reconciling innate and acquired immunity in atopic dermatitis. *J. Allergy Clin. Immunol.* **2020**, *145*, 1136–1137. [CrossRef] [PubMed]
2. Nakajima, S.; Tie, D.; Nomura, T.; Kabashima, K. Novel pathogenesis of atopic dermatitis from the view of cytokines in mice and humans. *Cytokine* **2021**, *148*, 155664. [CrossRef] [PubMed]
3. Kamata, M.; Tada, Y. Optimal use of jak inhibitors and biologics for atopic dermatitis on the basis of the current evidence. *JID Innov.* **2023**, *3*, 100195. [CrossRef]
4. Blauvelt, A.; Teixeira, H.D.; Simpson, E.L.; Costanzo, A.; De Bruin-Weller, M.; Barbarot, S.; Prajapati, V.H.; Lio, P.; Hu, X.; Wu, T.; et al. Efficacy and safety of Upadacitinib vs Dupilumab in adults with moderate-to-severe atopic dermatitis: A randomized clinical trial. *JAMA Dermatol.* **2021**, *157*, 1047–1055. [CrossRef] [PubMed]
5. Guttman-Yassky, E.; Teixeira, H.D.; Simpson, E.L.; Papp, K.A.; Pangan, A.L.; Blauvelt, A.; Thaçi, D.; Chu, C.Y.; Hong, H.C.; Katoh, N.; et al. Once-daily upadacitinib versus placebo in adolescents and adults with moderate-to-severe atopic dermatitis (Measure Up 1 and Measure Up 2): Results from two replicate double-blind, randomised controlled phase 3 trials. *Lancet* **2021**, *397*, 2151–2168. [CrossRef] [PubMed]
6. Reich, K.; Teixeira, H.D.; de Bruin-Weller, M.; Bieber, T.; Soong, W.; Kabashima, K.; Werfel, T.; Zeng, J.; Huang, X.; Hu, X.; et al. Safety and efficacy of upadacitinib in combination with topical corticosteroids in adolescents and adults with moderate-to-severe atopic dermatitis (AD UP): Results from a randomised, double-blind, placebo-controlled, phase 3 trial. *Lancet* **2021**, *397*, 2169–2181. [CrossRef] [PubMed]
7. Guttman-Yassky, E.; Thaçi, D.; Pangan, A.L.; Hong, H.C.; Papp, K.A.; Reich, K.; Beck, L.A.; Mohamed, M.F.; Othman, A.A.; Anderson, J.K.; et al. Upadacitinib in adults with moderate to severe atopic dermatitis: 16-week results from a randomized, placebo-controlled trial. *J. Allergy Clin. Immunol.* **2020**, *145*, 877–884. [CrossRef] [PubMed]
8. Chiricozzi, A.; Ortoncelli, M.; Schena, D.; Gori, N.; Ferrucci, S.M.; Babino, G.; Napolitano, M.; Fargnoli, M.C.; Stingeni, L.; Rossi, M.; et al. Long-term effectiveness and safety of upadacitinib for atopic dermatitis in a real-world setting: An interim analysis through 48 weeks of observation. *Am. J. Clin. Dermatol.* **2023**, *24*, 953–961. [CrossRef] [PubMed]
9. Kosaka, K.; Uchiyama, A.; Ishikawa, M.; Watanabe, G.; Motegi, S.I. Real-world effectiveness and safety of upadacitinib in Japanese patients with atopic dermatitis: A two-centre retrospective study. *Eur. J. Dermatol.* **2022**, *32*, 800–802. [CrossRef] [PubMed]
10. Gargiulo, L.; Ibba, L.; Piscazzi, F.; Alfano, A.; Cascio Ingurgio, R.; Valenti, M.; Costanzo, A.; Narcisi, A. Effectiveness and safety of upadacitinib for moderate-to-severe atopic dermatitis in a real-world setting: A 52-week retrospective study. *J. Eur. Acad. Dermatol. Venereol.* **2024**, *38*, e152–e154. [CrossRef] [PubMed]
11. Hagino, T.; Yoshida, M.; Hamada, R.; Fujimoto, E.; Saeki, H.; Kanda, N. Therapeutic effectiveness of upadacitinib on individual types of rash in Japanese patients with moderate-to-severe atopic dermatitis. *J. Dermatol.* **2023**, *50*, 1576–1584. [CrossRef] [PubMed]
12. Ständer, S.; Kwatra, S.G.; Silverberg, J.I.; Simpson, E.L.; Thyssen, J.P.; Yosipovitch, G.; Zhang, F.; Cameron, M.C.; Cella, R.R.; Valdez, H.; et al. Early itch response with abrocitinib is associated with later efficacy outcomes in patients with moderate-to-severe atopic dermatitis: Subgroup analysis of the randomized Phase III JADE COMPARE trial. *Am. J. Clin. Dermatol.* **2023**, *24*, 97–107. [CrossRef] [PubMed]
13. Hagino, T.; Yoshida, M.; Hamada, R.; Saeki, H.; Fujimoto, E.; Kanda, N. Early itch relief with upadacitinib predicts later skin clearance in Atopic dermatitis. *J. Dermatol. Treat.* **2024**, *35*, 2291317. [CrossRef] [PubMed]
14. Silverberg, J.I.; Simpson, E.L.; Wollenberg, A.; Bissonnette, R.; Kabashima, K.; DeLozier, A.M.; Sun, L.; Cardillo, T.; Nunes, F.P.; Reich, K. Long-term efficacy of baricitinib in adults with moderate to severe atopic dermatitis who were treatment responders or partial responders: An extension study of 2 randomized clinical trials. *JAMA Dermatol.* **2021**, *157*, 691–699. [CrossRef] [PubMed]
15. Hagino, T.; Yoshida, M.; Hamada, R.; Saeki, H.; Fujimoto, E.; Kanda, N. Predictive factors for responders to upadacitinib treatment in patients with atopic dermatitis. *J. Dermatol. Treat.* **2024**, *35*, 2310643. [CrossRef] [PubMed]
16. Armstrong, A.; Blauvelt, A.; Simpson, E.L.; Smith, C.H.; Herranz, P.; Kataoka, Y.; Seo, S.J.; Ferrucci, S.M.; Chao, J.; Chen, Z.; et al. Continued treatment with dupilumab is associated with improved efficacy in adults with moderate-to-severe atopic dermatitis not achieving optimal responses with short-term treatment. *Dermatol. Ther. (Heidelb.)* **2022**, *12*, 195–202. [CrossRef] [PubMed]
17. Ibba, L.; Gargiulo, L.; Vignoli, C.A.; Fiorillo, G.; Valenti, M.; Costanzo, A.; Narcisi, A. Practical Use of Upadacitinib in Patients with Severe Atopic Dermatitis in a Real-World Setting: A Systematic Review. *Clin. Cosmet. Investig. Dermatol.* **2024**, *17*, 593–604. [CrossRef] [PubMed]
18. Gargiulo, L.; Ibba, L.; Piscazzi, F.; Amoruso, F.; Balato, A.; Barei, F.; Bertello, M.; Burroni, A.G.; Caccavale, S.; Ferrucci, S.M.; et al. Upadacitinib improves symptoms of concomitant allergic rhinitis or allergic asthma in patients with severe atopic dermatitis: A 16-week multicentre retrospective study. *J. Eur. Acad. Dermatol. Venereol.* **2024**. *ahead of print*. [CrossRef] [PubMed]

19. Piscazzi, F.; Gargiulo, L.; Ibba, L.; Valenti, M.; Facheris, P.; Costanzo, A.; Narcisi, A. Upadacitinib for the treatment of atopic dermatitis in the elderly: An Italian case series of seven patients. *J. Dermatol. Treat.* **2023**, *34*, 2245510. [CrossRef] [PubMed]
20. Gargiulo, L.; Ibba, L.; Cortese, A.; Avagliano, J.; Valenti, M.; Costanzo, A.; Narcisi, A. Real-Life Effectiveness and Safety of Upadacitinib in Adults and Adolescents with Moderate-to-Severe Atopic Dermatitis: A Single-Center 16-Week Study. *Dermatol. Ther. (Heidelb.)* **2023**, *13*, 651–660. [CrossRef] [PubMed]

pharmaceuticals

MDPI

Article

Development of an Oral Isoliquiritigenin Self-Nano-Emulsifying Drug Delivery System (ILQ-SNEDDS) for Effective Treatment of Eosinophilic Esophagitis Induced by Food Allergy

Mingzhuo Cao [1,2], Yuan Wang [1,2], Heyun Jing [1], Zeqian Wang [1], Yijia Meng [2], Yu Geng [2], Mingsan Miao [1,*] and Xiu-Min Li [3,*]

[1] Academy of Chinese Medical Sciences, Henan University of Chinese Medicine, Zhengzhou 450058, China
[2] College of Pharmacy, Henan University of Chinese Medicine, Zhengzhou 450058, China
[3] Department of Pathology, Microbiology and Immunology, and Department of Otolaryngology, New York Medical College, Valhalla, NY 10595, USA
* Correspondence: miaomingsan@126.com (M.M.); xiumin_li@nymc.edu (X.-M.L.)

Abstract: Isoliquiritigenin (ILQ) is a natural flavonoid with various pharmacological activities. In this study, we optimized the preparation method of self-nano-emulsion-loaded ILQ to further improve its bioavailability based on our previous study. In addition, its effect on the treatment of eosinophilic esophagitis was also evaluated. Combined surfactants and co-surfactants were screened, and the optimal formulation of ILQ-SNEDDS was determined according to droplet size, droplet dispersity index (DDI), and drug loading. The formulation was composed of ethyl oleate (oil phase), Tween 80 & Cremophor EL (surfactant, 7:3), and PEG 400 & 1,2-propylene glycol (cosurfactant, 1:1), with a mass ratio of 3:6:1. Its physicochemical properties, including drug loading, droplets' size, Zeta potential, appearance, and Fourier transform infrared (FTIR) spectroscopy, were characterized. In vitro release profile, in situ intestinal absorption, and in vivo pharmacokinetics were applied to confirm the improvement of oral ILQ bioavailability by NEDDS. Finally, the efficacy of ILQ-SNEDDS in the treatment of food allergy-induced eosinophilic esophagitis (EOE) was further evaluated. When the ILQ drug loading was 77.9 mg/g, ILQ-SNEDDS could self-assemble into sub-spherical uniform droplets with an average size of about 33.4 ± 2.46 nm (PDI about 0.10 ± 0.05) and a Zeta potential of approximately -10.05 ± 3.23 mV. In situ intestinal absorption showed that optimized SNEDDS significantly increased the apparent permeability coefficient of ILQ by 1.69 times, and the pharmacokinetic parameters also confirmed that SNEDDS sharply increased the max plasma concentration and bioavailability of ILQ by 3.47 and 2.02 times, respectively. ILQ-SNEDDS also significantly improved the apparent signs, allergic index, hypothermia and body weight of EoE model mice. ILQ-SNEDDS treatment significantly reduced the levels of inflammatory cytokines, such as TNF-α, IL-4, and IL-5, and the level of PPE-s-IgE in serum, and significantly inhibited the expression of TGF-β1 in esophageal tissue. SNEDDS significantly improved the solubility and bioavailability of ILQ. Additionally, ILQ-SNEDDS treatment attenuated symptomatology of EoE model mice, which was associated with inhibiting the production of T_H2 inflammatory cytokines and PPE-s-IgE and the expression of TGF-β1. The above results shows that ILQ-SNEDDS has great potential as a good candidate for the treatment of eosinophilic esophagitis.

Keywords: eosinophilic esophagitis (EoE); isoliquiritigenin (ILQ); self-nano-emulsifying drug delivery system (SNEDDS); increased bioavailability

1. Introduction

Eosinophilic esophagitis (EoE) is a chronic esophageal inflammatory disease associated strongly with food allergy, characterized by significant esophageal eosinophils (Eos) and esophageal dysfunction, such as dysphagia and food impaction [1,2]. EoE imposes, on patients and their families, substantial negative impacts by causing emotional distress (fear and anxiety) and limiting social activities [3]. It has been documented that EoE has been rapidly increasing both in incidence and in prevalence over the last two decades, especially in Western countries [4]. EoE is currently the leading cause of dysphagia and bolus impaction and the second most common cause of chronic esophagitis after gastroesophageal reflux disease [2]. Despite increasing worldwide prevalence, EoE lacks sufficiently effective therapies. Due to the lack of sufficient understanding of the disease, there are no complete epidemiological data on EoE in China so far, but clinical reports of EoE case are gradually increasing significantly. Most EoE cases are in children (mainly 5–10 years old) and adults (mainly 30–50 years old) and clinical symptoms vary by age, with eosinophilic inflammation being seen in children and esophageal remodeling and fibrosis in adults [5,6]. This difference also supports the progression of EoE disease [2,7].

To date, the pharmacotherapy of EoE has highly relied on inhaled and swallowed corticosteroids. Despite their efficacy in suppressing EoE-related inflammation, concerns remain regarding long-term steroid use, such as esophageal candidiasis, abnormal bone mineral density, glaucoma, hyperglycemia, and other serious side effects [8]. It is urgent to find new, highly safe, and effective anti-inflammatory and anti-fibrosis agents for EoE.

Given the important roles of ongoing inflammation and fibrosis in the development of EoE disease, natural small-molecule compounds, such as polyphenols and flavonoids, with anti-inflammatory, antioxidant, and immunomodulatory effects have attracted increasing attention [9,10]. Isoliquiritigenin (ILQ, Figure 1) is a natural flavonoid compound with a chalcone structure, which has strong antioxidant, anti-inflammatory, anti-tumor, and anti-allergic effects [11–15]. In our previous study, we found that ILQ is one of the most potent flavonoids isolated from *Glycyrrhiza* to significantly suppress the Th2 type immune response and the production of eotaxin-1 [14,16,17], both of which greatly contribute to eosinophil inflammation in EoE. However, its poor solubility, fast elimination, and poor in vivo absorption hindered its further application in vivo [18]. Nanotechnology-based drug delivery systems have done good work in increasing the solubility and bioavailability of insoluble drugs in vivo, which has gradually become a consensus. Self-nano-emulsifying drug delivery systems (SNEDDS) have been paid extensive attention for their excellent properties for oral administration, such as spontaneous formation in the gastrointestinal tract, ease of manufacture, and low cost [19].

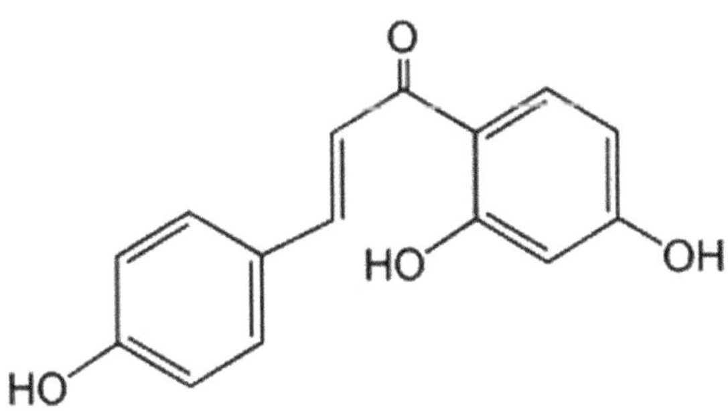

Figure 1. The structure of isoliquiritigenin (ILQ).

In our previous study, an oral self-nano-emulsified drug delivery system (SNEDDS)-loaded ILQ was designed to improve its solubility and in vivo bioavailability. However, the use of a high proportion of Tween 80 may result in an increased risk of hemolysis [20]. Currently, compatible surfactants and co-surfactants were used to optimize formulations for further improvement the safety and bioavailability of ILQ-SNEDDS. The appearance, average droplets' size, zeta potential, and morphology of the optimal ILQ-SNEDDS were characterized. Subsequently, the effects of different drug loadings on the in vitro release and in situ intestinal absorption of ILQ-SNEDDS were also investigated. Finally, the anti-inflammatory and anti-fibrosis effects of ILQ-SNEDDS were evaluated in a mouse model of eosinophilic esophagitis (EoE) induced by food allergy.

2. Results and Discussion

2.1. The Preparation and Characterization of ILQ-SNEDDS

In our previous study, by screening various excipients with high solubility of ILQ, oil phase, Tween 80, and PEG 400 were selected as oil phase, surfactant, and co-surfactant, respectively, with a weight ratio of 3:6:1. The high doses of Tween 80 in this formulation increase the risk of hemolysis toxicity of ILQ-SNEDDS administered in vivo. Therefore, in order to improve the safety of the nano-emulsion, this study intended to further improve the solubility of ILQ and decrease the dosage of Tween 80 without reducing the bioavailability of ILQ by screening other suitable mixed surfactants and co-surfactants.

Since the solubility of ILQ was nearly the same in Tween 80 and Cremophor EL, Cremophor EL was preferred as the mixed surfactant. The appropriate proportions between Tween 80 and Cremophor EL were further determined by a single factor factorial experiment. Maintaining the weight ratio of oil phase (ethyl oleate): mixed surfactant and co-surfactant (PEG-400) at 3:6:1, the ratios of Tween 80 and Cremophor EL were set at 9:1, 8:2, 7:3, 6:4, and 5:5. each ILQ-SNEDDS was prepared according to our previous method. The optimum ratio of Tween 80 to Cremophor EL was determined by comparing ILQ solubility, droplets' size, polydispersity index, and ξ potential. As shown in Figure 2A, each ILQ-SNEDDS showed both increased ILQ loading and droplets' size after the addition of Cremophor EL. When the ratio was 9:1, the drug loading of ILQ and its droplets' size were both the largest. As the Cremophor EL ratio continued to increase, the drug loading of ILQ and droplets' size both decreased a bit. The ratios of 8:2 and 7:3 showed high ILQ loading and small droplet size and polydispersity index, and was selected for the next experiment.

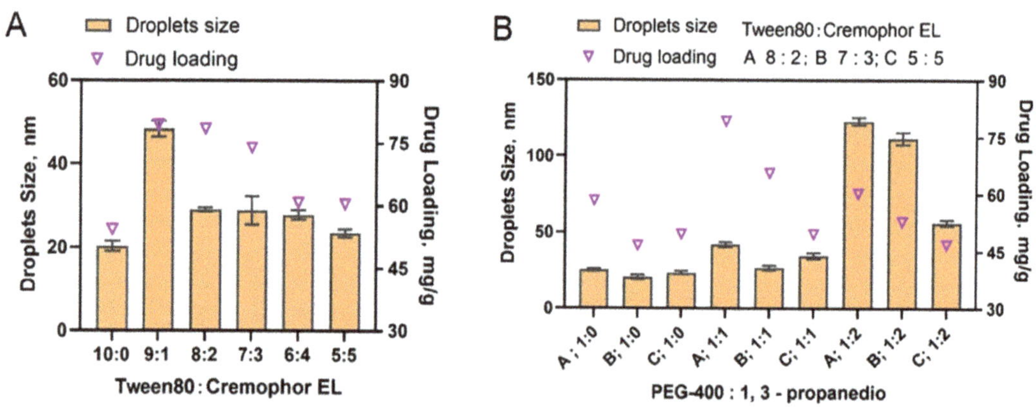

Figure 2. A single factor experiment was used to screen suitable mixed surfactant. (**A**) Screening of mixed surfactants; (**B**) screening of mixed co-surfactants.

Among the commonly used surfactants, the solubility of ILQ in 1,3-propanediol is the highest. However, droplet sizes of the nano-emulsion formed only with 1,2-propanediol as the cosurfactant were all more than 100 nm. Therefore, 1,2-Propanediol was considered to be used in combination with PEG 400 as a cosurfactant. A single factor experiment was used to further screen out the best ratio of the two. Ethyl oleate (oil phase):Tween80 and Cremophor EL (surfactant):1,2-propanediol and PEG 400 (cosurfactant) mass ratio was still set to 3:6:1, in which the ratios of Tween 80 to Cremophor EL (as co-surfactants) were set at 8:2, 7:3, and 5:5. The mass ratios of PEG 400 to 1,2-propanediol were set at 1.0, 1.1, and 1.2. The ILQ drug loading and droplet sizes of the prepared nano-emulsions are shown in Figure 2B. The results showed that the drug loading of ILQ increased when a certain proportion of

1,2-propanediol was added. But when the mass ratio of 1,2-propanediol to PEG 400 was set at 2:1, the droplet size of SNEDDS increased significantly to above 100 nm. Therefore, the mass ratio of 1,2-propanediol to PEG 400 (mixed cosurfactant) was determined to be 1:1.

Based on our previous study, a three-factor (Factor A, percentage of oil phase; Factor B, mass ratio of Tween80: Cremophor EL (mixed Surfactant); Factor C, the Km ratio of surfactant to co-surfactant) and three-level orthogonal experimental design were used to screen out the best formulation by comparing the drug loading of ILQ, droplets' size (polydispersity index and ξ potential) of the formed ILQ-SNEDDS. The results are shown in Table 1. The results of ILQ loading were analyzed first. The Km value of the ratio of surfactant and co-surfactant had the greatest influence on drug loading (R value was 19.91), followed by the percentage of oil phase (R value was 11.69). Mass ratio of Tween80 to Cremophor EL had the least effect on the results (R value of 4.83). Then, considering the droplets' size factor, when the Km value was 5:2, the droplets' sizes of the prepared nano-emulsion were not stable, which might be quite small (12 nm) or large (190 nm, 230 nm). Therefore, the finalized optimal SNEDDS formulation was oil phase (ethyl oleate), mixed surfactant (Tween 80: Cremophor EL, 7:3), and mixed cosurfactant (PEG 400:1, 2-propanediol = 1:1), with a mass ratio of 3:6:1. After 10-fold dilution with ultrapure water, they could quickly form a clear and transparent nano-emulsion in less than 2 min (Figure 3A–C). An interesting phenomenon was found during the study that the droplet size only increased slightly when the drug loading was lower than 80 mg/g under the optimized formulation conditions. The drug loading of ILQ-SNEDDS was 77.9 mg/g, and the encapsulation efficiency was 92.50% ± 0.45. As shown in Figure 3, the average droplet size was 33.40 ± 2.46 nm with a PDI of 0.10 ± 0.05 and its Zeta potential was −10.05 ± 3.23 mV. The results of TEM images of ILQ-SNEDDS (Figure 3D) were highly consistent with the DLS results. Most droplets were spherical in shape and uniform in size, ranging from 28–38 nm, with an average droplet size of 32.3 nm (Figure 3E). However, when the drug loading further increased, the droplet size was increased significantly and was positively correlated with drug loading. When the drug loading increased to 90 mg/g, the droplet size had increased to 140 nm with a broadened PDI, and when it further increased to 132 mg/g, the droplet size had increased to more than 240 nm.

Table 1. Orthogonal experiments of three factors and three levels. Factor A: Percentage of oil phase; Factor B: Mixed Surfactant (Tween80: Cremophor EL) mass ratio; Factor C: the mass ratio of surfactant and co-surfactant.

Num	Factor A	Factor B	Factor C	Drug Loading mg/g	Ave Size (nm)	Ave PDI	ζ Potential (mV)
1	25%	9:1	6	52.59	19.14	0.160	−6.74
2	25%	8:2	2.5	76.06	237.3	0.231	−5.28
3	25%	7:3	3.7	31.92	16.89	0.152	−9.27
4	30%	9:1	2.5	51.41	11.99	0.159	−8.34
5	30%	8:2	3.7	44.4	15.21	0.115	−8.61
6	30%	7:3	6	73.06	28.39	0.178	−10.11
7	35%	9:1	3.7	46.3	29.63	0.200	−9.79
8	35%	8:2	6	37.53	13.25	0.158	−3.47
9	35%	7:3	2.5	54.88	190.06	0.204	−4.39
Levels	A	B	C				
1	53.52	50.10	56.03				
2	57.93	52.66	40.87				
3	46.24	54.93	60.78				
R	11.69	4.83	19.91				
Ranking	2	3	1				

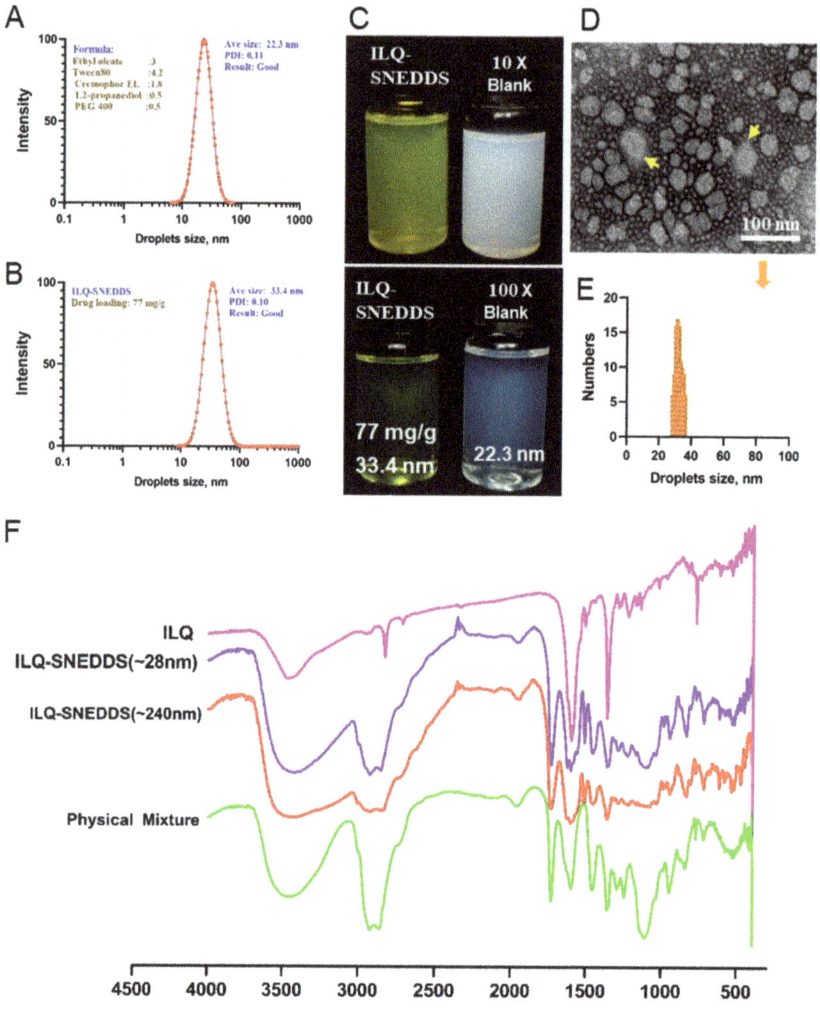

Figure 3. Physiochemistry characterization of ILQ-SNEDDS. (**A**) Blank SNEDDS droplet size distribution. (**B**) ILQ-SNEDDS droplet size distribution. (**C**) The appearance of freshly prepared Blank SNEDDS and ILQ-SNEDDS. (**D**) The TEM image of ILQ-SNEDDS (50 times dilution). The yellow arrows indicates that the droplets are at the edge of drug overload. (**E**) ILQ-SNEDDS droplet size distribution by TEM. (**F**) FTIR spectra of ILQ-SNEDDS (28 nm, 75 mg/g), ILQ-SNEDDS (240 nm, 135 mg/g), physical mixture (ILQ + SNEDDS), and ILQ.

On the FTIR spectrum (Figure 3F), the characteristic absorption peaks at 3426 cm^{-1} (O-H stretching vibration, disappeared), 2923 and 2858 cm^{-1} (νC-H stretching vibration, decreased), 1630 cm^{-1} (νC=C, increased), 1514 cm^{-1} (νC-H, increased), and 1110 cm^{-1} (νC-O stretching vibration, decreased) showed remarkable changes, indicating the increased interaction force between ILQ and SNEDDS.

2.2. In Vitro Release Profiles and Stability of ILQ-SNEDDS

In our previous study, we found that ILQ-SNEDDS showed robustness to dilution and good stability for storage. Therefore, we focused on the release behavior of ILQ-SNEDDS with different drug loading in the current study.

Figure 4A showed the release profiles of ILQ from a nano-emulsion with different drug loading. The results demonstrated that there was no significant difference in the cumulative release percentage for 12 h between ILQ-SNEDDS groups with different drug loading. More than 75% of ILQ were released from ILQ-SNEDD with a droplet size less than 33 nm. In addition, they were 20% higher than that of the ILQ suspension. However, ILQ-delayed release in simulated gastric juice was only observed in ILQ-SNEDDS groups with a droplet size of less than 33 nm and was negatively correlated with droplet sizes in comparison to the free ILQ-suspension. ILQ-SNEDDS with the largest droplet size (~240 nm) showed similar release characteristics with ILQ suspension in 1% Tween 80. Figure 4B showed the appearance of a nano-emulsion diluted 10 times and 100 times under different drug loading. These results suggested that ILQ-SNEDDS with small droplet size could successfully incorporate ILQ in bilayer emulsion droplets, thus contributing to much more ILQ release than the free ILQ suspension [21].

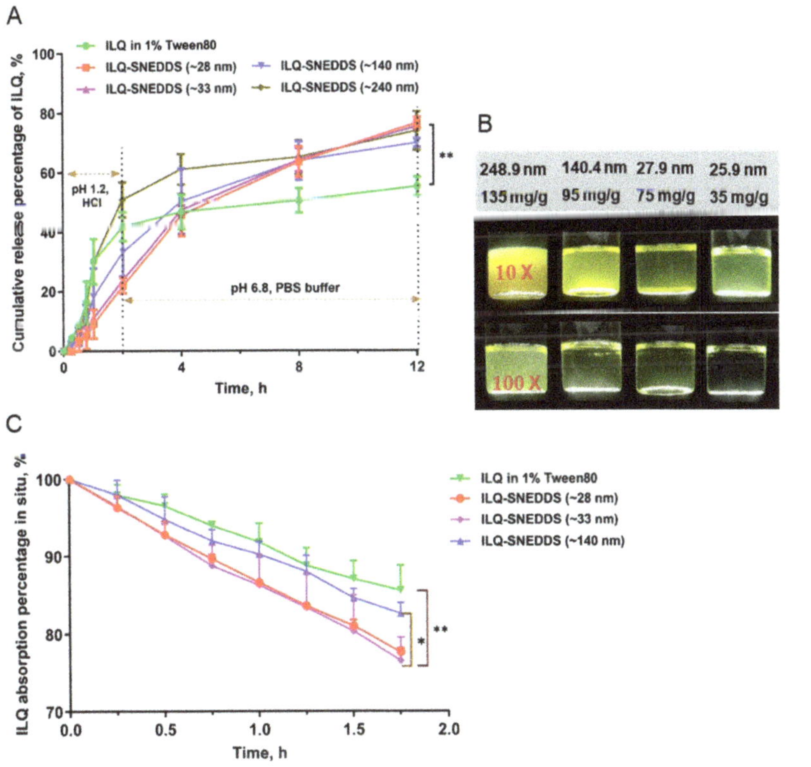

Figure 4. In vitro release profiles of ILQ from ILQ suspension and ILQ-SNEDDS with four different drug loading and their in-situ absorption. (**A**) In vitro release profiles of ILQ-SNEDDS in simulated gastric (pH 1.2, for the first 2 h) and intestinal (pH 6.8 PBS for the rest 22 h) fluid. (**B**) The appearance of freshly prepared ILQ-SNEDDS with different drug loading. (**C**) Absorption percentage curve of ILQ suspension or ILQ-SNEDDS with different drug loading in rats' proximal jejunum segment after perfusing 2 h with an ILQ dose of 200 μg/mL. Length of jejunum: 12~15 cm; Each value represents the mean ± SD, * $p < 0.05$ and, ** $p < 0.01$ (Prism Mann–Whitney test, n = 3~4).

SNEDDS is a thermodynamically stable system. The optimized ILQ-SNEDDS could withstand dilution with a large amount of simulated gastric juice (pH1.2 hydrochloric acid) and intestinal juice (pH 6.8 phosphate buffer), and its droplet size, PDI, and zeta potential showed minor changes under different harsh dilution conditions, indicating the good dilution stability of optimized ILQ-SNEDDS (Table 2). The optimized ILQ-SNEDDS was stored at 4 °C or 37 °C for more than one month, and its appearance did not show any change. However, with the extension of storage time to 2 months, it might coalesce, showing enlarged droplet sizes and reduced Zeta potentials (Table 2), especially under 37 °C.

Table 2. The results of stability of ILQ-SMEDDS at different storage conditions.

Items		Droplet Size (nm)	PDI	ζ-Potential (mV)
Freshly prepared (0 day)		27.93	0.151	−9.84
Dilution with pH 6.8 PBS		28.85	0.191	/
Dilution with 0.01 M HCl		28.33	0.204	/
1 month	at 4 °C	28.89	0.206	−8.34
	at 37 °C	29.30	0.211	−8.35
2 months	at 4 °C	140.41	0.224	−8.12
	at 37 °C	241.48	0.237	−4.41

2.3. Intestinal Absorption In Situ of ILQ-SNEDDS

In situ perfusion was used to evaluate the gastrointestinal absorption improvement potential of SNEDDS-ILQ preparations with different drug loading. As shown in Figure 4C, SNEDDS significantly increased the absorption of ILQ in the jejunum as expected, compared with free ILQ. However, ILQ drug loading could also significantly affect the absorption rate. The absorption rate of ILQ-SNEDDS with 75 mg/g was the highest and comparable to the drug loading of 35 mg/g, reaching 23.45%, which was 9.02% higher than that of free ILQ ($p < 0.01$), while ILQ-SNEDDS with 95 mg/g drug loading only increased by 3.03%. Parameters representing absorption enhancement, such as absorption rate constant (Ka), apparent permeability coefficient (Papp), and enhancement ratio (ER), were calculated and listed in Table 3. The results of in situ perfusion were consistent with the results of in vitro release, indicating that under the conditions of ensuring the small droplet size, properly increasing the drug loading would not affect the role of SNEDDS in promoting the absorption of ILQ. However, the excessive increase in drug loading would lead to a significant decrease in the absorption rate with the increase in droplet size.

Table 3. The absorption coefficient calculated in situ intestinal perfusion (n = 3 or 4).

Items	Globule Size and Drug Loading	Ap/%	Ka/h^{-1}	Papp·10^{-4}/h^{-1}·cm^2	Enhancement Ratio
ILQ-SNEDDS	28.9 nm (35 mg/g)	22.02 ± 0.39	0.144 ± 0.0043	29.58 ± 2.03	1.61
	33.6 nm (75 mg/g)	23.45 ± 2.96	0.149 ± 0.0060	30.97 ± 4.49	1.69
	140.4 nm (95 mg/g)	17.39 ± 1.34	0.104 ± 0.0107	20.14 ± 2.46	1.10
ILQ suspension	-	14.43 ± 3.27	0.086 ± 0.0080	18.34 ± 2.86	1.00

In a previous study, it was reported that a surfactant with an HLB value ranging from 10 to 17 in SNEDDS formulation plays a crucial role in enhancing drug absorption and intestinal penetration, which may be associated with the fact that surfactants could alter the mucus structure and enhance the hydrophilicity of the intestinal microenvironment [22,23]. In the current study, the co-surfactant of Tween 80 (with HLB 15) and Cremophor EL (with HLB 13.5) in the SNEDDS undoubtedly increased the absorption rate constant and apparent permeability coefficient of ILQ compared to free ILQ suspension. However, the droplet size was another important reason for the enhancement of ILQ permeation since the smaller droplet can easily permeate via the intestinal wall. If SNEDDS is overloaded with ILQ, its looser surfactant coating resulted in a larger droplet size and significantly lower permeability coefficient. Therefore, in the following experiments, the ILQ-SNEDDS with a drug loading of 75 mg/g was selected for in vivo experimental study.

2.4. Pharmacokinetic Study of ILQ-SNEDDS

Rats were given a single dose of 35 mg/kg free ILQ (dissolved in 1% Tween 80) and ILQ-SNEDDS (28.9 nm, equivalent to free ILQ). The plasma drug concentration–time profiles are presented in Figure 5, and the pharmacokinetic parameters were calculated by using a non-ventricular analysis and listed in Table 4. As shown in Figure 5, the maximum plasma concentration (C_{max}) of ILQ in the nano-emulsion group was 1.52 μg/mL, 3.47 times higher than that in the free ILQ group. Moreover, usage of SNEDDS led to a significant reduction in T_{max} (0.5 h vs. 0.75 h) and a statistically significant increase in $AUC_{0–t}$ compared to the free ILQ suspension.

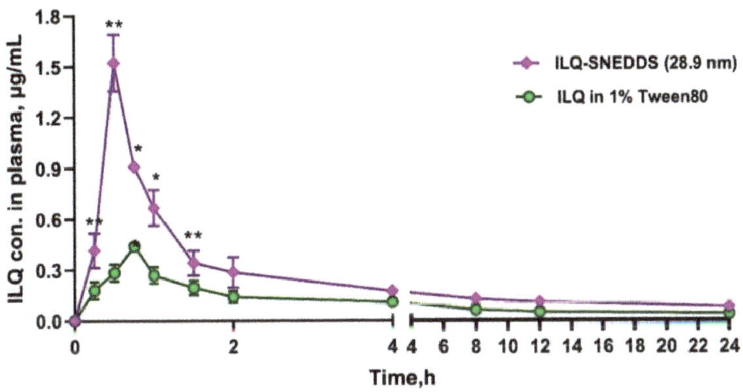

Figure 5. Mean plasma concentration–time profiles of ILQ in mice after oral administration of ILQ suspension or ILQ-SNEDDS (equivalent dose) at a dose of 35 mg/kg of ILQ. Each value represents the mean ± SD. * $p < 0.05$, ** $p < 0.01$. (Each time point, $n = 4$).

Table 4. Pharmacokinetic parameters after oral administration of free ILQ (35 mg/kg) or ILQ-SNEDDS (Equivalent Dose) in SD rats. (* $p < 0.05$.).

Items	Free ILQ Suspension	ILQ-SNEDDS
K_e, h^{-1}	0.4 ± 0.01	0.36 ± 0.01
$t_{1/2}$, h	1.79 ± 4.12	2.12 ± 6.87
T_{max}, h	0.75 ± 0.00	0.5 ± 0.00 *
C_{max}, μg/mL	0.43 ± 0.02	1.52 ± 0.13 *
AUC_{0-24}, μg/mL·h	1.86 ± 0.12	3.76 ± 0.38 *
Vz/F, L	320.32 ± 56.30	170.11 ± 13.11 *

Due to its poor dissolution capacity and low intestinal permeability, the free ILQ suspension showed poor bioavailability, while SNEDDS could improve the oral bioavailability of ILQ. The $AUC_{0–24}$ of the ILQ-SNEDDS was 3.80 μg·h·mL^{-1}, 2.02 times higher than that of free ILQ suspension, which was correlated with the result of the in vitro release study and in situ perfusion. In summary, the increased bioavailability of ILQ-SNEDDS was strongly associated with the following two factors: (i) SNEDDS could significantly increase the solubility of ILQ and ensure its dissolution, thereby improving the dissolution limiting step of ILQ [24,25]; (ii) the nano-emulsion with small droplet size could promote the intestinal lymphatic transport of ILQ [26,27]. Therefore, the C_{max} and $AUC_{0–24}$ of ILQ-SNEDDS increased by 3.47 times and 2.02 times, respectively, compared to the free ILQ suspension.

2.5. Hemolytic Toxicity of ILQ-SNEDDS

Tween-80 is widely used as a solubilizer and stabilizer in injection and oral preparations with a commonly used dosage of about 1–2%, including docetaxel and some vaccines. However, the hemolysis problem and other toxicities, including sensory neuropathy, nephrotoxicity, and hypersensitivity reactions caused by excessive use of Tween-80, have also attracted extensive attention, and the safe dosage of Tween-80 has become the focus of its use [20,28].

In this study, Tween-80 was still used as the major surfactant, but its dosage was reduced by more than 30% in the optimized formula. As shown in Figure 6, when the dose of ILQ-SNEDDS was under 50 µg/mL, no hemolysis could be observed. Within the effective therapeutic dose of ILQ-SNEDDS, the highest plasma concentration of ILQ was only about 1.65 µg/mL, the hemolysis toxicity caused by Tween 80 was unnoticeable. The single oral dose was even increased to 100 mg/kg and no obvious toxicity was found in rats. Since viable alternatives to Tween 80 remain unsolved, the toxicity caused by excessive use of Tween-80 should still be paid sufficient attention. The standardized use of Tween-80 is an essential method for the safe use of nano-emulsion.

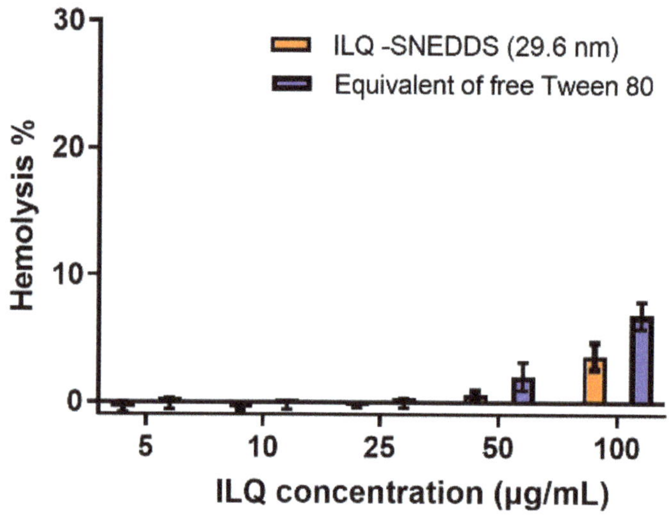

Figure 6. Hemolysis effect of ILQ-SNEDDS and equivalent amount of Tween-80 on rat RBC after incubation at 37 °C for 3 h ($n = 3$).

2.6. Pharmacodynamics Effects and Underlying Mechanism of ILQ-SNEDDS on EOE-Like Model Mice

2.6.1. ILQ-SNEDDS Alleviated Weight Loss and Hypothermia in EOE-Like Model Mice

A PPE-induced food allergy-like EOE mouse model was constructed according to the method (shown in Figure 7A) in a previous study [1] with minor modifications to evaluate the therapeutic effect of ILQ-SNEDDS. EOE mice daily received oral treatment with ILQ-SNEDDS at a 20 mg/kg equivalent ILQ dose for one month. In our previous study, ILQ-SMEDDS was developed to treat asthma, and the ILQ-SMEDDS group at the dose of 10 mg/kg showed a better anti-asthma effect than that of the ILQ suspension group at a dose of 20 mg/kg [29]. We made a first attempt to use ILQ to treat EOE, choosing ILQ-SNEDDS with higher bioavailability instead of free ILQ, which is also a limitation of the current study.

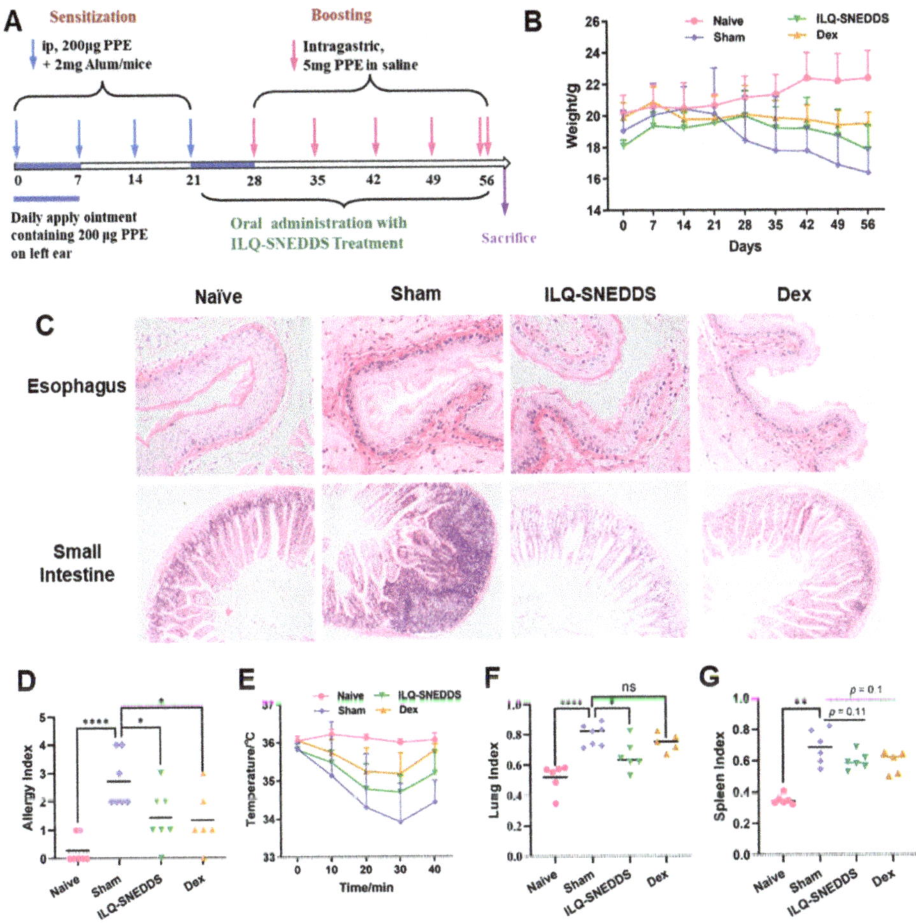

Figure 7. Daily oral treatment with ILQ-SNEDDS alleviated symptoms of food allergy-induced EoE-like disease mice. (**A**) Procedure for PPE-sensitized murine model of food allergy-induced EoE; (**B**) body weight; (**C**) H&E pathological section of esophagus (40×) and small intestine (20×) in each group. (**D**) Allergy index; (**E**) body temperature after the last challenge. (**F**) Spleen index, (**G**) lung index. Results are expressed as mean ± SD. *p* value was calculated by one-way ANOVA using Prism 9 software. * $p < 0.05$, ** $p < 0.01$, and **** $p < 0.0001$ compared to sham group.

We combined oral PPE challenge way and skin PPE challenge way to enhance the symptoms of experimental eosinophilic esophagitis. The PPE-induced EOE mouse model could well simulate the typical symptoms and pathological changes of EoE with typical characteristics of food allergy. Compared with the mice in the naïve group, all the model mice showed significant weight loss, decreased activity, poor hair luster, loose stool, spleen swelling, and responses of anaphylaxis, such as increased scratching behavior, hypothermia, cyanosis, difficulty breathing, and other severe hypersensitivity responses. In addition to the above allergic symptoms, the model mice also had symptoms of ear scabbing or even thickening. The above symptoms were mainly consistent with the clinicopathological changes of EoE. As shown in Figure 7B, the mean weight of sham-treated mice decreased significantly after each PPE challenge, which was 0.63 g lower than before the experiment after the first PPE challenge. Additionally, it had decreased by 2.71 g by the end of the experiment. Although the weight of the mice treated with ILQ-SNEDDS also decreased after PPE challenges, the weight of mice even increased by 0.63 g after four PPE challenges and only decreased by 0.29 g after the last high-dose PPE challenge. Furthermore, all sham-treated mice developed anaphylaxis with a mean symptom score of 2.71. Treatment with ILQ-SNEDDS could effectively reverse the pathogenesis of esophagitis and greatly alleviated these symptoms. The allergic symptom scores of mice treated with ILQ-SNEDDS were significantly lower than those of the sham mice ($p < 0.05$, Figure 7D), with no significant difference from dexamethasone-treated mice.

H&E staining results directly showed the pathological changes of EOE model mice. As shown in Figure 7C, the esophageal tissue of mice in the sham group was altered in association with the disease; the esophageal wall was significantly thickened, swollen, and congested, the lamina propria was elongated, the upper lamina propria was fibrotic, and the infiltration of inflammatory cells and eosinophils around the esophagus was significantly increased compared to the naïve mice. ILQ-SNEDDS and Dex treatment greatly relieved the above symptoms.

Figure 7E showed the changes in body temperature of all mice within 40 min after the last challenge. Core body temperature of all model mice dropped within 30 min after the challenge and recovered after 40 min. The mean body temperature of sham-treated mice was the lowest at 30 min, which was 33.92 ± 1.01 °C, and 2.08 °C lower than that of the naïve mice ($p < 0.001$). ILQ-SNEDDS and dexamethasone treatment could alleviate hypothermia in model mice, and their mean body temperature was 35.18 ± 0.54 °C and 34.84 ± 0.73 °C ($p < 0.05$, and $p = 0.15$, compared with the sham group). Anaphylaxis, such as food allergy and EoE, is a systemic disease triggered by the release of multiple inflammatory cells and might cause a variety of viscera damage [1]. The results of pathological section also showed that the intestinal structure of the sham mice was abnormal, damaged, and accompanied by a large number of inflammatory cells' infiltration. In addition, the sham mice also showed significant pulmonary inflammation and splenomegaly, with a significant increase in lung index (151.5%, $p < 0.001$, Figure 7F) and spleen index (208.0%, $p < 0.001$, Figure 7G) compared with the naïve mice. After treatment with ILQ-SNEDDS, the lung index and spleen index of mice decreased by 15.3% and 12.0%, respectively ($p < 0.05$, $p = 0.1$), indicating that ILQ-SNEDDS treatment could improve inflammation in the small intestine, spleen, and lung of mice to a certain extent.

2.6.2. ILQ-SNEDDS Reduced the Levels of IL-4, IL-5 and TNF-α in Peripheral Blood of EoE-Like Model Mice

Increasing evidence shows that EoE is the late manifestation of anaphylaxis progression, which usually starts from atopic dermatitis and develops into IgE-mediated food allergy, asthma, allergic rhinitis, and EoE [30]. Moreover, as a progressive disease, if not treated, the persistent inflammation generated during the active EoE will accelerate the progress of esophageal stenosis and fibrosis remodeling, leading to irreversible esophageal function damage in patients [31]. In the complex pathogenesis of EoE, multiple immune cells, such as T_H2 cells, eosinophils, and mast cells, are involved and jointly contribute to the inflammation produced in the active EoE [31,32].

As shown in Figure 8A–C, the levels of TNF-α, IL-4, and IL-5 in the serum of sham mice were sharply increased compared with those in naïve mice ($p < 0.0001$, $p < 0.0001$, and $p < 0.0001$). TNF-α is one of the earliest and most important inflammatory mediators in the process of inflammatory response [33]. TNF-α levels in the serum in the sham group reached 484.57 ng/mL. ILQ-SNEDDS and dexamethasone treatment could significantly reduce the above inflammatory cytokines compared with the sham group. The levels of TNF-α, IL-4, and IL-5 were decreased by 33.3% ($p < 0.05$), 56.7% ($p < 0.001$), and 39.6% ($p < 0.01$), respectively, after ILQ-SNEDDS treatment (Figure 8B,C).

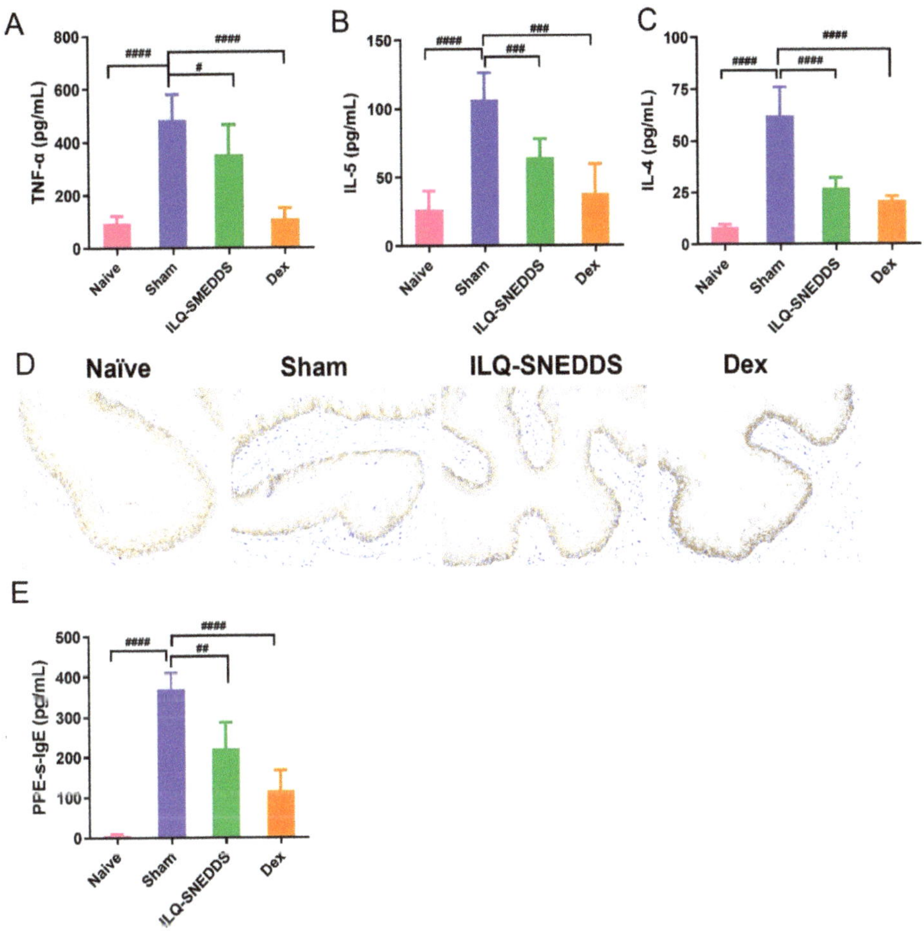

Figure 8. ILQ-SNEDDS treatment reduced the serum levels of the relevant Th2 inflammatory cytokines, TGF-β1 expression, and PPE-s-IgE. (**A**) TNF-α; (**B**) IL-4; (**C**) IL-5; (**D**) ICH for TGF-β1 expression (40×); (**E**) PPE-s-IgE. Results are expressed as mean ± SD. p value was calculated by one-way ANOVA using Prism 9 software., #, ##, ###, ####, $p < 0.05$, $p < 0.01$, $p < 0.001$, and $p < 0.0001$ as compared to the sham group.

2.6.3. ILQ-SNEDDS Suppressed the Expression of TGF-β1

In addition to the above inflammatory cytokines produced by immune cells, TGF-β1-mediated esophageal inflammation and fibrosis also played a critical role in the occurrence and development of EoE [5,34,35]. One study found that blocking TGF-β1 and MAPK signaling could inhibit the secretion of fibronectin and type I collagen by esophageal fibroblasts and muscle cells, thus relieving esophageal fibrosis [36]. As shown in Figure 8D, the TGF-β1 positive expression was yellowish brown and diffusely distributed in the cytoplasm of esophageal tissue. The TGF-β1 positive expression level in the sham group was much higher than that of the naïve group. After ILQ-SNEDDS treatment, the TGF-β1 positive expression level was obviously decreased.

2.6.4. ILQ-SNEDDS Reduced PPE-s-IgE Production in Peripheral Blood of EoE-Like Model Mice

Whether specific IgE plays an active role in the pathogenesis of disease or whether it is only a prognostic marker remains unclear. However, intensive studies have also confirmed that IgE is indeed closely associated with EoE [32].

Figure 8E showed the results of PPE-s-IgE levels measured by ELISA. Compared with the naïve group, the serum PPE-s-IgE in the sham group was significantly increased ($p < 0.0001$), with an average concentration of 369.89 ng/mL. ILQ-SNEDDS treatment could depress serum PPE-s-IgE production, which was significantly decreased by about 40% compared with that in the sham group ($p < 0.01$).

These physiological conditions and symptoms associated with EoE disease were gradually improved following the ILQ-SNEDDS treatment. However, although the safety of natural small molecule ILQ is significantly higher than that of dexamethasone, its improvement effect on EOE clinical symptoms is still inferior to that of dexamethasone. In view of the good anti-inflammatory and antioxidant effects of ILQ, it has significant potential in the treatment of asthma, food allergy, and EoE. We will continue to look for other phytonanotechnologies [37] that can improve the bioavailability of ILQ more efficiently in our subsequent research.

This study has several limitations. EoE is commonly associated with concomitant atopic diseases including atopic dermatitis, food allergy, and asthma. There were no significant differences between sexes in mid/proximal or distal esophageal eosinophil count in both adults and children [38]. Although EOE worldwide is predominant in male children and adults [38], we used female mice in our study according to the literature [1], because female mice experience more airway remodeling and T_H2 inflammation compared with male mice [39,40]. However, due to the differences in hormone levels and metabolism between men and women, to mice gender should be properly considered in EOE pathogenesis and drug absorption [41].

3. Materials and Methods

Isoliquiritigenin (ILQ, 98.0%) was purchased from Herb Purify Co., Ltd. (Chengdu, China). Ethyl oleate (EO), 1,3-propanediol, acetanilide Cremophor EL, urethane, and phenol red were purchased from Aladdin (Shanghai, China). Tween 80 and Al $(OH)_3$ gels were obtained from Sigma Aldrich (Shanghai, China). PEG 400 was obtained from Yipusheng Pharmaceutical Co., Ltd. (Ji'an, China).

3.1. Animals

Sprague Dawley (SD) rats (200 ± 20 g) and BALB/c mice (6–8 weeks old) were obtained from Shandong Laboratory Animal Center (Peng-Yue Laboratory Animals, Jinan, China). All mice were housed at 22 ± 2 °C in cages within laminar airflow hoods in a specific pathogen-free room with a 12-h light/12-h dark cycle and fed autoclaved chow and water ad libitum.

3.2. Preparation and Characterization of ILQ-SNEDDS

3.2.1. HPLC Method

The HPLC (e2695 system, Waters, Eschborn, Germany) method was established for the analysis of ILQ as previously reported with some modifications [16]. The detailed conditions were as follows: acetonitrile–water mixture (40/60, v/v) was used as mobile phase, with HPLC temperature set at 30 °C, wavelength at 372 nm, and flow rate 1.0 mL/min. The solubility of ILQ in surfactants was measured using the method reported in our previous study [29].

3.2.2. Optimization, Preparation, and Characterization of the ILQ-SNEDDS

In this study, we aimed to decrease the dosage of Tween 80. The use of mixed cosurfactants could directly reduce the dosage of Tween 80 on the one hand, and on the other hand, it could further indirectly reduce the dosage of Tween 80 by increasing the solubility of ILQ.

ILQ-SNEDDS was prepared using the method reported in our previous study. All emulsion components were mixed in pre-designed proportions and sonicated for 10 min to produce a homogeneous liquid. Then, excess ILQ was added to the above liquid and sonicated for 10 min. After that, the mixture was oscillated overnight at 100 rpm and 37 °C in an oscillation (Anjing Equipment, Shanghai, China). Finally, the undissolved ILQ precipitate was removed by centrifugation (Microfuge 20R, Beckman Coulter, Pasadena, CA, USA) at 8000 rpm for 30 min. Additionally, the transparent ILQ-SNEDDS was stirred gently with water (100-fold, v/v) drop by drop. The size, polydispersity index, and Zeta potential of ILQ-SNEDDS droplets were determined using a NanoBrook90PlusPALS meter (Brookhaven Instruments Corporation, Holtsville, NY, USA) at 25 °C.

Single-factor and orthogonal experimental designs were used to screen suitable ratios of mixed surfactants, mixed co-cosurfactants, and best prescription. Firstly, the weight ratio of ethyl oleate (EO, oil), Tween 80 (surfactant), and PEG-400 (co-surfactant) was fixed as 3:6:1, Tween 80 was replaced with different ratios of Tween 80 and Cremophor EL, and the droplets' size and drug loading were obtained using the above methods. Then, the optimal ratios of Tween 80 and Cremophor EL in the previous step were chosen for further screening of the optimum ratio of PEG-400 and 1,3-propanediol. Finally, a three-factor and three-level orthogonal experiment was performed to explore the best formulation.

The size and morphology of optimized ILQ-SNEDDS were obtained by transmission scanning electron microscope (TEM-1400, Tokyo, Japan) after staining with 2% phosphatotungstic acid (PTA). Drug encapsulation efficiency (EE) and drug loading (DL) were measured by the centrifugation method previously reported in the literature with some modification [42]. The new prepared ILQ-SNEDDS was diluted with methanol. The amount of ILQ was determined by HPLC after being filtered through a 0.22 μm filter membrane. The encapsulation efficiency and drug loading (DL) were calculated as follows:

$$EE(\%) = \frac{W_{\text{Loaded}}}{W_{\text{Total}-\text{added}}} \times 100\% \quad (1)$$

$$DL = \frac{W_{\text{Loaded}}}{W_{\text{Emulsion}}} \quad (2)$$

In which W_{loaded} and $W_{\text{total-added}}$ are the weight of encapsulated ILQ, the total amount of ILQ added, and the weight of emulsion added, respectively.

The IR spectra of ILQ-SNEDDS, ILQ, and mixture of ILQ and SNEDDS were acquired on the Fourier-transform infrared spectrometer (FT-IR) (Spectrum 100, Platinum Elmer, Waltham, MA, USA) by using a potassium bromide pressed disk method.

3.2.3. Stability of ILQ-SNEDDS

The stability of ILQ-SNEDDS under certain storage times and pH values was investigated, and the changes in emulsion appearance and droplets' size were recorded. ILQ-SNEDDS samples after dilution with 100 times ultra-pure water were stored in vials at 37 °C or 4 °C for 2 months. At a set time of 0, 0.5, 1, and 2 months, the droplets' size, PDIs, and zeta potentials were measured.

Tolerating the physiological pH of the gastrointestinal tract is very important for oral nano-emulsions to improve the bioavailability of drugs. The newly prepared ILQ-SNEDDS were diluted with simulated gastric fluid (pH 1.2 HCL) and intestinal fluid (pH 6.8 PBS) within a predetermined range, and the droplets' size, PDIs, and ζ potential were measured.

3.2.4. In Vitro Release Profile

The in vitro release of ILQ in ILQ-SNEDDS with different droplets' size in the simulated gastric and intestinal fluid was performed using the dialysis-diffusion method according to the Chinese Pharmacopoeia (2020) with slight modification. ILQ suspension

(5 mg ILQ in 2 mL of 2.0% Tween 80 liquid) and four ILQ-SNEDDSs (2 mL nano-emulsions with equivalent amount of ILQ) were placed in dialysis bags (weight cut-off 5000 Da). They were then placed in 250 mL release medium containing 1% Tween 80 (pH 1.2 HCl for the first 2 h and pH 6.8 PBS for the last 10 h) at 37 °C and oscillated at 150 rpm. Dialysate (2 mL each) was taken at scheduled time points and replenished quickly with fresh medium of equal volume. The release amount of ILQ in dialysate was determined by HPLC.

3.3. *Absorption In Situ and Pharmacokinetic In Vivo Studies*

Intestinal Absorption In Situ

The effects of different droplet sizes of ILQ-SNEDDS on the percent absorption (AP), absorption rate constant (Ka), and apparent permeability coefficient (Papp) of ILQ intestinal absorption were investigated using a rat in situ perfusion model according to the reported method with minor modifications [43,44]. Briefly, anesthetized rats were restrained in the supine position and maintained at normothermia using an infrared light. Upon confirmation of the loss of pain reflex, its abdomen was incised with an approximately 3 cm midline longitudinal incision. The distal jejunum was intubated immediately with two glass tubes (3.5 mm, OD) and ligated with surgical silk suture. Selected intestinal segments were gently rinsed with 5 mL of pre-warmed pH 7.4 PBS to remove fecal residue and debris, and then attached to the perfusion assembly consisting of a 2-head peristaltic pump (L100-1F/DG-2, Baoding Extended Precision Pump Co., Ltd., Baoding, China). One hundred milliliters of ILQ-SNEDDS with different droplets' size or ILQ suspension with an equivalent initial ILQ concentration were perfused through the selected intestinal segment at a flow rate of 6 mL/min for 10 min. The flow rate was subsequently adjusted to 3 mL/min, and after equilibration for an additional 15 min, the solution volume was recorded as the 0 min volume. Each perfusion experiment lasted for 1.75 h, and samples were taken at a preset interval of 15 min. At the end of the experiment, the radius and lengths of the perfused intestinal segment and the amount of ILQ remaining in each sample were measured. The absorption rate (AP), absorption rate constant (Ka, min^{-1}), apparent permeability coefficient (Papp, $\text{cm}^2{\cdot}\text{min}^{-1}$), and enhancement ratio (ER) of ILQ-SNEDDS with different droplets size or ILQ-Suspension were calculated as follows:

$$\text{AP} = \frac{C_0V_0 - C_0V}{C_0V_0} \times 100\% \tag{3}$$

$$\ln X_t = \ln X_0 - K_a \times t \tag{4}$$

$$P_{\text{app}} = K_\text{a}/\text{A} \tag{5}$$

$$\text{ER} = \frac{P_{\text{app}} \text{ of ILQ} - \text{SNEDDS}}{P_{\text{app}} \text{ of free ILQ Suspension}} \times 100\% \tag{6}$$

In which C_0 (or C_t) and V_0 (or V_t) were the concentration and volume of ILQ-SNEDDS (or free ILQ-suspension) in perfusate at 0 (or t) h, respectively. X_t and X_0 indicated the amounts of ILQ remaining in the perfusate at t h and 0 h, respectively. A (cm^2) was the surface area of the perfused intestinal segment (Length × diameter of intestinal).

3.4. *Pharmacokinetic Studies*

After one week of domestication, 20 female SD rats were randomly divided into two groups. All the animals were fasted overnight before the experiment with free access to water.

Rats were orally administered either free ILQ suspension (in PBS containing 1% Tween 80) or ILQ-SNEDDS (ILQ equivalent) at 35 mg/kg. We collected 0.5 mL of blood from the retro-orbital plexus at each set time point (0, 0.25, 0.5, 0.75, 1, 1.5, 2, 4, 8, 12, 24 h) after administration. Plasma was obtained by centrifugation at 3000 rpm for 15 min and stored at −80 °C for further HPLC analysis. Then, 100 μL of plasma sample was mixed with

15 μL of acetanilide (50 μg/mL, internal standard) and deproteinized by adding 600 μL of acetonitrile for 15 min. After centrifugation at 12,000 rpm for 25 min, the supernatant was dried at room temperature in a concentrator (Eppendorf, Hamburg, Germany). The samples were dissolved in mobile phase and analyzed by HPLC.

Non-compartmental analysis was performed using PK Solver 2.0 software (a plug-in program for pharmacokinetic analysis in Microsoft Excel) to obtain key pharmacokinetic parameters, including Lambda_z (h^{-1}, terminal elimination rate constant), T_{max} (h, time to reach maximum plasma concentration), C_{max} ($\mu g \cdot mL^{-1}$, maximum plasma concentration), AUC_{0-24} ($\mu g \cdot mL^{-1}$, area under the plasma concentration time curve), Vz/F ($L \cdot kg^{-1}$, apparent volume of distribution), and $T_{1/2}$ (h, half-life).

3.5. Hemolytic Toxicity of ILQ-SNEDDS

We prepared 5×10^8 /mL Red Blood Cells (RBC) suspension according to the method reported in our previous study [29,45]. First, 0.5 mL of 5, 10, 25, 50 μg/mL ILQ-SNEDDS and equivalent of Tween 80 were added to equal volume of RBC suspension, and 1% Triton X100 and PBS were used as positive and negative controls, respectively (n = 3). After gently shaking, the RBC suspension was incubated at 37 °C for 3 h. Afterwards, each sample was centrifuged at 3500 rpm/min at room temperature for 5 min. Then, 100 μL of supernatant of each sample was transferred to a 96-well plate and the absorbance at 570 nm was recorded using a microplate reader (SpectraMax iD3, Molecular Devices, San Jose, CA, USA). Percentage of hemolysis was calculated with the following equation:

$$\text{Hemolysis\%} = (OD_{sample} - OD_{PBS})/(OD_{1\%\ Triton\text{-}100} - OD_{PBS}) \times 100\% \quad (7)$$

3.6. Establishment of PPE-Induced EOE Model

The peanut protein extract (PPE)-induced EoE model was established using a previously reported method with minor modification [1,34]. The BALB/c mice were randomly divided into four groups according to the random number table method after adaptive feeding for 1 week, which were designated as naïve group, sham group, dexamethasone control group, and nano-emulsion treatment group, respectively. PPE was prepared by PBS extraction after completely degreasing with acetone, following the method used in our laboratory before.

Except for the naïve group, the BALB/c mice were sensitized by intraperitoneal (i.p.) injections of 0.2 mg PPE adsorbed to 2 mg Alum adjuvant in 200μL PBS on the 0th, 7th, 14th, and 21st days. Meanwhile, they were sensitized by applying 20 mg of calcipotriol ointment containing 1% PPE to the left ear from the days 1–7 and 21–28. Then, they were challenged orally with 5 mg PPE in 100 μL PBS on days 28, 35, 42, and 49, and 10 mg PPE in 100 μL PBS on day 56 (for a total of 5 challenges). All mice were intragastrically treated for 5 weeks. The naïve group was injected, applied, or treated with an equal volume of PBS.

3.7. Pharmacodynamic Effect Evaluation

General epigenetic indications' observation, serum PPE-specific-IgE (PPE-s-IgE), IL-4, IL-5, TNF-α cytokines, and esophagus, small intestine, lung histopathological analyses were used to evaluate the pharmacodynamic effect of ILQ-SNEDDS on food allergy-induced EoE.

Epigenetic indications included body weight, other behaviors during the entire experiment, rectal temperature, and allergy index after the last challenges, as well as spleen and lung index after sacrifice.

Allergy indices were observed over 40 min and grades 0–5 was used to score the reactions by blind method as previously described [46,47] with minor modifications. The criteria were as follows: 0—asymptomatic; 1—head and nose disturbance; 2—diarrhea, edema around eyes and mouth, erect hair, and decreased activity frequency; 3—cyanosis, dyspnea and decreased activity frequency, and drop in temperature; 4—no reaction or only mild reaction, hypothermia, tremor, and spasm; 5—death. Rectal temperatures were measured using a rectal probe at 0, 10, 20, 30, and 40 min.

Blood was collected at the end of the experiment. The levels of PPE-s-IgE, IL-4, IL-5, and TNF-α (pharmingen, BD Biosciences, New York, USA) were determined by ELISA according to the manufacturer's instructions. The mice were sacrificed, the tissues of esophagus and small intestine were taken and fixed with 4% paraformaldehyde, paraffin-embedded, and sectionalized in 5μm thick sections using a Leica RM2235 microtome (Leica, Nussloch, Germany). The pathological specimens were stained with hematoxylin and eosin (H&E). The inflammatory infiltration, tissue damage, villus deformation, and edema of intestinal epithelial cells in the tissues were observed by an inverted microscope (Nikon, Tokyo, Japan).

TGF-β1 Immunohistochemistry: The paraffin section of the esophagus tissue was dewaxed and fixed, incubated with TGF-β1 antibody (Immunoway, Wuhan, China), and then antibody II, and then the slices were stained and sealed. The positive expression of TGF-β1 was observed with an inverted microscope.

3.8. Statistical Analysis

All data were represented as mean ± standard deviation (SD). All inter-group statistical analyses were performed by using unpaired *t* test (Mann–Whitney test, *p* smaller than 0.05 considered statistically significant) by GraphPad Prism 9 software (GraphPad Software, Inc., La Jolla, CA, USA).

4. Conclusions

In our previous study, the good properties of ILQ-SNEDDS improved the bioavailability and anti-asthma activity of ILQ. In the current study, and we further optimized the formulation of SNEDDS to reduce the Tween 80 dosage and made a first attempt to use ILQ to treat EOE. The optimized formula of ILQ-SNEDDS consisted of an oil phase (ethyl oleate), surfactant (Tween 80: Cremophor EL = 7:3), and cosurfactant (PEG 400:1, 2-propylene glycol = 1:1), with a mass ratio of 3:6:1, and it showed good biophysical properties, including small droplet size, appropriate negative Zeta potential, high drug content, and good stability. These favorable properties of ILQ-SNEDDS improve the bioavailability of ILQ and made ILQ show excellent anti-EoE activity by inhibiting the production of T_H2-inflammatory cytokines and PPE-s-IgE, and the expression of TGF-β1 in EoE model mice. This study provides a promising new drug candidate for the treatment of eosinophilic esophagitis.

Author Contributions: Conceptualization, M.C. and X.-M.L.; methodology, M.C. and Y.G.; validation, Y.W., H.J. and Y.M.; investigation, Y.W., Z.W. and Y.M.; data curation, M.C. and Y.W.; Writing—original draft preparation, M.C.; writing—review and editing, M.M. and X.-M.L.; supervision, M.M.; funding acquisition, M.M., M.C. and X.-M.L. All authors have read and agreed to the published version of the manuscript.

Funding: This work was funded by M.C., grants number: 222102310662 (Henan Province Science and Technology Research Project) and BSJJ2022-13 (Henan University of Chinese Medicine), and M.M. and X.L., grants number: GZS2019006 (Henan Outstanding Foreign Scientist Project). and ORA LOG NO.: 012318-101 (Henan University of Chinese Medicine and New York Medical College).

Institutional Review Board Statement: The study was conducted in accordance with the NIH guidelines for the care and use of laboratory animals, and was approved by the Animal Care and Use Committee (Approval No. DWLL202105101S) of Henan University of Chinese Medicine.

Informed Consent Statement: Not applicable.

Data Availability Statement: Data is contained within the article.

Conflicts of Interest: The authors declare no conflict of interest.

References

1. Lianto, P.; Han, S.; Li, X.; Ogutu, F.O.; Zhang, Y.; Fan, Z.; Che, H. Quail egg homogenate alleviates food allergy induced eosinophilic esophagitis like disease through modulating PAR-2 transduction pathway in peanut sensitized mice. *Sci. Rep.* **2018**, *8*, 1049. [CrossRef] [PubMed]
2. Dellon, E.S. Epidemiology of eosinophilic esophagitis. *Gastroenterol. Clin. N. Am.* **2014**, *43*, 201–218. [CrossRef] [PubMed]
3. Kanikowska, A.; Hryhorowicz, S.; Rychter, A.M.; Kucharski, M.A.; Zawada, A.; Iwanik, K.; Eder, P.; Slomski, R.; Dobrowolska, A.; Krela-Kazmierczak, I. Immunogenetic, Molecular and Microbiotic Determinants of Eosinophilic Esophagitis and Clinical Practice-A New Perspective of an Old Disease. *Int. J. Mol. Sci.* **2021**, *22*, 10830. [CrossRef] [PubMed]
4. Dellon, E.S.; Jensen, E.T.; Martin, C.F.; Shaheen, N.J.; Kappelman, M.D. Prevalence of eosinophilic esophagitis in the United States. *Clin. Gastroenterol. Hepatol.* **2014**, *12*, 589–596.e1. [CrossRef] [PubMed]
5. Nhu, Q.M.; Hsieh, L.; Dohil, L.; Dohil, R.; Newbury, R.O.; Kurten, R.; Moawad, F.J.; Aceves, S.S. Antifibrotic Effects of the Thiazolidinediones in Eosinophilic Esophagitis Pathologic Remodeling: A Preclinical Evaluation. *Clin. Transl. Gastroenterol.* **2020**, *11*, e00164. [CrossRef]
6. Iuliano, S.; Minelli, R.; Vincenzi, F.; Gaiani, F.; Ruberto, C.; Leandro, G.; Bizzarri, B.; Nouvenne, A.; Di Mario, F.; De'Angelis, G.L. Eosinophilic esophagitis in pediatric age, state of the art and review of the literature. *Acta Biomed.* **2018**, *89*, 20–26. [CrossRef]
7. Dellon, E.S.; Kim, H.P.; Sperry, S.L.; Rybnicek, D.A.; Woosley, J.T.; Shaheen, N.J. A phenotypic analysis shows that eosinophilic esophagitis is a progressive fibrostenotic disease. *Gastrointest. Endosc.* **2014**, *79*, 577–585.e4. [CrossRef]
8. Noti, M.; Wojno, E.D.; Kim, B.S.; Siracusa, M.C.; Giacomin, P.R.; Nair, M.G.; Benitez, A.J.; Ruymann, K.R.; Muir, A.B.; Hill, D.A.; et al. Thymic stromal lymphopoietin-elicited basophil responses promote eosinophilic esophagitis. *Nat. Med.* **2013**, *19*, 1005–1013. [CrossRef]
9. Ho, S.C.; Kuo, C.T. Hesperidin, nobiletin, and tangeretin are collectively responsible for the anti-neuroinflammatory capacity of tangerine peel (Citri reticulatae pericarpium). *Food Chem. Toxicol. Int. J. Publ. Br. Ind. Biol. Res. Assoc.* **2014**, *71*, 176–182. [CrossRef]
10. Salinas, E.; Reyes-Pavon, D.; Cortes-Perez, N.G.; Torres-Maravilla, E.; Bitzer-Quintero, O.K.; Langella, P.; Bermudez-Humaran, L.G. Bioactive Compounds in Food as a Current Therapeutic Approach to Maintain a Healthy Intestinal Epithelium. *Microorganisms* **2021**, *9*, 1634. [CrossRef]
11. Yu, D.; Liu, X.; Zhang, G.; Ming, Z.; Wang, T. Isoliquiritigenin Inhibits Cigarette Smoke-Induced COPD by Attenuating Inflammation and Oxidative Stress via the Regulation of the Nrf2 and NF-kappaB Signaling Pathways. *Front. Pharmacol.* **2018**, *9*, 1001. [CrossRef]
12. Liu, C.; Yang, N.; Chen, X.; Tversky, J.; Zhan, J.; Chehade, M.; Miller, R.L.; Li, X.M. The Flavonoid 7,4′-Dihydroxyflavone Prevents Dexamethasone Paradoxical Adverse Effect on Eotaxin Production by Human Fibroblasts. *Phytother. Res.* **2017**, *31*, 449–458. [CrossRef]
13. Alshangiti, A.M.; Togher, K.L.; Hegarty, S.V.; Sullivan, A.M.; O'Keeffe, G.W. The dietary flavonoid isoliquiritigenin is a potent cytotoxin for human neuroblastoma cells. *Neuronal Signal.* **2019**, *3*, NS20180201. [CrossRef]
14. Liu, B.; Yang, J.; Wen, Q.; Li, Y. Isoliquiritigenin, a flavonoid from licorice, relaxes guinea-pig tracheal smooth muscle in vitro and in vivo: Role of cGMP/PKG pathway. *Eur. J. Pharmacol.* **2008**, *587*, 257–266. [CrossRef]
15. Yu, H.; Li, H.; Li, Y.; Li, M.; Chen, G. Effect of isoliquiritigenin for the treatment of atopic dermatitis-like skin lesions in mice. *Arch. Dermatol. Res.* **2017**, *309*, 805–813. [CrossRef]
16. Jayaprakasam, B.; Doddaga, S.; Wang, R.; Holmes, D.; Goldfarb, J.; Li, X.M. Licorice flavonoids inhibit eotaxin-1 secretion by human fetal lung fibroblasts in vitro. *J. Agric. Food Chem.* **2009**, *57*, 820–825. [CrossRef]
17. Yang, N.; Patil, S.; Zhuge, J.; Wen, M.C.; Bolleddula, J.; Doddaga, S.; Goldfarb, J.; Sampson, H.A.; Li, X.M. Glycyrrhiza uralensis flavonoids present in anti-asthma formula, ASHMI, inhibit memory Th2 responses in vitro and in vivo. *Phytother. Res.* **2013**, *27*, 1381–1391. [CrossRef]
18. Lee, Y.K.; Chin, Y.W.; Bae, J.K.; Seo, J.S.; Choi, Y.H. Pharmacokinetics of isoliquiritigenin and its metabolites in rats: Low bioavailability is primarily due to the hepatic and intestinal metabolism. *Planta Med.* **2013**, *79*, 1656–1665. [CrossRef]
19. Spernath, A.; Aserin, A. Microemulsions as carriers for drugs and nutraceuticals. *Adv. Colloid Interface Sci.* **2006**, *128–130*, 47–64. [CrossRef]
20. Korolev, D.; Shumilo, M.; Shulmeyster, G.; Krutikov, A.; Golovkin, A.; Mishanin, A.; Gorshkov, A.; Spiridonova, A.; Domorad, A.; Krasichkov, A.; et al. Hemolytic Activity, Cytotoxicity, and Antimicrobial Effects of Human Albumin- and Polysorbate-80-Coated Silver Nanoparticles. *Nanomaterials* **2021**, *11*, 1484. [CrossRef]
21. Liu, W.; Liu, J.; Salt, L.J.; Ridout, M.J.; Han, J.; Wilde, P.J. Structural stability of liposome-stabilized oil-in-water pickering emulsions and their fate during in vitro digestion. *Food Funct.* **2019**, *10*, 7262–7274. [CrossRef] [PubMed]
22. Verma, S.; Singh, S.K.; Verma, P.R. Fabrication of lipidic nanocarriers of loratadine for facilitated intestinal permeation using multivariate design approach. *Drug Dev. Ind. Pharm.* **2016**, *42*, 288–306. [CrossRef] [PubMed]
23. Shrivastava, N.; Parikh, A.; Dewangan, R.P.; Biswas, L.; Verma, A.K.; Mittal, S.; Ali, J.; Garg, S.; Baboota, S. Solid Self-Nano Emulsifying Nanoplatform Loaded with Tamoxifen and Resveratrol for Treatment of Breast Cancer. *Pharmaceutics* **2022**, *14*, 1486. [CrossRef] [PubMed]
24. Chen, L.; Liu, C.S.; Chen, Q.Z.; Wang, S.; Xiong, Y.A.; Jing, J.; Lv, J.J. Characterization, pharmacokinetics and tissue distribution of chlorogenic acid-loaded self-microemulsifying drug delivery system. *Eur. J. Pharm. Sci.* **2017**, *100*, 102–108. [CrossRef] [PubMed]

25. Sawatdee, S.; Atipairin, A.; Sae Yoon, A.; Srichana, T.; Changsan, N.; Suwandecha, T. Formulation Development of Albendazole-Loaded Self-Microemulsifying Chewable Tablets to Enhance Dissolution and Bioavailability. *Pharmaceutics* **2019**, *11*, 134. [CrossRef]
26. Zhang, X.; Qiao, H.; Zhang, T.; Shi, Y.; Ni, J. Enhancement of gastrointestinal absorption of isoliquiritigenin by nanostructured lipid carrier. *Adv. Powder Technol.* **2014**, *25*, 1060–1068. [CrossRef]
27. Han, W.; Xie, B.; Li, Y.; Shi, L.; Wan, J.; Chen, X.; Wang, H. Orally Deliverable Nanotherapeutics for the Synergistic Treatment of Colitis-Associated Colorectal Cancer. *Theranostics* **2019**, *9*, 7458–7473. [CrossRef]
28. Singh, A.; Thakur, S.; Singh, H.; Singh, H.; Kaur, S.; Kaur, S.; Dudi, R.; Mondhe, D.M.; Jain, S.K. Novel Vitamin E TPGS based docetaxel nanovesicle formulation for its safe and effective parenteral delivery: Toxicological, pharmacokinetic and pharmacodynamic evaluation. *J. Liposome Res.* **2021**, *31*, 365–380. [CrossRef]
29. Cao, M.; Zhan, M.; Wang, Z.; Wang, Z.; Li, X.M.; Miao, M. Development of an Orally Bioavailable Isoliquiritigenin Self-Nanoemulsifying Drug Delivery System to Effectively Treat Ovalbumin-Induced Asthma. *Int. J. Nanomed.* **2020**, *15*, 8945–8961. [CrossRef]
30. Hill, D.A.; Grundmeier, R.W.; Ramos, M.; Spergel, J.M. Eosinophilic Esophagitis Is a Late Manifestation of the Allergic March. *J. Allergy Clin. Immunology. Pract.* **2018**, *6*, 1528–1533. [CrossRef]
31. Spergel, J.; Aceves, S.S. Allergic components of eosinophilic esophagitis. *J. Allergy Clin. Immunol.* **2018**, *142*, 1–8. [CrossRef]
32. Blanchard, C.; Simon, D.; Schoepfer, A.; Straumann, A.; Simon, H.U. Eosinophilic esophagitis: Unclear roles of IgE and eosinophils. *J. Intern. Med.* **2017**, *281*, 448–457. [CrossRef]
33. Liu, C.; Yang, N.; Song, Y.; Wang, L.; Zi, J.; Zhang, S.; Dunkin, D.; Busse, P.; Weir, D.; Tversky, J.; et al. Ganoderic acid C1 isolated from the anti-asthma formula, ASHMI suppresses TNF-alpha production by mouse macrophages and peripheral blood mononuclear cells from asthma patients. *Int. Immunopharmacol.* **2015**, *27*, 224–231. [CrossRef]
34. Cho, J.Y.; Doshi, A.; Rosenthal, P.; Beppu, A.; Miller, M.; Aceves, S.; Broide, D. Smad3-deficient mice have reduced esophageal fibrosis and angiogenesis in a model of egg-induced eosinophilic esophagitis. *J. Pediatr. Gastroenterol. Nutr.* **2014**, *59*, 10–16. [CrossRef]
35. Nguyen, N.; Fernando, S.D.; Biette, K.A.; Hammer, J.A.; Capocelli, K.E.; Kitzenberg, D.A.; Glover, L.E.; Colgan, S.P.; Furuta, G.T.; Masterson, J.C. TGF-β1 alters esophageal epithelial barrier function by attenuation of claudin-7 in eosinophilic esophagitis. *Mucosal Immunol.* **2018**, *11*, 415–426. [CrossRef]
36. Rieder, F.; Nonevski, I.; Ma, J.; Ouyang, Z.; West, G.; Protheroe, C.; DePetris, G.; Schirbel, A.; Lapinski, J.; Goldblum, J.; et al. T-helper 2 cytokines, transforming growth factor beta1, and eosinophil products induce fibrogenesis and alter muscle motility in patients with eosinophilic esophagitis. *Gastroenterology* **2014**, *146*, 1266–1277.e9. [CrossRef]
37. Javed, R.; Ghonaim, R.; Shathili, A.; Khalifa, S.A.; El-Seedi, H.R. Phytonanotechnology: A greener approach for biomedical applications. In *Biogenic Nanoparticles for Cancer Theranostics*; Elsevier: Amsterdam, The Netherlands, 2021; pp. 43–86. [CrossRef]
38. Moawad, F.J.; Dellon, E.S.; Achem, S.R.; Ljuldjuraj, T.; Green, D.J.; Maydonovitch, C.L.; Brizuela, D.R.; Gupta, S.K.; Chehade, M. Effects of Race and Sex on Features of Eosinophilic Esophagitis. *Clin. Gastroenterol. Hepatol.* **2016**, *14*, 23–30. [CrossRef]
39. Takeda, M.; Tanabe, M.; Ito, W.; Ueki, S.; Konnno, Y.; Chihara, M.; Itoga, M.; Kobayashi, Y.; Moritoki, Y.; Kayaba, H.; et al. Gender difference in allergic airway remodelling and immunoglobulin production in mouse model of asthma. *Respirology* **2013**, *18*, 797–806. [CrossRef]
40. Rossi, A.; Roviezzo, F.; Sorrentino, R.; Riemma, M.A.; Cerqua, I.; Bilancia, R.; Spaziano, G.; Troisi, F.; Pace, S.; Pinto, A.; et al. Leukotriene-mediated sex dimorphism in murine asthma-like features during allergen sensitization. *Pharmacol. Res.* **2019**, *139*, 182–190. [CrossRef]
41. Kralovicova, J.; Bartunek, A.; Hofmann, J.; Krizek, T.; Kozlik, P.; Rousarova, J.; Rysanek, P.; Sima, M.; Slanar, O. Pharmacokinetic Variability in Pre-Clinical Studies: Sample Study with Abiraterone in Rats and Implications for Short-Term Comparative Pharmacokinetic Study Designs. *Pharmaceutics* **2022**, *14*, 643. [CrossRef]
42. Zhang, K.; Wang, Q.; Yang, Q.; Wei, Q.; Man, N.; Adu-Frimpong, M.; Toreniyazov, E.; Ji, H.; Yu, J.; Xu, X. Enhancement of Oral Bioavailability and Anti-hyperuricemic Activity of Isoliquiritigenin via Self-Microemulsifying Drug Delivery System. *AAPS PharmSciTech* **2019**, *20*, 218. [CrossRef] [PubMed]
43. Li, H.; Zhao, X.; Ma, Y.; Zhai, G.; Li, L.; Lou, H. Enhancement of gastrointestinal absorption of quercetin by solid lipid nanoparticles. *J. Control. Release* **2009**, *133*, 238–244. [CrossRef] [PubMed]
44. Xiong, Y.; Zou, Y.; Chen, L.; Xu, Y.; Wang, S. Development and In Vivo Evaluation of Ziyuglycoside I-Loaded Self-Microemulsifying Formulation for Activity of Increasing Leukocyte. *AAPS PharmSciTech* **2019**, *20*, 101. [CrossRef] [PubMed]
45. Greco, I.; Molchanova, N.; Holmedal, E.; Jenssen, H.; Hummel, B.D.; Watts, J.L.; Hakansson, J.; Hansen, P.R.; Svenson, J. Correlation between hemolytic activity, cytotoxicity and systemic in vivo toxicity of synthetic antimicrobial peptides. *Sci. Rep.* **2020**, *10*, 13206. [CrossRef]
46. Harris, M.B.; Chang, C.C.; Berton, M.T.; Danial, N.N.; Zhang, J.; Kuehner, D.; Ye, B.H.; Kvatyuk, M.; Pandolfi, P.P.; Cattoretti, G.; et al. Transcriptional Repression of Stat6-Dependent Interleukin-4-Induced Genes by BCL-6: Specific Regulation of IεTranscription and Immunoglobulin E Switching. *Mol. Cell. Biol.* **1999**, *19*, 7264–7275. [CrossRef]
47. Cao, M.; Liu, C.; Srivastava, K.D.; Lin, A.; Lazarski, C.; Wang, L.; Maskey, A.; Song, Y.; Chen, X.; Yang, N.; et al. Anti-IgE effect of small-molecule-compound arctigenin on food allergy in association with a distinct transcriptome profile. *Clin. Exp. Allergy* **2022**, *52*, 250–264. [CrossRef]

pharmaceuticals

MDPI

Review

Therapies for Chronic Spontaneous Urticaria: Present and Future Developments

Riccardo Asero [1], Paolo Calzari [2], Silvia Vaienti [3] and Massimo Cugno [4,*]

1. Clinica San Carlo, Ambulatorio di Allergologia, 20037 Paderno Dugnano, Italy; r.asero@libero.it
2. Department of Pathophysiology and Transplantation, Scuola di Specializzazione, Allergologia e Immunologia Clinica, Università degli Studi di Milano, 20122 Milan, Italy; paolo.calzari@unimi.it
3. Section of Dermatology and Venereology, Department of Medicine, University of Verona, 37126 Verona, Italy; silvia.vaienti@hotmail.it
4. Department of Pathophysiology and Transplantation, Internal Medicine, Fondazione IRCCS Ca' Granda Ospedale Maggiore Policlinico, Università degli Studi di Milano, 20122 Milan, Italy

* Correspondence: massimo.cugno@unimi.it; Tel.: +39-0255035340

Abstract: Chronic spontaneous urticaria (CSU) is a complex dermatological condition characterized by recurrent wheals and/or angioedema lasting for more than six weeks, significantly impairing patients' quality of life. According to European guidelines, the first step in treatment involves second-generation H1-antihistamines (sgAHs), which block peripheral H1 receptors to alleviate symptoms. In cases with inadequate responses, the dose of antihistamines can be increased by up to fourfold. If symptoms persist despite this adjustment, the next step involves the use of omalizumab, a monoclonal anti-IgE antibody, which has shown efficacy in the majority of cases. However, a subset of patients remains refractory, necessitating alternative treatments such as immunosuppressive agents like cyclosporine or azathioprine. To address these unmet needs, several new therapeutic targets are being explored. Among them, significant attention is being given to drugs that block Bruton's tyrosine kinase (BTK), such as remibrutinib, which reduces mast cell activation. Therapies like dupilumab, which target the interleukin-4 (IL-4) and IL-13 pathways, are also under investigation. Additionally, molecules targeting the Mas-related G protein-coupled receptor X2 (MRGPRX2), and those inhibiting the tyrosine kinase receptor Kit, such as barzolvolimab, show promise in clinical studies. These emerging treatments offer new options for patients with difficult-to-treat CSU and have the potential to modify the natural course of the disease by targeting key immune pathways, helping to achieve longer-term remission. Further research is essential to better elucidate the pathophysiology of CSU and optimize treatment protocols to achieve long-term benefits in managing this condition. Altogether, the future of CSU treatments that target pathogenetic mechanisms seems promising.

Keywords: chronic spontaneous urticaria; antihistamines; omalizumab; corticosteroids; cyclosporin; dupilumab; barzolvolimab; CDX-0159; Tezepelumab; vixarelimab; mepolizumab; UB-221; remibrutinib; rilzabrutinib; TAS 5315; TLL-018; povorcitinib; EP 262

1. Introduction

Urticaria is clinically characterized by the appearance of wheals (hives), which can be accompanied by angioedema. When the spontaneous recurrence of short-lived wheals, angioedema, or both lasts for more than 6 weeks, this is defined as chronic spontaneous urticaria (CSU) [1]. CSU has an estimated prevalence of 0.5% to 1% and female predominance (female/male ratio: 2/1) [2]. CSU symptoms significantly affect many aspects of patients' health-related quality of life, and the health status scores of CSU patients have been reported to be comparable with those of patients with coronary artery disease in terms of work performance, sleep disruption, emotional reactions, and social interactions [3]. Evaluating CSU can be difficult, and the Weekly Urticaria Activity Score (UAS7) is one of the most commonly used methods to accomplish this. This tool relies on the patient's daily self-assessment of key symptoms, including wheals and itching. Each symptom is rated on a scale from 0 to 3, where 0 indicates no intensity and 3 represents severe intensity. Patients record their scores every day for seven days, with the total score ranging from 0 to 42 [1]. The international guidelines recommend treating patients until a complete clinical response is achieved. Currently, a three-step approach is suggested. The first step consists of using second-generation H1-antihistamines (sgAHs) at the licensed dosage. The second step involves increasing the use of sgAHs up to four times the licensed dosage. The third step consists of the addition of the anti-IgE monoclonal antibody, omalizumab [1] (Table 1). Although most patients with CSU achieve complete or partial control of the disease with stepwise treatment, some remain unresponsive. In such cases, switching to immunosuppressive therapy is suggested, with cyclosporine being the most studied and frequently prescribed option. Azathioprine, methotrexate (MTX) and mycophenolate mofetil (MMF) have also been proposed as alternative treatments. In the case of acute exacerbation, the guidelines suggest considering a short course of systemic glucocorticosteroids. Other therapies are being developed to target the pathomechanisms of CSU. In particular, these target the mast cells [4], whose activation leads to wheal formation via the release of vasoactive substances such as histamine. The sequence of events responsible for mast cell activation is not completely defined and involves autoimmunity [5,6], autoallergy [7–9], the complement system, and coagulation [10–13], with the participation of other cells [14] such as eosinophils, endothelial cells, basophils, B lymphocytes, T lymphocytes, and monocytes.

Table 1. The first approach to the therapeutic treatment of chronic spontaneous urticaria (CSU).

Drug	Type of Molecule	Administration	Mechanism of Action	Response	
Second-generation H1-antihistamines (standard dose)	Second-generation H1-antihistamine	Oral, standard dosage (varies by drug)	Selective peripheral H1 receptor antagonist	Significant reduction in UAS7 score, fewer sedative effects compared to first-generation antihistamines	Step 1
		Oral, up to 4× standard dosage		Improved efficacy in non-responders to standard doses, increased risk of somnolence but still well-tolerated	Step 2
Omalizumab	Humanized monoclonal anti-IgE antibody	Subcutaneous, 300 mg every 4 weeks	Binds free IgE, preventing attachment of FcεRI to mast cells and basophils	Significant reduction in urticaria activity and angioedema, especially in patients unresponsive to antihistamines	Step 3
Cyclosporin	Immunosuppressant,	Oral, 3.5–5 mg/kg per day	Inhibits calcineurin/NFAT and JNK/p38 signaling pathways	Effective in patients unresponsive to antihistamines and omalizumab, dose-dependent safety profile	Step 4
Corticosteroids	Anti-inflammatory, immunosuppressant	Oral or intravenous, 20–50 mg/day, up to 10 days	Inhibits pro-inflammatory cytokines and immune response, binds glucocorticoid receptor	Short-term relief of acute exacerbations; not recommended for long-term use due to side effects such as hypertension, osteoporosis, and immunosuppression	Acute phase

According to European guidelines [1], the treatment of CSU begins with a standard dose of second-generation H1-antihistamines (step 1). If needed, the dose can be increased by up to fourfold (step 2). The third step involves the addition of omalizumab (step 3). When a good clinical response is achieved, a step-down approach can be considered. If the patient does not respond adequately, an immunosuppressant such as cyclosporine may be added (step 4). A short course of corticosteroids may be considered in the case of acute exacerbation.

An improvement in the understanding of CSU pathogenesis and the consequent development of new therapies has led to the definition of disease-modifying treatments (DMTs). These treatments are designed not only to alleviate symptoms but also to alter the underlying mechanisms driving the disease. DMTs aim to prevent or delay disease progression, achieve long-lasting remission without ongoing therapy, and directly target the core disease mechanisms.

DMTs include therapies that reduce the production of autoantibodies or target specific cytokines involved in inflammation and symptom manifestation: these drugs are reported in Table 2 (monoclonal antibodies) and in Table 3 (small molecules) [15].

Table 2. Breakthrough treatments for chronic spontaneous urticaria (CSU): monoclonal antibodies.

Drug	Target	Mechanism of Action	Administration	Response	Clinical Trial Phase	References
Dupilumab	IL-4 R á (IL-4; IL-13)	The block of the alpha subunit of the IL-4 receptor, which is shared with the IL-13 receptor, thereby inhibiting both IL-4 and IL-13 signaling pathways	Subcutaneous	A significant reduction in UAS7; showed efficacy in biologic-naïve patients but limited efficacy in omalizumab-refractory patients	Phase III	NCT04180488, (LIBERTY-CUPID CSU) [16,17]
Barzolvolimab (CDX-0159)	Kit	The inhibition of Kit receptor, reducing mast cell survival and activation	Intravenous	Although the phase III study is still ongoing, in phase II a reduction in activity and quality of life scores has been reported	Phase III	NCT06445023; NCT06455202 [18]
Tezepelumab	TSLP	The inhibition of TSLP, a key initiator of type 2 inflammation	Subcutaneous	Preliminary results indicate a good response; however, the final data of phase II study are still not available	Phase II	NCT04833855 [19]
Vixarelimab	IL-31 R	The block of the IL-31 and oncostatin M signaling pathways, reducing pruritus and inflammation	Subcutaneous	Although the phase II study in CSU is still ongoing, its promising results in the treatment of prurigo nodularis suggest potential benefits for CSU	Phase II	NCT03858634
Mepolizumab	IL-5	The inhibition of IL-5, reducing eosinophil migration and activation	Subcutaneous	Effective in reducing CSU symptoms, especially in patients with eosinophilic diseases	Phase I	NCT03494881 [20,21]
UB-221	IgE	Binding to IgE with high affinity, preventing interaction with mast cells and basophils	Intravenous	Although the phase II study in CSU is still ongoing, the drug appears to be promising due to its safety and its superior effectiveness in reducing IgE levels compared to omalizumab	Phase II	NCT05298215 [22]

IgE: immunoglobulin E; IL: interleukin; Kit: tyrosine kinase receptor Kit; R: receptor; TSLP: thymic stromal lymphopoietin; UAS7: Weekly Urticaria Activity Score.

Table 3. Breakthrough treatments for chronic spontaneous urticaria (CSU): small molecules.

Drug	Target	Mechanism of Action	Administration	Response	Clinical Trial Phase	References
Remibrutinib	BTK	The inhibition of BTK, a key component of FcεRI signaling in mast cells and basophils, thereby reducing the release of inflammatory mediators like histamine.	Oral	Rapid and sustained symptom control, good safety profile in antihistamine-refractory CSU	Phase III	NCT03926611, NCT05114057 [23–25]
Rilzabrutinib	BTK		Oral	Results of the phase II studies are still pending. However, given their mechanism of action, which closely mirrors that of remibrutinib, their potential effectiveness in CSU seems likely.	Phase II	NCT05107115
TAS 5315	BTK		Oral		Phase II	NCT05335499 [26]
TLL-018	JAK1	The selective inhibition of JAK1, reducing cytokine-driven inflammation.	Oral	Despite being in the early phase of study, its inhibitory effects on JAK 1 suggest it could be a promising therapeutic option for CSU.	Phase I	NCT06396026
Povorcitinib	JAK1, JAK2, TYK2	The inhibition of JAK1, JAK2, and TYK2, disrupting cytokine signaling.	Oral	Although the results of the phase I and II studies are still pending, their broad spectrum of action makes these molecules appear promising.	Phase II	NCT05373355 NCT05936567
EP 262	MRGPRX2	The block of MRGPRX2 (the non-IgE mast cell receptor)	Oral	Given the emerging role of MRGPRX2 in CSU pathophysiology, blocking this receptor makes the drug a highly promising candidate, although the results from the phase II trial are still pending.	Phase II	NCT06077773

BTK: Bruton tyrosine kinase; FcεRI: high-affinity receptor for the fragment crystallizable region of immunoglobulin E; JAK: Janus kinase; MRGPRX2: Mas-related G protein-coupled receptor X2; TYK: tyrosine kinase.

Here, we review the current and potential treatments for CSU based on the latest understanding of its pathogenesis. The therapeutic approaches are categorized according to the mechanisms of action of the different drugs: blocking mast cell mediators, inhibiting mast cell activation, silencing mast cells, depleting mast cells, targeting shared enzymatic pathways (Figure 1), and possibly using miscellaneous immunosuppressants.

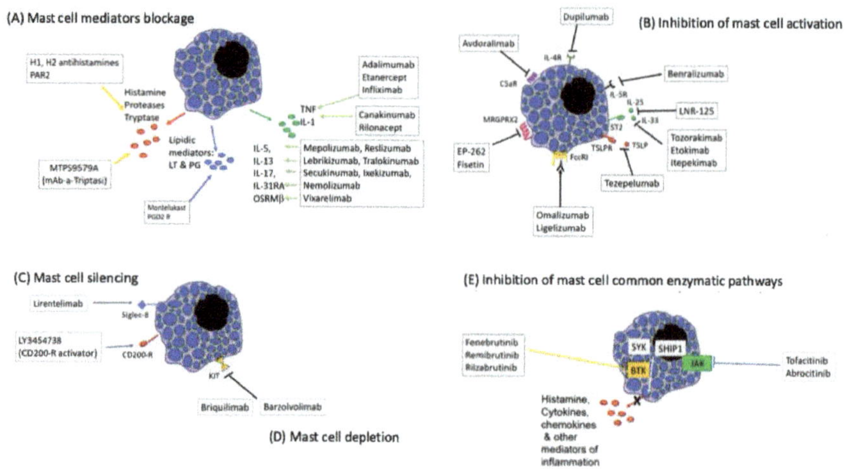

Figure 1. Mechanisms of action of currently used and potentially effective drugs in chronic spontaneous urticaria treatment.BTK: Bruton tyrosine kinase; C5aR: C5 a receptor; CD200 R: CD 200 receptor; FcεRI: high-affinity receptor for the fragment crystallizable region of immunoglobulin E; IL: Interleukin; IL 4R: interleukin 4 receptor; IL 5R: interleukin 5 receptor; IL 31RA: interleukin 31 receptor A; JAK: Janus kinase; Kit: tyrosine kinase receptor Kit; LT: leukotriene; mAb: monoclonal antibody; MRGPRX2: Mas-related G protein–coupled receptor X2; OSMRβ: Oncostatin-M specific receptor subunit beta; PAR2: Protease activated receptor 2; PG: prostaglandins, PGD2R: Prostaglandin D receptor; Siglec-8: Sialic acid-binding Ig-like lectin 8; SHIP 1: Src homology 2 (SH2) domain containing inositol polyphosphate 5-phosphatase 1; SYK: Tyrosine-protein kinase SYK; ST2: suppression of tumorigenicity 2; TNF: tumor necrosis factor; TSLP: thymic stromal lymphopoietin.

Search Methodology

The PubMed and Google Scholar databases were screened using 'chronic spontaneous urticaria' and 'treatment', examining research published between 1990 and 2024. We also searched the ClinicalTrials.gov database for recent and ongoing randomized clinical trials in CSU using the keyword "chronic spontaneous urticaria".

BTK: Bruton tyrosine kinase; C5aR: C5 a receptor; CD200 R: CD 200 receptor; FcεRI: high-affinity receptor for the fragment crystallizable region of immunoglobulin E; IL: interleukin; IL 4R: interleukin 4 receptor; IL 5R: interleukin 5 receptor; IL 31RA: interleukin 31 receptor A; JAK: Janus kinase; Kit: tyrosine kinase receptor Kit; LT: leukotriene; mAb: monoclonal antibody; MRGPRX2: Mas-related G protein-coupled receptor X2; OSMRβ: oncostatin M-specific receptor subunit beta; PAR2: protease-activated receptor 2; PG: prostaglandins, PGD2R: prostaglandin D receptor; Siglec-8: sialic acid-binding Ig-like lectin 8; SHIP 1: Src homology 2 (SH2) domain containing inositol polyphosphate 5-phosphatase 1; SYK: tyrosine-protein kinase SYK; ST2: suppression of tumorigenicity 2; TNF: tumor necrosis factor; TSLP: thymic stromal lymphopoietin.

2. Mast Cell Mediators Blockage

2.1. Second-Generation H1-Antihistamines

The use of SgAHs is the first step in the treatment of CSU [1]. Their mechanism of action involves the highly selective blockade of peripheral H1 receptors (a G protein-coupled receptor—GPCR), preventing the histamine effectives of vasodilation and an increase in vascular permeability [27,28]. The blockade of peripheral H1 receptors occurs through inverse regulation, achieved by positioning a common phenyl group within the hydrophobic cavity [28]. Secondary ligand-binding sites in H1R, characterized by several polar residues, are novel targets which could be effectively blocked using optimized derivative groups [28].

The molecules most used to treat CSU are as follows: ebastine, bilastine, loratadine, desloratadine, rupatadine, cetirizine, and levocetirizine [1]. Compared to first-generation antihistamines, these drugs have a better therapeutic profile, selectively blocking peripheral histamine receptors, which leads to fewer side effects such as sedation and anticholinergic effects [29].

The choice between various antihistamines in CSU treatment often depends on the patient's profile and preferences, as there is no conclusive clinical evidence demonstrating significant differences in terms of their efficacy [30–32]. However, a recent Indian study found that bilastine caused a more significant reduction in the mean total symptom score (MTSS) and pruritus scale within one week of administration compared to cetirizine. Moreover, bilastine had fewer sedative side effects than cetirizine, making it a preferable option for many patients [33]. Another study compared bilastine, fexofenadine, and levocetirizine in terms of treating CSU. At week 4, bilastine demonstrated a statistically significant improvement in urticaria symptoms compared to levocetirizine ($p < 0.05$). Additionally, bilastine enhanced the quality of life (QoL) of patients, as measured by the CU-Q2oL questionnaire ($p < 0.05$), significantly more than both fexofenadine and levocetirizine. Bilastine was also associated with significantly lower somnolence compared to fexofenadine and levocetirizine, even after up-dosing ($p < 0.05$). Regarding adverse events, bilastine had the fewest, with the most common being sedation, headache, nausea, and fatigue [34]. These findings are further supported by another study, showing a significant reduction in UAS7 scores in subjects treated with bilastine compared to those treated with levocetirizine ($p = 0.03$) [35].

In the case of standard doses of sgAHs lacking efficacy, guidelines allow the use of up to fourfold standard doses [1]. Studies have demonstrated the safety and efficacy of off-label high-dose sgAH therapy, including the use of bilastine, cetirizine, desloratadine, ebastine, fexofenadine, levocetirizine, and rupatadine, at doses up to four times the recommended daily amount [36–41]. However, increased doses of sgAHs are associated with a higher risk of somnolence compared to standard doses (relative risk of 3.28; 95% confidence interval of 1.55–6.95; $p = 0.002$) [42]. Typically, a 2-week period is sufficient to assess the effects of antihistamine adjustments in CSU treatment [43]. Approximately 61% of CSU patients do not respond to standard licensed doses of sgAHs. Of these non-responders, only about 63% benefit from an increased dose [36]; the others can benefit from a therapeutic step up with regard to omalizumab.

2.2. Histamine Human Immunoglobulin

Histamine human immunoglobulin (histaglobulin, a combination of human normal immunoglobulin and histamine dihydrochloride that elicits the production of histamine-binding antibodies) is going to be studied in China. The study is currently not yet recruiting and will start in March 2025. The study should be closed by the end of 2025. A preliminary prospective study carried out in India found that the weekly subcutaneous administration of histaglobulin was able to reduce the UAS7 scores by >80% after 8 weeks and 45% of patients attained a complete remission without relevant side effects. [44]. A more recent case report confirmed these observations [45].

2.3. Leukotriene Receptor Antagonists

Leukotriene receptor antagonists (LRAs) block cysteinyl leukotrienes, which are potent pro-inflammatory mediators [46]. The potential role of LRAs in the treatment of CSU was described for the first time in 2000 in a case report [47]. This study reported that NSAID-induced exacerbations in a patient with CSU were successfully prevented with montelukast (10 mg once a day for 3 weeks) and zafirlukast (20 mg twice daily for 3 weeks) treatment.

The effectiveness of LRAs was further investigated one year later by the same group [48] in a 12-patient sample with steroid-dependent CSU. The team administered montelukast, 10 mg, once a day or zafirlukast, 20 mg, twice daily for 3 weeks. One patient was excluded because of intolerance (severe headache) and 6/11 patients reached the remission stage.

In a single-blind, placebo-controlled, and crossover clinical study in 2002, montelukast treatment outcomes were superior to placebo outcomes [49].

An Indian double-blind, randomized, and controlled trial published in 2017 [50] compared treatment with 10 mg of levocetirizine to treatment with a combination of 5 mg of levocetirizine and 10 mg of montelukast. Both therapies were effective in terms of disease control, but the addition of montelukast was useful in terms of reducing the dosage of cetirizine and its side effects, such as dizziness. Other studies reported the usefulness of montelukast as an added therapy [51,52].

In contrast to the studies mentioned, there is evidence that indicates the absence of an advantage of treating with LRAs compared to treating with antihistamines in a monotherapy setting [53,54].

Finally, a case report described a paradoxical exacerbation of CSU in a patient under treatment with antihistamines and montelukast [55].

In a systematic review considering 10 randomized controlled trials, no significant adverse effects or change in laboratory were observed in patients treated with LRAs [46].

2.4. *Anti-Cytokine Therapies*

2.4.1. Canakinumab

Canakinumab is a human anti-IL-1 beta monoclonal antibody that is currently approved by the European Medicines Agency for treating periodic fever syndromes, Still's disease, and gouty arthritis. In fact, IL-1beta plays a role in the pathogenesis of neutrophilic diseases. Moreover, many periodic fever syndromes can lead to cutaneous manifestations, such as urticaria. [56]. A phase II randomized double-blind placebo-controlled single-center study [57] investigated the efficacy of canakinumab compared to a placebo. Canakinumab was administered subcutaneously at a dosage of 150 mg once at baseline, but after 4 weeks, it was not superior to the placebo, suggesting the limited relevance of IL-1beta in the pathophysiology of CSU.

2.4.2. Mepolizumab

Mepolizumab is a monoclonal antibody, targeting IL-5, that is approved for use in severe eosinophilic asthma, chronic rhinosinusitis with nasal polyposis, eosinophilic granulomatosis with polyangiitis, and hypereosinophilic syndrome. Since IL-5 appears to play an important role in CSU, mediating eosinophil migration to the skin during the period of active disease [58,59], this cytokine could be a new therapeutic target.

Two case reports, the first one including one patient and the second one, more recent, including three asthmatic patients with CSU, described the achievement of complete symptom resolution following mepolizumab treatment, with UCT scores reaching 15 after the first dose and symptom-free periods extending for up to six months [20,59]. Moreover, a phase I trial is currently underway to evaluate mepolizumab's effectiveness in treating CSU (NCT03494881). There are still no data available on urticaria treatment with mepolizumab, which has shown a good safety profile for the treatment of other diseases.

2.4.3. Reslizumab

Reslizumab is a monoclonal antibody targeting IL-5 approved for use in severe eosinophilic asthma. In a case report, it demonstrated significant effectiveness treating asthma, CSU, and cold urticaria [19].

2.4.4. Secukinumab

Patients with CSU showed elevated serum levels of IL-17 and IL-23, which have been associated with disease activity, and a positive autologous serum skin test, an indicator of autoimmune CSU (aiCSU) [60]. Additionally, IL-17A expression was significantly higher in both lesional and non-lesional skin of CSU patients compared to the skin of healthy controls, where IL-17A expression was minimal or absent [61]. The preliminary findings indicated that all eight patients with antihistamine-resistant and omalizumab-resistant CSU who were treated with the anti-IL-17A mAb, secukinumab, experienced significant improvements in disease activity. In particular, the reduction in disease activity, assessed by UAS7, was 55% at 30 days and 82% at 90 days [61].

2.4.5. Tildrakizumab

Since serum levels of IL-23 are increased in CSU patients, the anti-IL-23 mAb tildrakizumab has been administrated to treat patients with CSU refractory to omalizumab. Good control of the disease was obtained after four weeks in two out of three CSU patients. After 90 days, the overall reduction in disease activity from the baseline values ranged from 19% to 75% [62].

2.4.6. Vixarelimab

Vixarelimab, a human mAb that targets the beta subunit of the oncostatin M receptor, inhibits the signaling pathways of IL-31 and oncostatin M, both of which contribute to pruritus. Vixarelimab has been successfully used in prurigo nodularis [63] and is currently undergoing a phase II trial to assess its efficacy in CSU (NCT03858634).

3. Inhibition of Mast Cell Activation

3.1. Anti IgE

3.1.1. Omalizumab

Mechanism of Action

Omalizumab, a humanized monoclonal anti-IgE antibody, was initially developed to treat allergic respiratory disorders like asthma. It works by binding free IgE to the binding site of the high-affinity receptor for the fragment crystallizable region of immunoglobulin E (FcεRI) [43], preventing IgE from attaching to FcεRI on mast cells and halting the immunological cascade. In vitro experiments with basophils demonstrate that omalizumab is able to detach IgE from high-affinity IgE receptors [64]. Its potential for treating CSU was recognized in 2005 [65,66]. Phase II studies confirmed omalizumab's efficacy for autoallergic CSU, particularly in patients with IgE autoantibodies to thyroperoxidase [67]. While the exact mechanism in CSU is not fully understood, omalizumab reduces free IgE levels and downregulates FcεRI expression in skin cells and basophils [68,69]. Other contributing mechanisms may include changes in mast cells, autoantibodies, coagulation abnormalities, and inflammatory cytokine levels [70,71]. Patients with type IIb autoimmunity, characterized by IgG and IgM antibodies that act against IgE receptors, experience more severe CSU and respond less effectively to omalizumab [72].

Clinical Response

The efficacy of omalizumab in treating CSU is supported by several phase III studies, including ASTERIA I, ASTERIA II, and GLACIAL [73–75]. These studies confirmed that omalizumab significantly outperformed placebos in terms of reducing urticaria activity and itch severity in patients aged 12–75 with moderate to severe CSU unresponsive to H1-antihistamines [76]. A meta-analysis of seven randomized controlled trials validated these findings, showing significant reductions in itch and wheal scores, particularly administering a 300 mg dosage every four weeks [77]. Additionally, the phase III trials highlighted that omalizumab increased the proportion of angioedema-free days [78].

Omalizumab is both well tolerated and effective across different patient populations, including children, adolescents, and older adults [79–83]. Despite CSU being more prevalent in females, both sexes respond similarly to omalizumab treatment, although relapses are more common in males [84]. The phase III POLARIS study [85] also demonstrated significant decreases in itch severity for omalizumab compared to placebos in patients affected by CSU with an inducible component [86]. Furthermore, there is limited information on omalizumab's use in pregnant subjects with cancer or those undergoing treatment with other biological therapies [87,88].

Omalizumab significantly improves QoL, sleep, sexual function, anxiety, and work productivity in CSU patients, as demonstrated by patient-reported outcomes, which are assessed by UAS7 and the Urticaria Control Test (UCT) [89–94]. The phase IV SUNRISE and EXTEND-CIU studies show that disease control is achieved by week 12 (assessed by the UCT and UAS7), with sustained improvements in various patient-reported outcomes for 48 weeks [95–97].

Additionally, omalizumab benefits patients with CSU and angioedema, as evidenced by the X-ACT study [98,99]. However, more research is needed to assess its effectiveness treating isolated angioedema.

The response to omalizumab varies among patients, who can be classified into four categories: 'early responders' (ER), who experience a swift and comprehensive recovery within less than one month; 'late responders' (LR), who show complete improvement only after several months of therapy; 'partial responders' (PR), who exhibit some improvement but not a complete response; and 'non-responders' (NR), who do not respond at all [100–102]. Kaplan et al. [101] found a median time to complete response of 8–10 weeks with 300 mg of omalizumab, but responses occurred at times ranging from the first injection to up to 24 weeks. About half of the non-responders at week 12 responded by week 24. Early responders showed a rapid decrease in IgE and basophil FcεRI levels.

The treatment plans depend on the initial response. Non-responders and partial responders may need up-dosing and re-evaluation after three months, while good responders might benefit from lower dosing after 3–6 months [103]. Several studies found that up-dosing (to 450 mg or 600 mg, or at an increased frequency) is safe and effective in up to 60% of refractory patients, especially those with angioedema, basophil activation, high BMI values, prior cyclosporin treatment, greater ages, lower UCT scores, associate chronic inducible urticaria (CIndU), or lower IgE levels [104–107]. However, such an approach is not allowed in all countries by regulatory agencies.

A Korean group of researchers found that a low dose of omalizumab (150 mg/month) is effective at managing chronic spontaneous urticaria (CSU), offering a cost-effective option in settings where higher doses are not feasible due to financial constraints. Better responses to low-dose omalizumab treatment were observed in patients with mild disease activity, the absence of atopic comorbidities, and current smoking status [108].

About 50% of CSU patients achieve long-term remission (over 4 years) after one to two courses of omalizumab [109]. However, relapse can occur, particularly in those with high baseline UAS score or slow symptom decrease [110]. A retrospective cohort study conducted in Poland found that relapses commonly occurred within the first 6 weeks after discontinuing omalizumab treatment, with each additional point gained in terms of the UAS7 score increasing the risk of relapse by 5.4% [111]. Fortunately, re-treatment is as effective as the initial treatment, as shown in a study where 88% of patients re-treated after relapse regained control [112].

Furthermore, another therapeutic strategy is to extend the dosing interval in responders in which this seems to help with discontinuation [113].

Predictors of Response

The most reliable predictor of omalizumab response in CSU is the total IgE level [100,114–120]. Studies consistently show that non-responders typically have low baseline total IgE levels. These are typically lower than 40 IU/mL, and in some cases lower than 20 IU/mL. Early responders generally have IgE levels above 70 IU/mL. Ertas et al. [114,121] demonstrated that the best predictor of the response is the ratio of week 4 IgE levels to baseline IgE levels. Non-responders had a significantly lower ratio than partial and complete responders. This finding was supported by the work of Esteves Caldeira et al. [122]. Another predictor of a good response to omalizumab is the presence of elevated sFcεRI serum levels [115,123,124]. In a recent paper, Ji et al. found increased levels of Gal-9+ eosinophils and basophils in patients with high disease activity and a good response to omalizumab treatment. Omalizumab effectively reduces these levels in responders, suggesting that Gal-9+ cells may serve as predictors of treatment response [125].

Other response indicators include serum omalizumab trough levels [126], eosinopenia [127], antinuclear antibodies [128], and IL-31 [115,116].

A poor response was associated with basophil CD203c activity [129], higher anti-FcεRI IgG autoantibody levels [130], psychiatric disease, and thyroid antibodies [131]. Patients with poor or delayed responses to omalizumab often have a type IIb autoimmune form of CSU, characterized by IgG autoantibodies targeting IgE or its receptor (FcεRI) on mast cells. This leads to persistent cell activation and histamine release, which omalizumab may not adequately suppress, as its primary mechanism targets free IgE. [132,133].

Predictors of relapse after stopping omalizumab treatment include high IgE levels, high initial UAS7 scores, and an early response to treatment [110,114,116].

Safety

Omalizumab has demonstrated excellent safety over 20 years of various uses and dosages [134], as confirmed by both clinical trials and real-world studies [135]. A meta-analysis of 67 real-world studies indicated a 4% adverse event rate, matching the safety profile observed in clinical trials [136]. Nine-year long-term data showed no increase in side effects with extended omalizumab use [137,138]. Reports of anaphylaxis are very rare, with incidences between 0% and 0.09%, which are lower than the rates seen with most other biologics [139]. The US FDA reported more severe anaphylaxis cases in asthma patients than in those with urticaria [140,141].

The safety of omalizumab was further supported by a recent multinational cohort study that analyzed its long-term effectiveness and safety in treating chronic urticaria across 14 centers in 10 countries. The study involved 2325 patients and revealed an overall drug survival rate of 76% at 1 year, decreasing to 39% at 7 years. The primary reason for discontinuation was well-controlled disease (65%) [142]. However, a minority of patients discontinued treatment due to a lack of efficacy; in these cases, current guidelines suggest immunosuppressive therapy, with cyclosporin being the most commonly used.

3.1.2. Ligelizumab

Ligelizumab is a second-generation anti-IgE monoclonal antibody, with 50 times higher affinity for IgE than omalizumab. It was developed for patients with CSU who were unresponsive to standard treatments. Initial studies showed that it provided rapid and effective relief with a long-lasting effect [143,144]. However, phase III trials (PEARL-1 and PEARL-2) were halted because ligelizumab, while superior to the placebo, did not significantly outperform omalizumab. The safety was consistent with that seen in previous studies [144].

3.1.3. UB-221

UB-221 binds to IgE with high affinity, preventing IgE from interacting with the FcεRI receptor on mast cells and basophils. Additionally, UB-221 can bind to the IgE that is already bound to the CD23 receptor on B cells. This interaction promotes the CD23-mediated downregulation of IgE production. Unlike omalizumab, UB-221 can freely bind to CD23-bound IgE and form complexes with CD23, enhancing its ability to reduce IgE synthesis and the overall IgE levels in the body [22]. Based on the results of the phase I study (NCT03632291), UB-221 was well tolerated without serious adverse events. Currently, a phase II study is recruiting patients (NCT05298215).

3.1.4. Miscellaneous Drugs Targeting IgE

Quilizumab, a monoclonal antibody targeting membrane-bound IgE, did not show any visible improvement in patients with CSU [145]. Another drug, UCB8600, was investigated for use treating CSU patients (NCT04444466), but the study was terminated by the company for reasons unrelated to safety. Furthermore, the IgE-Trap protein (YH35324), which has a high affinity for serum-free IgE, is currently being investigated in a phase I trial (NCT05960708) involving patients with chronic spontaneous urticaria (CSU) and cold urticaria.

3.2. Dupilumab

Dupilumab is a monoclonal antibody that blocks the alpha subunit of the interleukin-4 (IL-4) and interleukin-13 (IL-13) receptors, thereby inhibiting their signaling pathways. It is currently indicated for the treatment of type 2 inflammatory conditions such as atopic dermatitis, asthma, and chronic rhinosinusitis with nasal polyposis. Dupilumab's efficacy in treating CSU was demonstrated in the placebo-controlled phase 3 clinical trial, LIBERTY-CSU CUPID Study A. This study investigated 138 biologic-naïve patients with CSU refractory to antihistamines and observed a significant reduction in UAS7, pruritus, and urticaria at week 24 [16]. These findings are also supported by a real-life study on 33 patients affected by CSU and treated with dupilumab [17]. However, another phase 3 study including 83 patients refractory to omalizumab, LIBERTY-CUPID Study B, was discontinued due to a lack of efficacy as it did not achieve statistical significance for the primary endpoints [16]. Additional papers have described a total of 25 patients with refractory CSU who responded positively to dupilumab [146–159].

Furthermore, by targeting B cells and reducing IgE levels, which in turn affects IgE receptor expression, dupilumab has shown potential in modifying the course of CSU. A case report indicated that 67% of patients maintained the remission of CSU for up to 22 months after discontinuing therapy with dupilumab [160]. These findings underscore the potential of dupilumab as a disease-modifying treatment in CSU [15]. The safety results were generally consistent with the known safety profile of dupilumab in its approved dermatological indications, with no differences with the placebo group [16].

3.3. Benralizumab

Benralizumab, a monoclonal antibody targeting the IL-5 receptor, has shown potential in treating CIndU, as evidenced by a case report where a patient with severe chronic symptomatic dermographism benefited from the treatment [21,161]. Although preliminary study results were promising, the drug demonstrated limited efficacy in a placebo-controlled randomized clinical trial, leading to the discontinuation of the development program (NCT04612725). Furthermore, a case report showed that in some cases, benralizumab can worsen CSU, although the exact mechanism behind this remains unclear [162].

3.4. Tezepelumab

Thymic stromal lymphopoietin (TSLP), an epithelial cell-derived cytokine, plays a critical role in initiating type 2 inflammation through both innate and adaptive immune pathways. Tezepelumab, an anti-TSLP mAb, has been shown to be safe, well tolerated, and effective in improving asthma control, also reducing the incidence of exacerbation and hospitalization in patients with severe asthma [163]. Increased levels of Th2-initiating cytokines, including TSLP, have been observed in the lesional skin of CSU patients [164]. A phase II trial of Tezepelumab for CSU has been completed (NCT04833855), with results pending publication.

3.5. MRGPRX2 Antagonists

Mas-related G protein-coupled receptor X2 (MRGPRX2) overexpression was observed in allergic and skin diseases, as CSU [165], and its downregulation in human or mice mast cells, leads to a reduction in mast cells degranulation [166]. MRGPRX2 is an important non-IgE-mediated pathway for mast cell activation and a potential therapeutic target for CSU [167,168]. Moreover, a recent study proposed that serum MRGPX2 may be a potential biomarker reflecting CSU activity, especially in naïve patients [169].

Some novel small molecules, designed through a computational approach and targeting MRGPRX2, were reported in a study published in 2023 [170]. In particular, the effects of the novel MRGPRX2 antagonists were assessed in vitro and in vivo using a mouse model of acute allergy and systemic anaphylaxis. It was observed that the small molecules inhibited both the early and the late phases of mast cell activation.

The therapeutic potential of MRGPRX2 antagonists was confirmed in a recent study [171] in which the molecules were tested on multiple functional assays in cell lines overexpressing human MRGPRX2, including isolated skin mast cells.

Two highly selective small molecule antagonists of MRGPRX2 are in trials for chronic spontaneous urticaria (EVO756, phase 1; EP262, phase 2 NCT06077773) and chronic inducible urticaria (EP262, phase 1b NCT06050928), but the results are still pending.

3.6. Complement Pathway Inhibitors

Another promising therapeutic target is the C5a/C5aR pathway. In CSU, the degranulation of mast cells by IgG autoantibodies requires them to bind to the IgE receptor and the activation of the classical complement cascade [172,173]. Another source of complement activation is the extrinsic coagulation pathway, which operates via the production of complement C5a, acting on the C5a receptor (C5aR) present on mast cells. Experimental studies have confirmed that the process may be inhibited by the C5aR antagonist, W-54011; however, studies in humans are still lacking to date [13,172].

4. Mast Cell Silencing

Lirentelimab

Lirentelimab is a monoclonal antibody that targets the receptor of sialic acid-binding immunoglobulin-like lectin-8 (Siglec-8) on eosinophils and mast cells. Its effect leads to the depletion of eosinophils via apoptosis and the silencing of mast cells [173]. In preliminary clinical studies, lirentelimab showed improved disease control in both omalizumab-naïve and omalizumab-refractory patients with CSU, as well as in patients with CIndU. These improvements were assessed by the evaluation of the increases in UCT and UAS7 score [174]. However, in January 2024, the company announced that the primary endpoints of the phase II CSU trial were not met, and further development of the drug is unlikely [174,175].

5. Mast Cell Depletion

5.1. Barzolvolimab

The main regulators of mast cell biology are the tyrosine kinase receptor Kit (CD117), which is highly expressed by mast cells, and its ligand stem cell factor (SCF). The bond between the two molecules leads to the differentiation, chemotaxis, maturation, and survival of mast cells [176,177]. By preventing SCF from binding to Kit, the critical survival signals cease, and the mast cell undergoes apoptosis.

Barzolvolimab (CDX-0159) is a humanized immunoglobulin G1 kappa (IgG1κ) monoclonal antibody that binds to the extracellular domain of Kit with high specificity and sub-nanomolar affinity, preventing the activation by SCF [178].

It was demonstrated that mice deficient in either Kit or SCF [179] and patients under treatment with imatinib [180], a tyrosine kinase inhibitor, have significantly reductions in mast cell burden. Then, Alvarado et al. in 2022 demonstrated that barzolvolimab (CDX-0159) induces mast cell suppression [178].

A single-center, open-label phase 1b study (NCT04548869; EUDRA-CT 2020-002792-35 [18]) in 2022 presented preliminary results concerning the tolerability and the effectiveness of barzolvolimab in the treatment of chronic inducible urticaria. Adults between 18 and 75 years of age with a diagnosis of cold-induced urticaria or spontaneous dermographism for $\geq$3 months were included. A single dose of 3 mg/kg of barzolvolimab was administered intravenously on day 1 with a 12-week follow up. The drug exhibited a terminal half-life of 20.1 $\pm$ 7.1 days. No severe adverse event was detected; however, hair color changes (areas of hair lightening) and infusion-related reactions were often observed. All patients saw an improvement by week 12 in terms of disease control (UCT, TempTest®, FricTest®), quality of life (DLQI), serum parameters (tryptase, SCF) and histopathological features (mast cells in non-lesional skin). The trial is still ongoing, and the results will be available once the study is complete.

Two global phase 3 trials (randomized, double-blind, placebo-controlled) are still ongoing, investigating the efficacy, safety, and tolerability of barzolvolimab in adult participants with CSU (EMBARQ-CSU 1 and 2 [NCT06445023; NCT06455202]).

5.2. Briquilimab

Briquilimab (JSP191) is an unconjugated, aglycosilated anti-cKit monoclonal antibody that functionally blocks the interaction between cKit and SCF. The studies in phase 1b/2a SPOTLIGHT (NCT06353971) and BEACON (NCT06162728) are investigating the effect of subcutaneous Briquilimab in adults with cold urticaria and chronic spontaneous urticaria, respectively. Results are expected at the end of 2025.

6. Inhibition of Mast Cell Common Enzymatic Pathways

6.1. Bruton Tyrosine Kinase Inhibitors

Bruton tyrosine kinase (BTK) is a central player in the pathogenesis of CSU due to its critical role in FcεRI-mediated signaling, which is essential for mast cell and basophil activation. BTK facilitates the downstream signaling required for the activation and degranulation of these cells, leading to the release of inflammatory mediators like histamine, which contribute to CSU symptoms [26,181]. Additionally, BTK is involved in B-cell receptor (BCR) signaling, which is crucial to the production of autoantibodies by B cells [26].

By inhibiting BTK, it is possible to block both the FcεRI and BCR signaling pathways, thereby targeting the two key mechanisms driving CSU [26]. This finding makes BTK inhibitors promising therapeutic options for patients with antihistamine-refractory CSU.

BTK inhibitors (BTKis) are employed to treat several inflammatory and autoimmune conditions, as well as in cancer treatment [182]. Early-generation BTK inhibitors, like ibrutinib, were developed to treat B-cell malignancies but had limitations due to off-target effects and safety concerns (e.g., atrial fibrillation and bleeding) [26,183–185]. Newer BTK inhibitors, such as remibrutinib and fenebrutinib, are more selective, offering improved safety profiles while retaining efficacy [186]. Four oral BTKis—fenebrutinib, remibrutinib, rilzabrutinib, and TAS5315—have been or are currently being evaluated for use in chronic urticaria [26].

6.1.1. Fenebrutinib

Fenebrutinib, a potent and highly selective reversible BTKi, has been shown to block IgE-mediated histamine release from mast cells in vitro [181]. In a recent double-blind, placebo-controlled phase II trial, fenebrutinib was effective in reducing disease activity in patients with sgAH-resistant CSU [187]. The drug was generally well tolerated, though some patients experienced reversible grade 2 to 3 alanine aminotransferase/aspartate transaminase (ALT/AST) abnormalities, particularly at higher doses. These findings were consistent across studies in rheumatoid arthritis and lupus patients as well [188,189]. The potential role of fenebrutinib in CSU was supported by Metz et al. [187]; however, the follow-up study (NCT03693625) was discontinued [190].

6.1.2. Remibrutinib

Remibrutinib (LOU064), a novel, irreversible, and covalent BTKi, has demonstrated high selectivity and potency for BTK inhibition [26]. In phase II studies, remibrutinib showed good clinical efficacy and a favorable safety profile in patients with sgAHs-refractory CSU across a dose range of 10 to 200 mg daily [23]. The 25 mg twice-daily dose was particularly effective compared to placebos, reducing itching and hives as early as the first week of treatment, with effects sustained through week 12. Phase III trials confirmed these findings, meeting all primary and secondary endpoints and demonstrating rapid symptom control with a good safety profile [24,25]. Thus, remibrutinib appears to be a promising new treatment option for patients with sgAH-refractory CSU.

6.1.3. Rilzabrutinib

Rilzabrutinib, a reversible, covalent, and selective BTKi, has shown efficacy and good tolerability in clinical trials for several autoimmune disorders, including chronic immune thrombocytopenia [26,191]. Its activity in CSU has been evaluated in a phase II trial (NCT05107115), although the results are not yet available.

6.1.4. TAS5315

TAS5315, another highly potent and selective BTKi, has also been evaluated for treatment CSU in a phase II trial (NCT05335499), but, similarly, the results are still pending [26].

6.2. JAK-STAT Inhibitors

In the attempt to downregulate the expression of pro-inflammatory cytokines, some preliminary studies have considered employing JAK/STAT inhibitors in CSU treatment.

The Janus kinase–signal transducer and activator of transcription (JAK-STAT) is an intracellular pathway involved in the signaling of many inflammatory cytokines and other effector molecules. The JAK family of kinases includes JAK1, JAK2, JAK3, and tyrosine kinase 2 (Tyk2) [192]. JAK inhibitors are small molecules with anti-inflammatory and immunomodulatory properties that are currently employed to treat autoimmune and chronic inflammatory conditions [192]. Tofacitinib, a JAK1/3 inhibitor, caused a reduction in symptoms in four patients with CSU and was well tolerated [193]. Additionally, ruxolitinib, which inhibits JAK1/2, has also demonstrated efficacy in CSU treatment [194]. Ongoing investigations include TLL-018, a dual JAK1/Tyk2 inhibitor, and povorcitinib, a JAK1 inhibitor, both of which are being evaluated in phase I and II studies for CSU (NCT06396026, NCT05373355, and NCT05936567).

7. Miscellaneous Immunosuppressants

7.1. Corticosteroids

Systemic corticosteroids act as anti-inflammatory and immunomodulatory molecules. In particular, they diffuse passively across the cellular membrane and bind to the intracellular glucocorticoid receptor-creating complex, which is then translocated into the nucleus. This complex, binding to DNA sequences called glucocorticoid-responsive elements (GREs), blocks the promoter sites of pro-inflammatory genes (e.g., activator protein-1 and nuclear factor κB) [195] and those of the synthesis of cytokines [196]. On the other hand, it recruits sequences coding for anti-inflammatory molecules (e.g., lipocortin I and p11 and calpactin-binding protein) [197,198]. Moreover, glucocorticoids inhibit the secretion of inflammatory cytokines by affecting post-translational events [199].

According to the most recent European guidelines [1], systemic corticosteroids are a symptomatic short-term therapy, and they should not represent a first-line option. In particular, the appropriate dosage in adults should be between 20 and 50 mg/d of prednisone, the equivalent of up to 10 days of treatment. This regimen should be considered a rescue therapy for acute urticaria and should be used for acute exacerbations of CSU to reduce the disease duration/activity [200,201]. The main reasons for limiting therapy to the acute phase are the long-term side effects associated with corticosteroids, such as skin thinning, striae, hypertension, hirsutism, immunosuppression, hyperglycemia, osteoporosis, obesity, impaired wound healing, and mood disorders [197]. Moreover, there is a lack [202,203] of randomized controlled trials.

Finally, it should be mentioned that, according to evidence in the French literature, the administration of systemic corticosteroids for the treatment of CSU as first-line treatment induces resistance to anti-H1 and a rebound effect at each interruption [204,205].

7.2. Cyclosporin

Cyclosporin is a cyclic undecapeptide derived from a fungus, Tolypocladium inflatum, and is widely used as an anti-inflammatory and immunosuppressant. In particular, it acts by inhibiting the calcineurin/NFAT pathway and the JNK and p38 signaling pathway [206].

The vast majority of studies concerning the efficacy of cyclosporin in the treatment of CSU date back to the introduction of omalizumab in order to find a long-term treatment for patients who are refractory to antihistamines in monotherapy [207–209].

According to the most recent European urticaria guidelines [1], cyclosporin, with a dosage of 3.5–5 mg/kg per day [208,210], is reserved for patients who have not responded to high doses of SgAHs and omalizumab [211,212].

It was reported that cyclosporin, in association with cetirizine, is significantly more effective than placebos and cetirizine alone in reducing the severity of CSU after 8 weeks [213].

Cyclosporin is considered effective, and its safety is dose-dependent. It cannot be considered a first-line treatment because of its side effects, such as hypertension, nephrotoxicity, dyslipidemia, electrolytes alterations, hypertrichosis, higher rates of infection and neoplastic risk, and gingival hyperplasia [214].

In one study, patients that responded well to cyclosporine had high CRP levels before the treatment [215]; on the other hand, another study reveals that there are no positive predictive factors [210].

In 2020, Maoz Segal et al. [216] proposed the use of an intensified protocol with omalizumab plus an immune-suppressive agent to treat patients refractory to one of these drugs when used in monotherapy. The immunosuppressor most commonly combined with omalizumab in the protocol was cyclosporin. The authors concluded that an association protocol is safe and effective for recalcitrant CSU and may be indicated in patients with low baseline IgE levels.

7.3. Traditional Immunosuppressors/Immunomodulators Other than Cyclosporin

Although the evidence from publications is scarce, clinical experience suggests that traditional immunosuppressants other than cyclosporine, such as azathioprine, methotrexate, dapsone, hydroxychloroquine, and mycophenolate mofetil, may be useful in certain contexts.

Since omalizumab has drastically modified treatment paradigms for CSU, the use of traditional immunosuppressors is currently limited to cases refractory to multiple therapies. However, they still have an important role in developing countries due to their low cost.

7.3.1. Azathioprine

Azathioprine acts as immunosuppressor through inhibition in intracellular purine synthesis, which results in decreased numbers of circulating B and T lymphocytes, reduced immunoglobulin synthesis, and diminished interleukin 2 (IL-2) secretion [217].

Azathioprine was found to be effective at a dosage of 150 mg/day in 2 patients [218] affected by CSU resistant to other immunosuppressors. Moreover, its efficacy, at a dosage of 50 mg/day, was confirmed in a single-blind randomized control trial in patients with autologous serum skin test-positive CSU [219]. Finally, in 2019, a randomized prospective study on 80 antihistamine-refractory patients concluded the non-inferiority of azathioprine compared to cyclosporin [220].

The most common side effects of azathioprine at the doses typically used in the treatment of rheumatic diseases include gastrointestinal intolerance and bone marrow suppression [217].

7.3.2. Methotrexate

Methotrexate is an antimetabolite agent, highly similar to folic acid, that targets critical folate-dependent enzymatic steps in the de novo synthesis of purines and pyrimidines, resulting in a reduction in circulating leukocytes [221].

A systematic review published in 2022 [222] concluded that methotrexate may be a therapeutic agent in recalcitrant or steroid-dependent cases of CSU, but there is no evidence of its superiority to other first-line molecules, in particular antihistamines [223]. Methotrexate might be considered a further option in omalizumab-resistant patients [224] and can be used in combination with omalizumab itself [225]. Regarding what is reported in the literature, the maximal dose of methotrexate in CSU treatment is 25 mg/week [222].

The main side effects of methotrexate are gastrointestinal and hematologic toxicity, which can be controlled by a small amount of folic acid supplementation [226].

7.3.3. Dapsone

Dapsone is an antibiotic that is effective in leprosy infection but also effective in skin inflammatory conditions interfering with the migration of neutrophils.

Dapsone has been described as effective [227–229] and superior to antihistamines in monotherapy [230]. In a double-blind placebo-controlled study, dapsone administration, at a dosage of 100 mg/day, saw superior results to placebos in patients that failed antihistamine treatment [231].

The most important side effects are hematologic; in particular, there is an augmented metahemoglobine level [232].

7.3.4. Hydroxychloroquine

Hydroxychloroquine is an antimalaric drug commonly used as an immunomodulator and is anti-inflammatory when used in several autoimmune diseases [233].

In 2017, Boonpiyathad et al. [234]. conducted a randomized single-blinded placebo-controlled trial and an open-label comparison study to investigate the efficacy of hydroxychloroquine, administered at a dosage of 400 mg/day, in the treatment of antihistamine-refractory CSU. They reported the efficacy of hydroxychloroquine and its superiority to placebos and leukotriene receptor antagonist if added to the fourfold dose of H1-antihistamines. A real-world retrospective study in 2022 [235] investigated the effectiveness of the add-on therapy with omalizumab and hydroxychloroquine in patients refractory to antihistamines. The authors concluded that although omalizumab was superior, hydroxychloroquine was effective in two-thirds of treated patients and should be considered as a safe add-on option in monotherapy for CSU patients refractory to antihistamines.

The main adverse effect is retinopathy and for this reason patients treated with hydroxychloroquine should be periodically monitored [233].

7.3.5. Mycophenolate Mofetil

Mycophenolate mofetil is a prodrug of mycophenolic acid which inhibits the enzyme inosine-5′-monophosphate dehydrogenase, leading to lymphocyte-selective immunosuppression [236].

The use of mycophenolate mofetil in CSU is mentioned in the literature by a few studies. In an open-label, uncontrolled trial [237], nine patients affected with CSU who were poorly responsive to antihistamines and/or corticosteroids were successfully treated with mycophenolate mophetil at a dosage of 1000 mg twice daily. The efficacy of mycophenolate mofetil (at the initial dose of 500 mg twice daily with progressive increments) was confirmed in another retrospective study in 2012 [238]. Although the adverse effect profile of MMF is comparatively benign, gastrointestinal adverse effects are a major concern [239].

7.3.6. Rituximab

Rituximab is a chimeric murine/human monoclonal antibody against CD20 that has been investigated by a few authors for the treatment of selected recalcitrant CSU patients. The available data are contradictory. In some cases, rituximab was effective [240–243], while it was ineffective in others [244]. Moreover, in one case, rituximab triggered urticaria in a young patient treated for pemphigus vulgaris [245].

In conclusion, a high level of evidence concerning the use of rituximab in urticaria is lacking and it should be highlighted that its main side effect consists of long-term deep immunosuppression.

7.3.7. Tranexamic Acid

Tranexamic acid is a synthetic derivative of lysine capable of inhibiting the conversion of plasminogen into plasmin. It is commonly used as an anti-hemorrhagic drug. The rationale for the use of tranexamic acid in the treatment of CSU comes from the evidence that the disease is often characterized by the activation of the coagulation cascade as well as fibrinolysis, with often high levels of D-dimer. A pilot study conducted on 68 patients in 2010 [246] reported that an elevated D-dimer level was associated with a more severe disease and with resistance to antihistamines. In this study, 5/8 cases with elevated D-dimer showed marked improvements regarding tranexamic acid in association with nadroparin.

The data concerning the correlation between D-dimer level, disease severity, and resistance to conventional therapies were confirmed by an Indian retrospective study in 2021 [247]. Nausea and diarrhea are the most common adverse events [248].

8. Conclusions

Chronic spontaneous urticaria (CSU) is a complex, long-lasting disease that significantly impacts on patients' quality of life. In this review, we present a comprehensive overview of CSU treatments, including evidence on both established drugs and new promising molecules that have been the subject of preliminary studies. We also discuss therapies that, despite being linked to CSU's pathomechanisms, have not demonstrated significant clinical outcomes.

Currently, omalizumab remains the best treatment option for most patients, representing a revolution that has dramatically improved disease outcomes and patients' quality of life. No treatment currently surpasses omalizumab in terms of efficacy and tolerability. At present, only antihistamines and omalizumab are approved for the treatment of CSU, with no additional approved options available for patients resistant to omalizumab.

Traditional immunosuppressants and immunomodulators may be considered in cases where first-line therapy fails, either as alternatives or for use in combination with other treatments. However, these drugs tend to be less well tolerated compared to antihistamines and omalizumab.

The key pathways in chronic spontaneous urticaria are mast cell activation and degranulation, leading to the release of mediators like histamine, which causes itching, redness, and swelling. In addition to autoimmunity, autoallergy, the complement system, and coagulation, with the participation of other cells such as eosinophils, endothelial cells, basophils, B lymphocytes, T lymphocytes, and monocytes, mast cell activation potentially involves additional mechanisms. The role of epithelial-derived alarmins, which activate the group 2 innate lymphoid cells (ILC2 cells), promoting TH2 cytokines and allergen-specific IgE, thus triggering mast cell activation, is under investigation. Targets for current and future therapies include key receptors (FcεRI, C5aR, MRGPRX2), signaling pathways (BTK, SYK), and mediators (IL-4, IL-17, IL-31).

Among the molecules targeting various pathogenic pathways currently under study, the emerging drugs are represented by BTKis, like remibrutinib; monoclonal antibodies targeting IL-4 and IL-13, such as dupilumab; and anti-Kit agents, such as barzolvolimab, JAK inhibitors, and MRGPRX2 antagonists (Tables 2 and 3). If these findings are confirmed, they may lead to the introduction of new disease-modifying drugs.

Funding: This work was partially supported by the Italian Ministry of Health—grant number: RC 2024 and University of Milan, thought the APC initiative.

Conflicts of Interest: R.S.A. has recently been speaker and or advisor for Novartis, GSK, Astra Zeneca, Lofarma, Hal Allergy, Smart Practice, Allergy Therapeutics, Menarini, Malesci, Sanofi and Jasper Therapeutics all outside the submitted work. P.C. has recently been speaker for Almirall all outside the submitted work. S.V. and M.C. have no conflicts of interest.

References

1. Zuberbier, T.; Abdul Latiff, A.H.; Abuzakouk, M.; Aquilina, S.; Asero, R.; Baker, D.; Ballmer-Weber, B.; Bangert, C.; Ben-Shoshan, M.; Bernstein, J.A.; et al. The international EAACI/GA2LEN/EuroGuiDerm/APAACI guideline for the definition, classification, diagnosis, and management of urticaria. *Allergy* **2022**, *77*, 734–766. [CrossRef] [PubMed]
2. Maurer, M.; Weller, K.; Bindslev-Jensen, C.; Giménez-Arnau, A.; Bousquet, P.J.; Bousquet, J.; Canonica, G.W.; Church, M.K.; Godse, K.V.; Grattan, C.E.H.; et al. Unmet clinical needs in chronic spontaneous urticaria. A GA2LEN task force report. *Allergy* **2011**, *66*, 317–330. [CrossRef] [PubMed]
3. O'Donnell, B.F.; Lawlor, F.; Simpson, J.; Morgan, M.; Greaves, M.W. The impact of chronic urticaria on the quality of life. *Br. J. Dermatol.* **1997**, *136*, 197–201. [CrossRef]
4. Church, M.K.; Kolkhir, P.; Metz, M.; Maurer, M. The role and relevance of mast cells in urticaria. *Immunol. Rev.* **2018**, *282*, 232–247. [CrossRef]
5. Grattan, C.E.H.; Francis, D.M.; Hide, M.; Greaves, M.W. Detection of circulating histamine releasing autoantibodies with functional properties of anti-IgE in chronic urticaria. *Clin. Exp. Allergy* **1991**, *21*, 695–704. [CrossRef]
6. Hide, M.; Francis, D.M.; Grattan, C.; Hakimi, J.; Kochan, J.P.; Greaves, M.W. Autoantibodies against the high-affinity IgE receptor as a cause of histamine release in chronic urticaria. *N. Engl. J. Med.* **1993**, *328*, 1599–1604. [CrossRef]

7. Altrichter, S.; Peter, H.J.; Pisarevskaja, D.; Metz, M.; Martus, P.; Maurer, M. IgE mediated autoallergy against thyroid peroxidase—A novel pathomechanism of chronic spontaneous urticaria? *PLoS ONE* **2011**, *6*, e14794. [CrossRef]
8. Schmetzer, O.; Lakin, E.; Topal, F.A.; Preusse, P.; Freier, D.; Church, M.K.; Maurer, M. IL-24 is a common and specific autoantigen of IgE in patients with chronic spontaneous urticaria. *J. Allergy Clin. Immunol.* **2018**, *142*, 876–882. [CrossRef]
9. Asero, R.; Marzano, A.; Ferrucci, S.; Lorini, M.; Carbonelli, V.; Cugno, M. Co-occurrence of IgE and IgG autoantibodies in patients with chronic spontaneous urticaria. *Clin. Exp. Immunol.* **2020**, *200*, 242–249. [CrossRef]
10. Asero, R.; Tedeschi, A.; Riboldi, P.; Cugno, M. Plasma of patients with chronic urticaria shows signs of thrombin generation, and its intradermal injection causes wheal-and-flare reactions much more frequently than autologous serum. *J. Allergy Clin. Immunol.* **2006**, *117*, 1113–1117. [CrossRef]
11. Asero, R.; Tedeschi, A.; Coppola, R.; Griffini, S.; Paparella, P.; Riboldi, P.; Marzano, A.V.; Fanoni, D.; Cugno, M. Activation of the tissue factor pathway of blood coagulation in patients with chronic urticaria. *J. Allergy Clin. Immunol.* **2007**, *119*, 705–710. [CrossRef] [PubMed]
12. Cugno, M.; Marzano, A.V.; Tedeschi, A.; Fanoni, D.; Venegoni, L.; Asero, R. Expression of tissue factor by eosinophils in patients with chronic urticaria. *Int. Arch. Allergy Immunol.* **2009**, *148*, 170–174. [CrossRef] [PubMed]
13. Yanase, Y.; Matsuo, Y.; Takahagi, S.; Kawaguchi, T.; Uchida, K.; Ishii, K.; Tanaka, A.; Matsubara, D.; Ozawa, K.; Hide, M. Coagulation factors induce human skin mast cell and basophil degranulation via activation of complement 5 and the C5a receptor. *J. Allergy Clin. Immunol.* **2021**, *147*, 1101–1104.e7. [CrossRef] [PubMed]
14. Giménez-Arnau, A.M.; de Montjoye, L.; Asero, R.; Cugno, M.; Kulthanan, K.; Yanase, Y.; Hide, M.; Kaplan, A.P. The Pathogenesis of Chronic Spontaneous Urticaria: The Role of Infiltrating Cells. *J. Allergy Clin. Immunol. Pract.* **2021**, *9*, 2195–2208. [CrossRef] [PubMed]
15. Maurer, M.; Kolkhir, P.; Pereira, M.P.; Siebenhaar, F.; Witte-Händel, E.; Bergmann, K.; Bonnekoh, H.; Buttgereit, T.; Fluhr, J.W.; Frischbutter, S.; et al. Disease modification in chronic spontaneous urticaria. *Allergy* **2024**, *79*, 2396–2413. [CrossRef]
16. Maurer, M.; Casale, T.B.; Saini, S.S.; Ben-Shoshan, M.; Giménez-Arnau, A.M.; Bernstein, J.A.; Yagami, A.; Stjepanovic, A.; Radin, A.; Staudinger, H.W.; et al. Dupilumab in patients with chronic spontaneous urticaria (LIBERTY-CSU CUPID): Two randomized, double-blind, placebo-controlled, phase 3 trials. *J. Allergy Clin. Immunol.* **2024**, *154*, 184–194. [CrossRef]
17. Kudlaty, E.; Newell, P.; Chovatiya, R. Dupilumab as Add-on Therapy for Management of Chronic Spontaneous Urticaria. *J. Clin. Aesthet. Dermatol.* **2024**, *17*, 10–12.
18. Terhorst-Molawi, D.; Hawro, T.; Grekowitz, E.; Kiefer, L.; Merchant, K.; Alvarado, D.; Thomas, L.J.; Hawthorne, T.; Crowley, E.; Heath-Chiozzi, M.; et al. Anti-KIT antibody, barzolvolimab, reduces skin mast cells and disease activity in chronic inducible urticaria. *Allergy* **2023**, *78*, 1269–1279. [CrossRef]
19. Maurer, M.; Altrichter, S.; Metz, M.; Zuberbier, T.; Church, M.; Bergmann, K.C. Benefit from reslizumab treatment in a patient with chronic spontaneous urticaria and cold urticaria. *J. Eur. Acad. Dermatol. Venereol.* **2018**, *32*, e112–e113. [CrossRef]
20. Antonicelli, L.; Tontini, C.; Garritani, M.S.; Piga, M.A.; Bilò, M.B. Efficacy of Mepolizumab in Patients With Severe Eosinophilic Asthma and Concomitant Severe Chronic Urticaria: An Example of Personalized Medicine? *J. Investig. Allergol. Clin. Immunol.* **2023**, *33*, 54–56.
21. Bergmann, K.C.; Altrichter, S.; Maurer, M. Benefit of benralizumab treatment in a patient with chronic symptomatic dermographism. *J. Eur. Acad. Dermatol. Venereol.* **2019**, *33*, e413–e415. [CrossRef] [PubMed]
22. Kuo, B.S.; Li, C.H.; Chen, J.B.; Shiung, Y.Y.; Chu, C.Y.; Lee, C.H.; Liu, Y.J.; Kuo, J.H.; Hsu, C.; Su, H.W.; et al. IgE-neutralizing UB-221 mAb, distinct from omalizumab and ligelizumab, exhibits CD23-mediated IgE downregulation and relieves urticaria symptoms. *J. Clin. Investig.* **2022**, *132*, e157765. [CrossRef] [PubMed]
23. Maurer, M.; Berger, W.; Giménez-Arnau, A.; Hayama, K.; Jain, V.; Reich, A.; Haemmerle, S.; Lheritier, K.; Walsh, P.; Xia, S.; et al. Remibrutinib, a novel BTK inhibitor, demonstrates promising efficacy and safety in chronic spontaneous urticaria. *J. Allergy Clin. Immunol.* **2022**, *150*, 1498–1506.e2. [CrossRef] [PubMed]
24. Novartis. Novartis Phase III Data Confirm Sustained Efficacy and Long-Term Safety of Oral Remibrutinib in Chronic Spontaneous Urticaria. Available online: https://www.novartis.com/news/media-releases/novartis-phase-iii-data-confirm-sustained-efficacy-and-long-term-safety-oral-remibrutinib-chronic-spontaneous-urticaria (accessed on 15 September 2024).
25. Jain, V.; Giménez-Arnau, A.; Hayama, K.; Reich, A.; Carr, W.; Tillinghast, J.; Dahale, S.; Lheritier, K.; Walsh, P.; Zharkov, A.; et al. Remibrutinib demonstrates favorable safety profile and sustained efficacy in chronic spontaneous urticaria over 52 weeks. *J. Allergy Clin. Immunol.* **2024**, *153*, 479–486.e4. [CrossRef] [PubMed]
26. Bernstein, J.A.; Maurer, M.; Saini, S.S. BTK signaling—A crucial link in the pathophysiology of chronic spontaneous urticaria. *J. Allergy Clin. Immunol.* **2024**, *153*, 1229–1240. [CrossRef]
27. Xiang, Y.-K.; Fok, J.S.; Podder, I.; Yücel, M.B.; Özkoca, D.; Thomsen, S.F.; Kocatürk, E. An update on the use of antihistamines in managing chronic urticaria. *Expert. Opin. Pharmacother.* **2024**, *25*, 551–569. [CrossRef]
28. Wang, D.; Guo, Q.; Wu, Z.; Li, M.; He, B.; Du, Y.; Zhang, K.; Tao, Y. Molecular mechanism of antihistamines recognition and regulation of the histamine H1 receptor. *Nat. Commun.* **2024**, *15*, 84. [CrossRef] [PubMed] [PubMed Central]
29. He, L.; Yi, W.; Huang, X.; Long, H.; Lu, Q. Chronic Urticaria: Advances in Understanding of the Disease and Clinical Management. *Clin. Rev. Allergy Immunol.* **2021**, *61*, 424–448. [CrossRef]
30. Sánchez, J.; Zakzuk, J.; Cardona, R. Prediction of the Efficacy of Antihistamines in Chronic Spontaneous Urticaria Based on Initial Suppression of the Histamine-Induced Wheal. *J. Investig. Allergol. Clin. Immunol.* **2016**, *26*, 177–184. [CrossRef]

31. Recto, M.T.; Gabriel, M.T.; Kulthanan, K.; Tantilipikorn, P.; Aw, D.C.-W.; Lee, T.H.; Chwen, C.C.; Mutusamy, S.; Hao, N.T.; Quang, V.T.; et al. Selecting optimal second-generation antihistamines for allergic rhinitis and urticaria in Asia. *Clin. Mol. Allergy* **2017**, *15*, 19. [CrossRef]
32. Xiao, X.; Xue, P.; Shi, Y.; Yao, J.; Cao, W.; Zhang, L.; Zou, Z.; Zhou, S.; Wang, C.; Chen, M.; et al. The efficacy and safety of high-dose nonsedating antihistamines in chronic spontaneous urticaria: A systematic review and meta-analysis of randomized clinical trials. *BMC Pharmacol. Toxicol.* **2023**, *24*, 23. [CrossRef] [PubMed]
33. Sinha, V.V.; Kalikar, M.V.; Mukhi, J.I.; Giradkar, A.B.; Sontakke, S. Comparative study of efficacy and safety of cetirizine and bilastine in patients of chronic spontaneous urticaria: Open-label, randomized, parallel-group study. *Perspect. Clin. Res.* **2023**, *14*, 180–186. [CrossRef] [PubMed]
34. Shah, B.; Dhoot, D.; Choudhary, A.; Jangid, N.; Mistry, D.; Shah, S.; Kamat, S.; Barkate, H. A Comparative, Three-Arm, Randomized Clinical Trial to Evaluate the Effectiveness and Tolerability of Bilastine vs Fexofenadine vs Levocetirizine at the Standard Dose and Bilastine vs Fexofenadine at Higher Than the Standard Dose (Up-Dosing) vs Levocetirizine and Hydroxyzine (in Combination) in Patients with Chronic Spontaneous Urticaria. *Clin. Cosmet. Investig. Dermatol.* **2022**, *15*, 261–270. [PubMed]
35. Podder, I.; Das, A.; Ghosh, S.; Biswas, D.; Sengupta, S.; Chowdhury, S.N. Effectiveness, safety, and tolerability of bilastine 20 mg vs levocetirizine 5 mg for the treatment of chronic spontaneous urticaria: A double-blind, parallel group, randomized controlled trial. *Dermatol. Ther.* **2020**, *33*, e13946. [CrossRef]
36. Guillén-Aguinaga, S.; Presa, I.J.; Aguinaga-Ontoso, E.; Guillén-Grima, F.; Ferrer, M. Updosing nonsedating antihistamines in patients with chronic spontaneous urticaria: A systematic review and meta-analysis. *Br. J. Dermatol.* **2016**, *175*, 1153–1165. [CrossRef]
37. Zuberbier, T.; Münzberger, C.; Haustein, U.; Trippas, E.; Burtin, B.; Mariz, S.; Henz, B. Double-blind crossover study of high-dose cetirizine in cholinergic urticaria. *Dermatology* **1996**, *193*, 324–327. [CrossRef]
38. Staevska, M.; Popov, T.A.; Kralimarkova, T.; Lazarova, C.; Kraeva, S.; Popova, D.; Church, D.S.; Dimitrov, V.; Church, M.K. The effectiveness of levocetirizine and desloratadine in up to 4 times conventional doses in difficult-to-treat urticaria. *J. Allergy Clin. Immunol.* **2010**, *125*, 676–682. [CrossRef]
39. Siebenhaar, F.; Degener, F.; Zuberbier, T.; Martus, P.; Maurer, M. High-dose desloratadine decreases wheal volume and improves cold provocation thresholds compared with standard-dose treatment in patients with acquired cold urticaria: A randomized, placebo-controlled, crossover study. *J. Allergy Clin. Immunol.* **2009**, *123*, 672–679. [CrossRef]
40. Giménez-Arnau, A.; Izquierdo, I.; Maurer, M. The use of a responder analysis to identify clinically meaningful differences in chronic urticaria patients following placebo-controlled treatment with rupatadine 10 and 20 mg. *J. Eur. Acad. Dermatol. Venereol.* **2009**, *23*, 1088–1091. [CrossRef]
41. Cataldi, M.; Maurer, M.; Taglialatela, M.; Church, M.K. Cardiac safety of second-generation H1-antihistamines when updosed in chronic spontaneous urticaria. *Clin. Exp. Allergy* **2019**, *49*, 1615–1623. [CrossRef]
42. Zhou, P.; Zeng, S.; Fu, L.; Chen, H.; Li, L. Efficacy and Safety of Intensive Nonsedating Antihistamines for Chronic Spontaneous Urticaria: A Meta-Analysis of Randomized Controlled Trials. *Int. Arch. Allergy Immunol.* **2022**, *183*, 796–803. [CrossRef] [PubMed]
43. Presta, L.G.; Lahr, S.J.; Shields, R.L.; Porter, J.P.; Gorman, C.M.; Fendly, B.M.; Jardieu, P.M. Humanization of an antibody directed against IgE. *J. Immunol.* **1993**, *151*, 2623–2632. [CrossRef]
44. Rajesh, G.; Keerthi, S.; Karthikeyan, K.; Venkatesan, M. Weekly injection of histaglobulin produces long-term remission in chronic urticaria: A prospective clinical study. *Indian. J. Pharmacol.* **2016**, *48*, 292–297. [CrossRef] [PubMed] [PubMed Central]
45. Kim, H.S.; Noh, G. Induction of remission in 205 chronic urticaria by immunotherapy using immunoglobulin/histamine complex 206 (Histobulin™): A case report. *Allergy Asthma Clin. Immunol.* **2021**, *17*, 116. [CrossRef]
46. de Silva, N.L.; Damayanthi, H.; Rajapakse, A.C.; Rodrigo, C.; Rajapakse, S. Leukotriene receptor antagonists for chronic urticaria: A systematic review. *Allergy Asthma Clin. Immunol.* **2014**, *10*, 24. [CrossRef]
47. Asero, R. Leukotriene receptor antagonists may prevent NSAID-induced exacerbations in patients with chronic urticaria. *Ann. Allergy Asthma Immunol.* **2000**, *85*, 156–157. [CrossRef]
48. Asero, R.; Tedeschi, A.; Lorini, M. Leukotriene receptor antagonists in chronic urticaria. *Allergy* **2001**, *56*, 456–457. [CrossRef]
49. Erbagci, Z. The leukotriene receptor antagonist montelukast in the treatment of chronic idiopathic urticaria: A single-blind, placebo-controlled, crossover clinical study. *J. Allergy Clin. Immunol.* **2002**, *110*, 484–488. [CrossRef]
50. Sarkar, T.K.; Sil, A.; Pal, S.; Ghosh, C.; Das, N.K. Effectiveness and safety of levocetirizine 10 mg versus a combination of levocetirizine 5 mg and montelukast 10 mg in chronic urticaria resistant to levocetirizine 5 mg: A double-blind, randomized, controlled trial. *Indian. J. Dermatol. Venereol. Leprol.* **2017**, *83*, 561–568.
51. Alkeraye, S.; AlRuhaimi, D.K. The Addition of Montelukast for the Treatment of Chronic Idiopathic Urticaria. *Cureus* **2021**, *13*, e16137. [CrossRef]
52. Khan, S.; Lynch, N. Efficacy of montelukast as added therapy in patients with chronic idiopathic urticaria. *Inflamm. Allergy Drug Targets.* **2012**, *11*, 235–243. [CrossRef] [PubMed]
53. Di Lorenzo, G.; Pacor, M.L.; Mansueto, P.; Esposito Pellitteri, M.; Lo Bianco, C.; Ditta, V.; Martinelli, N.; Rini, G.B. Randomized placebo-controlled trial comparing desloratadine and montelukast in monotherapy and desloratadine plus montelukast in combined therapy for chronic idiopathic urticaria. *J. Allergy Clin. Immunol.* **2004**, *114*, 619–625. [CrossRef] [PubMed]
54. Godse, K.V. Oral montelukast monotherapy is ineffective in chronic idiopathic urticaria: A comparison with oral cetirizine. *Indian. J. Dermatol. Venereol. Leprol.* **2006**, *72*, 312–314. [CrossRef] [PubMed]

55. Tedeschi, A. Paradoxical exacerbation of chronic urticaria by H1-antihistamines and montelukast. *Eur. Ann. Allergy Clin. Immunol.* **2009**, *41*, 187–189.
56. Haas, N.; Küster, W.; Zuberbier, T.; Henz, B.M. Muckle-Wells syndrome: Clinical and histological skin findings compatible with cold air urticaria in a large kindred. *Br. J. Dermatol.* **2004**, *151*, 99–104. [CrossRef]
57. Maul, J.T.; Distler, M.; Kolios, A.; Maul, L.V.; Guillet, C.; Graf, N.; Imhof, L.; Lang, C.; Navarini, A.A.; Schmid-Grendelmeier, P. Canakinumab Lacks Efficacy in Treating Adult Patients with Moderate to Severe Chronic Spontaneous Urticaria in a Phase II Randomized Double-Blind Placebo-Controlled Single-Center Study. *J. Allergy Clin. Immunol. Pract.* **2021**, *9*, 463–468.e3. [CrossRef]
58. Antosz, K.; Batko, J.; Błażejewska, M.; Gawor, A.; Sleziak, J.; Gomułka, K. Insight into IL-5 as a Potential Target for the Treatment of Allergic Diseases. *Biomedicines* **2024**, *12*, 1531. [CrossRef]
59. Magerl, M.; Terhorst, D.; Metz, M.; Altrichter, S.; Zuberbier, T.; Maurer, M.; Bergmann, K.C. Benefit of mepolizumab treatment in a patient with chronic spontaneous urticaria. *J. Dtsch. Dermatol. Ges.* **2018**, *16*, 477–478. [CrossRef]
60. Atwa, M.A.; Emara, A.S.; Youssef, N.; Bayoumy, N.M. Serum concentration of IL-17, IL-23 and TNF-α among patients with chronic spontaneous urticaria: Association with disease activity and autologous serum skin test. *J. Eur. Acad. Dermatol. Venereol.* **2014**, *28*, 469–474. [CrossRef]
61. Sabag, D.A.; Matanes, L.; Bejar, J.; Sheffer, H.; Barzilai, A.; Church, M.K.; Toubi, E.; Maurer, M.; Vadasz, Z. Interleukin-17 is a potential player and treatment target in severe chronic spontaneous urticaria. *Clin. Exp. Allergy* **2020**, *50*, 799–804. [CrossRef]
62. Bonnekoh, H.; Kiefer, L.; Buttgereit, T.; Kolkhir, P.; Lütke-Eversloh, M.; Scheffel, J.; Maurer, M.; Metz, M. Anti-IL-23 treatment with tildrakizumab can be effective in omalizumab-refractory chronic spontaneous urticaria: A case series. *J. Allergy Clin. Immunol. Pract.* **2023**, *11*, 2578–2580.e1. [CrossRef] [PubMed]
63. Sofen, H.; Bissonnette, R.; Yosipovitch, G.; Silverberg, J.I.; Tyring, S.; Loo, W.J.; Zook, M.; Lee, M.; Zou, L.; Jiang, G.-L.; et al. Efficacy and safety of vixarelimab, a human monoclonal oncostatin M receptor β antibody, in moderate-to-severe prurigo nodularis: A randomised, double-blind, placebo-controlled, phase 2a study. *EClinicalMedicine* **2023**, *57*, 101826. [CrossRef] [PubMed]
64. Maggi, L.; Rossettini, B.; Montaini, G.; Matucci, A.; Vultaggio, A.; Mazzoni, A.; Palterer, B.; Parronchi, P.; Maggi, E.; Liotta, F.; et al. Omalizumab dampens type 2 inflammation in a group of long-term treated asthma patients and detaches IgE from FcεRI. *Eur. J. Immunol.* **2018**, *48*, 2005–2014. [CrossRef] [PubMed]
65. Mankad, V.S.; Burks, A.W. Omalizumab: Other indications and unanswered questions. *Clin. Rev. Allergy Immunol.* **2005**, *29*, 17–30. [CrossRef]
66. Kaplan, A.P. Chronic urticaria: Pathogenesis and treatment. *J. Allergy Clin. Immunol.* **2004**, *114*, 465–474, quiz 475. [CrossRef]
67. Maurer, M.; Altrichter, S.; Bieber, T.; Biedermann, T.; Bräutigam, M.; Seyfried, S.; Brehler, R.; Grabbe, J.; Hunzelmann, N.; Jakob, T.; et al. Efficacy and safety of omalizumab in patients with chronic urticaria who exhibit IgE against thyroperoxidase. *J. Allergy Clin. Immunol.* **2011**, *128*, 202–209.e5. [CrossRef]
68. Metz, M.; Staubach, P.; Bauer, A.; Brehler, R.; Gericke, J.; Kangas, M.; Ashton-Chess, J.; Jarvis, P.; Georgiou, P.; Canvin, J.; et al. Clinical efficacy of omalizumab in chronic spontaneous urticaria is associated with a reduction of FcεRI-positive cells in the skin. *Theranostics* **2017**, *7*, 1266–1276. [CrossRef]
69. Kaplan, A.P.; Giménez-Arnau, A.M.; Saini, S.S. Mechanisms of action that contribute to efficacy of omalizumab in chronic spontaneous urticaria. *Allergy* **2017**, *72*, 519–533. [CrossRef]
70. Zhou, B.; Li, J.; Liu, R.; Zhu, L.; Peng, C. The Role of Crosstalk of Immune Cells in Pathogenesis of Chronic Spontaneous Urticaria. *Front. Immunol.* **2022**, *13*, 879754. [CrossRef]
71. Hoşgören-Tekin, S.; Eyüboğlu, I.P.; Akkiprik, M.; Giménez-Arnau, A.M.; Salman, A. Inflammatory cytokine levels and changes during omalizumab treatment in chronic spontaneous urticaria. *Arch. Dermatol. Res.* **2024**, *316*, 261. [CrossRef]
72. Gericke, J.; Metz, M.; Ohanyan, T.; Weller, K.; Altrichter, S.; Skov, P.S.; Falkencrone, S.; Brand, J.; Kromminga, A.; Hawro, T.; et al. Serum autoreactivity predicts time to response to omalizumab therapy in chronic spontaneous urticaria. *J. Allergy Clin. Immunol.* **2017**, *139*, 1059–1061.e1. [CrossRef] [PubMed]
73. Kaplan, A.; Ledford, D.; Ashby, M.; Canvin, J.; Zazzali, J.L.; Conner, E.; Veith, J.; Kamath, N.; Staubach, P.; Jakob, T.; et al. Omalizumab in patients with symptomatic chronic idiopathic/spontaneous urticaria despite standard combination therapy. *J. Allergy Clin. Immunol.* **2013**, *132*, 101–109. [CrossRef] [PubMed]
74. Maurer, M.; Rosén, K.; Hsieh, H.-J.; Saini, S.; Grattan, C.; Gimenéz-Arnau, A.; Agarwal, S.; Doyle, R.; Canvin, J.; Kaplan, A.; et al. Omalizumab for the treatment of chronic idiopathic or spontaneous urticaria. *N. Engl. J. Med.* **2013**, *368*, 924–935. [CrossRef] [PubMed]
75. Saini, S.S.; Bindslev-Jensen, C.; Maurer, M.; Grob, J.-J.; Baskan, E.B.; Bradley, M.S.; Canvin, J.; Rahmaoui, A.; Georgiou, P.; Alpan, O.; et al. Efficacy and safety of omalizumab in patients with chronic idiopathic/spontaneous urticaria who remain symptomatic on H1 antihistamines: A randomized, placebo-controlled study. *J. Investig. Dermatol.* **2015**, *135*, 67–75. [CrossRef]
76. Giménez-Arnau, A.M. Omalizumab for treating chronic spontaneous urticaria: An expert review on efficacy and safety. *Expert. Opin. Biol. Ther.* **2017**, *17*, 375–385. [CrossRef]
77. Zhao, Z.-T.; Ji, C.-M.; Yu, W.-J.; Meng, L.; Hawro, T.; Wei, J.-F.; Maurer, M. Omalizumab for the treatment of chronic spontaneous urticaria: A meta-analysis of randomized clinical trials. *J. Allergy Clin. Immunol.* **2016**, *137*, 1742–1750.e4. [CrossRef]

78. Zazzali, J.L.; Kaplan, A.; Maurer, M.; Raimundo, K.; Trzaskoma, B.; Solari, P.G.; Antonova, E.; Mendelson, M.; Rosén, K.E. Angioedema in the omalizumab chronic idiopathic/spontaneous urticaria pivotal studies. *Ann. Allergy Asthma Immunol.* **2016**, *117*, 370–377.e1. [CrossRef]
79. Dekkers, C.; Aghdam, M.A.; Graaf, M.; Knulst, A.C.; Meijer, Y.; Reek, J.M.P.; Stadermann, M.B.; Röckmann, H. Safety and effectiveness of omalizumab for the treatment of chronic urticaria in pediatric patients. *Pediatr. Allergy Immunol.* **2021**, *32*, 720–726. [CrossRef]
80. Ari, A.; Levy, Y.; Segal, N.; Maoz-Segal, R.; Benor, S.; Broides, A.; Horev, A.; Epstein-Rigbi, N.; Agmon-Levin, N.; Marcus, N. Efficacy of omalizumab treatment for pediatric chronic spontaneous urticaria: A multi-center retrospective case series. *Pediatr. Dermatol.* **2020**, *37*, 1051–1054. [CrossRef]
81. Ocak, M.; Soyer, O.; Buyuktiryaki, B.; Sekerel, B.E.; Sahiner, U.M. Omalizumab treatment in adolescents with chronic spontaneous urticaria: Efficacy and safety. *Allergol. Immunopathol.* **2020**, *48*, 368–373. [CrossRef]
82. Song, X.T.; Chen, Y.D.; Yu, M.; Liu, B.; Zhao, Z.T.; Maurer, M. Omalizumab in children and adolescents with chronic urticaria: A 16-week real-world study. *Allergy* **2021**, *76*, 1271–1273. [CrossRef] [PubMed]
83. Martina, E.; Damiani, G.; Grieco, T.; Foti, C.; Pigatto, P.D.M.; Offidani, A. It is never too late to treat chronic spontaneous urticaria with omalizumab: Real-life data from a multicenter observational study focusing on elderly patients. *Dermatol. Ther.* **2021**, *34*, e14841. [CrossRef] [PubMed]
84. Sirufo, M.M.; Bassino, E.M.; De Pietro, F.; Ginaldi, L.; De Martinis, M. Sex differences in the efficacy of omalizumab in the treatment of chronic spontaneous urticaria. *Int. J. Immunopathol. Pharmacol.* **2022**, *35*, 20587384211065870. [CrossRef]
85. Hide, M.; Park, H.-S.; Igarashi, A.; Ye, Y.-M.; Kim, T.-B.; Yagami, A.; Roh, J.; Lee, J.-H.; Chinuki, Y.; Youn, S.W.; et al. Efficacy and safety of omalizumab in Japanese and Korean patients with refractory chronic spontaneous urticaria. *J. Dermatol. Sci.* **2017**, *87*, 70–78. [CrossRef]
86. Skander, D.; Allenova, A.; Maurer, M.; Kolkhir, P. Omalizumab is effective in patients with chronic spontaneous urticaria plus multiple chronic inducible urticaria. *Eur. Ann. Allergy Clin. Immunol.* **2021**, *53*, 91–93. [CrossRef]
87. González-Medina, M.; Curto-Barredo, L.; Labrador-Horrillo, M.; Giménez-Arnau, A. Omalizumab use during pregnancy for chronic spontaneous urticaria (CSU): Report of two cases. *J. Eur. Acad. Dermatol. Venereol.* **2017**, *31*, e245–e246. [CrossRef]
88. Türk, M.; Carneiro-Leão, L.; Kolkhir, P.; Bonnekoh, H.; Buttgereit, T.; Maurer, M. How to Treat Patients with Chronic Spontaneous Urticaria with Omalizumab: Questions and Answers. *J. Allergy Clin. Immunol. Pract.* **2020**, *8*, 113–124. [CrossRef]
89. Finlay, A.Y.; Kaplan, A.P.; Beck, L.A.; Antonova, E.N.; Balp, M.M.; Zazzali, J.; Khalil, S.; Maurer, M. Omalizumab substantially improves dermatology-related quality of life in patients with chronic spontaneous urticaria. *J. Eur. Acad. Dermatol. Venereol.* **2017**, *31*, 1715–1721. [CrossRef]
90. Gimenéz-Arnau, A.M.; Spector, S.; Antonova, E.; Trzaskoma, B.; Rosén, K.; Omachi, T.A.; Stull, D.; Balp, M.M.; Murphy, T. Improvement of sleep in patients with chronic idiopathic/spontaneous urticaria treated with omalizumab: Results of three randomized, double-blind, placebo-controlled studies. *Clin. Transl. Allergy* **2016**, *6*, 32. [CrossRef]
91. Maurer, M.; Sofen, H.; Ortiz, B.; Kianifard, F.; Gabriel, S.; Bernstein, J.A. Positive impact of omalizumab on angioedema and quality of life in patients with refractory chronic idiopathic/spontaneous urticaria: Analyses according to the presence or absence of angioedema. *J. Eur. Acad. Dermatol. Venereol.* **2017**, *31*, 1056–1063. [CrossRef]
92. Durmaz, K.; Ataseven, A.; Temiz, S.A.; Isik, B.; Dursun, R. Does omalizumab use in chronic spontaneous urticaria results in improvement in sexual functions? *J. Cosmet. Dermatol.* **2022**, *21*, 4877–4881. [CrossRef] [PubMed]
93. Porter, E.; Tierney, E.; Byrne, B.; Basheer-O'Dwyer, S.; Kanaan, A.; Ramsay, B.; Field, S. "It has given me my life back": A qualitative study exploring the lived experience of patients with chronic spontaneous urticaria on omalizumab. *Clin. Exp. Dermatol.* **2022**, *47*, 2032–2034. [CrossRef] [PubMed]
94. Tan, M.G.; Bailey, A.M.J.; Dorus, B.; Kirchhof, M.G. Clinical Impacts of Omalizumab on the Psychiatric Comorbidities of Chronic Spontaneous Urticaria: A Systematic Review and Meta-Analysis. *J. Drugs Dermatol.* **2024**, *23*, e116–e117. [CrossRef]
95. Bérard, F.; Ferrier Le Bouedec, M.C.; Bouillet, L.; Reguiai, Z.; Barbaud, A.; Cambazard, F.; Milpied, B.; Pelvet, B.; Kasujee, I.; Gharbi, H.; et al. Omalizumab in patients with chronic spontaneous urticaria nonresponsive to H1-antihistamine treatment: Results of the phase IV open-label SUNRISE study. *Br. J. Dermatol.* **2019**, *180*, 56–66. [CrossRef]
96. Casale, T.B.; Win, P.H.; Bernstein, J.A.; Rosén, K.; Holden, M.; Iqbal, A.; Trzaskoma, B.L.; Yang, M.; Antonova, E.N.; Murphy, T.; et al. Omalizumab response in patients with chronic idiopathic urticaria: Insights from the XTEND-CIU study. *J. Am. Acad. Dermatol.* **2018**, *78*, 793–795. [CrossRef]
97. Casale, T.B.; Murphy, T.R.; Holden, M.; Rajput, Y.; Yoo, B.; Bernstein, J.A. Impact of omalizumab on patient-reported outcomes in chronic idiopathic urticaria: Results from a randomized study (XTEND-CIU). *J. Allergy Clin. Immunol. Pract.* **2019**, *7*, 2487–2490.e1. [CrossRef]
98. Goswamy, V.P.; Lee, K.E.; McKernan, E.M.; Fichtinger, P.S.; Mathur, S.K.; Viswanathan, R.K. Omalizumab for treatment of idiopathic angioedema. *Ann. Allergy Asthma Immunol.* **2022**, *129*, 605–611.e1. [CrossRef]
99. Staubach, P.; Metz, M.; Chapman-Rothe, N.; Sieder, C.; Bräutigam, M.; Canvin, J.; Maurer, M. Effect of omalizumab on angioedema in H1-antihistamine-resistant chronic spontaneous urticaria patients: Results from X-ACT, a randomized controlled trial. *Allergy* **2016**, *71*, 1135–1144. [CrossRef]
100. Asero, R.; Ferrucci, S.M.; Calzari, P.; Consonni, D.; Cugno, M. Thyroid Autoimmunity in CSU: A Potential Marker of Omalizumab Response? *Int. J. Mol. Sci.* **2023**, *24*, 7491. [CrossRef]

101. Kaplan, A.; Ferrer, M.; Bernstein, J.A.; Antonova, E.; Trzaskoma, B.; Raimundo, K.; Rosén, K.; Omachi, T.A.; Khalil, S.; Zazzali, J.L. Timing and duration of omalizumab response in patients with chronic idiopathic/spontaneous urticaria. *J. Allergy Clin. Immunol.* **2016**, *137*, 474–481. [CrossRef]
102. Syrigos, N.; Grapsa, D.; Zande, M.; Tziotou, M.; Syrigou, E. Treatment response to omalizumab in patients with refractory chronic spontaneous urticaria. *Int. J. Dermatol.* **2018**, *57*, 417–422. [CrossRef] [PubMed]
103. Giménez Arnau, A.M.; Valero Santiago, A.; Bartra Tomás, J.; Jáuregui Presa, I.; Labrador Horrillo, M.; Miquel Miquel, F.J.; Ortiz de Frutos, J.; Sastre, J.; Silvestre Salvador, J.F.; Ferrer Puga, M. Therapeutic Strategy According to Differences in Response to Omalizumab in Patients with Chronic Spontaneous Urticaria. *J. Investig. Allergol. Clin. Immunol.* **2019**, *29*, 338–348. [CrossRef] [PubMed]
104. Metz, M.; Vadasz, Z.; Kocatürk, E.; Giménez-Arnau, A.M. Omalizumab Updosing in Chronic Spontaneous Urticaria: An Overview of Real-World Evidence. *Clin. Rev. Allergy Immunol.* **2020**, *59*, 38–45. [CrossRef] [PubMed]
105. Brás, R.; Costa, C.; Limão, R.; Caldeira, L.E.; Paulino, M.; Pedro, E. Omalizumab in Chronic Spontaneous Urticaria (CSU): Real-Life Experience in Dose/Interval Adjustments and Treatment Discontinuation. *J. Allergy Clin. Immunol. Pract.* **2023**, *11*, 2392–2402. [CrossRef]
106. Chen, Q.; Wang, W.; Yang, X.; Li, S.; Deng, S.; Wang, H.; Liu, W.; Ni, B.; Song, Z. Characteristics and Clinical Significance of Atopy in Chronic Spontaneous Urticaria: A Cross-Sectional Observational Study. *Int. Arch. Allergy Immunol.* **2024**, 1–6. [CrossRef]
107. Pierrard, G.; Bernier, C.; Du-Thanh, A.; Bara, C.; Soria, A.; Castelain, F.; Boccon-Gibod, I.; Hacard, F.; Delaunay, J.; de Montjoye, L.; et al. Characterization of omalizumab updosing patterns and predictive factors in chronic spontaneous urticaria: A prospective multicentric observational study. *Allergy* **2024**, *79*, 2448–2457. [CrossRef]
108. Kim, M.J.; Kim, B.R.; Kim, S.H.; Chang, Y.S.; Youn, S.W. Clinical Response to Low-dose Omalizumab Treatment in Chronic Spontaneous Urticaria: A Retrospective Study of 179 Patients. *Acta Derm. Venereol.* **2023**, *103*, adv11627. [CrossRef]
109. Di Bona, D.; Nettis, E.; Bilancia, M.; Ridolo, E.; Minenna, E.; Nizi, M.C.; Albanesi, M.; Caiaffa, M.F.; Macchia, L. Duration of chronic spontaneous urticaria remission after omalizumab discontinuation: A long-term observational study. *J. Allergy Clin. Immunol. Pract.* **2021**, *9*, 2482–2485.e2. [CrossRef]
110. Ferrer, M.; Giménez-Arnau, A.; Saldana, D.; Janssens, N.; Balp, M.-M.; Khalil, S.; Risson, V. Predicting Chronic Spontaneous Urticaria Symptom Return After Omalizumab Treatment Discontinuation: Exploratory Analysis. *J. Allergy Clin. Immunol. Pract.* **2018**, *6*, 1191–1197.e5. [CrossRef]
111. Kucharczyk, A.; Marczyk, K.; Kucharczyk, B.; Plisko, R.; Perkowska, I.; Owczarek, W.; Jahnz-Różyk, K. Predicting relapse in chronic spontaneous urticaria: A retrospective cohort study evaluating omalizumab withdrawal regimens. *Allergy* **2024**, *79*, 2554–2557. [CrossRef]
112. Sussman, G.; Hébert, J.; Gulliver, W.; Lynde, C.; Yang, W.H.; Papp, K.; Gooderham, M.; Chambenoit, O.; Khalil, S.; DeTakacsy, F.; et al. Omalizumab Re-Treatment and Step-Up in Patients with Chronic Spontaneous Urticaria: OPTIMA Trial. *J. Allergy Clin. Immunol. Pract.* **2020**, *8*, 2372–2378.e5. [CrossRef] [PubMed]
113. Salman, A.; Aktas, M.; Apti Sengun, O. Remission of chronic spontaneous urticaria following omalizumab with gradually extended dosing intervals: Real-life data. *Australas. J. Dermatol.* **2021**, *62*, 398–402. [CrossRef] [PubMed]
114. Ertas, R.; Ozyurt, K.; Atasoy, M.; Hawro, T.; Maurer, M. The clinical response to omalizumab in chronic spontaneous urticaria patients is linked to and predicted by IgE levels and their change. *Allergy* **2018**, *73*, 705–712. [CrossRef] [PubMed]
115. Fok, J.S.; Kolkhir, P.; Church, M.K.; Maurer, M. Predictors of treatment response in chronic spontaneous urticaria. *Allergy* **2021**, *76*, 2965–2981. [CrossRef]
116. Marzano, A.V.; Genovese, G.; Casazza, G.; Fierro, M.T.; Dapavo, P.; Crimi, N.; Ferrucci, S.; Pepe, P.; Liberati, S.; Pigatto, P.D.; et al. Predictors of response to omalizumab and relapse in chronic spontaneous urticaria: A study of 470 patients. *J. Eur. Acad. Dermatol. Venereol.* **2019**, *33*, 918–924. [CrossRef]
117. Straesser, M.D.; Oliver, E.; Palacios, T.; Kyin, T.; Patrie, J.; Borish, L.; Saini, S.S.; Lawrence, M.G. Serum IgE as an immunological marker to predict response to omalizumab treatment in symptomatic chronic urticaria. *J. Allergy Clin. Immunol. Pract.* **2018**, *6*, 1386–1388.e1. [CrossRef]
118. Weller, K.; Ohanyan, T.; Hawro, T.; Ellrich, A.; Sussman, G.; Koplowitz, J.; Gimenez-Arnau, A.M.; Peveling-Oberhag, A.; Staubach, P.; Metz, M.; et al. Total IgE levels are linked to the response of chronic spontaneous urticaria patients to omalizumab. *Allergy* **2018**, *73*, 2406–2408. [CrossRef]
119. Yu, M.; Terhorst-Molawi, D.; Altrichter, S.; Hawro, T.; Chen, Y.D.; Liu, B.; Song, X.T.; Zhao, Z.T.; Maurer, M. Omalizumab in chronic inducible urticaria: A real-life study of efficacy, safety, predictors of treatment outcome and time to response. *Clin. Exp. Allergy* **2021**, *51*, 730–734. [CrossRef]
120. Maurer, M.; Kolkhir, P.; Moñino-Romero, S.; Metz, M. The Crucial Role of IgE as a Predictor of Treatment Response to Omalizumab in Chronic Spontaneous Urticaria. *J. Allergy Clin. Immunol. Pract.* **2023**, *11*, 2390–2391. [CrossRef]
121. Asero, R. Clinical variables of severe chronic spontaneous urticaria from total IgE standpoint: A retrospective study. *Eur. Ann. Allergy Clin. Immunol.* **2022**, *54*, 30–33. [CrossRef]
122. Caldeira, L.E.; Bernardino, A.; Paulino, M.; Costa, C. Four-week total IgE/baseline total IgE ratio: Biomarker for omalizumab good response in chronic spontaneous urticaria real-life patients. *J. Allergy Clin. Immunol. Pract.* **2023**, *11*, 3808–3811. [CrossRef] [PubMed]

123. Deza, G.; Bertolín-Colilla, M.; Sánchez, S.; Soto, D.; Pujol, R.M.; Gimeno, R.; Giménez-Arnau, A.M. Basophil FcεRI expression is linked to time to omalizumab response in chronic spontaneous urticaria. *J. Allergy Clin. Immunol.* **2018**, *141*, 2313–2316.e1. [CrossRef] [PubMed]
124. Moñino-Romero, S.; Kolkhir, P.; Ohanyan, T.; Szépfalusi, Z.; Weller, K.; Metz, M.; Scheffel, J.; Maurer, M.; Altrichter, S. Elevated baseline soluble FcεRI may be linked to early response to omalizumab treatment in chronic spontaneous urticaria. *J. Eur. Acad. Dermatol. Venereol.* **2024**, *38*, 167–174. [CrossRef]
125. Ji, J.; Tang, M.; Zhao, Y.; Zhang, C.; Shen, Y.; Zhou, B.; Liu, C.; Maurer, M.; Jiao, Q. In chronic spontaneous urticaria, increased Galectin-9 expression on basophils and eosinophils is linked to high disease activity, endotype-specific markers, and response to omalizumab treatment. *Allergy* **2024**, *79*, 2435–2447. [CrossRef]
126. Ghazanfar, M.N.; Bartko, E.A.; Arildsen, N.S.; Poulsen, L.K.; Jensen, B.M.; Enevold, C.; Holm, J.G.; Woetmann, A.; Ødum, N.; Thomsen, S.F. Omalizumab serum levels predict treatment outcomes in patients with chronic spontaneous urticaria: A three-month prospective study. *Clin. Exp. Allergy* **2022**, *52*, 715–718. [CrossRef]
127. Kolkhir, P.; Church, M.K.; Altrichter, S.; Skov, P.S.; Hawro, T.; Frischbutter, S.; Metz, M.; Maurer, M. Eosinopenia, in Chronic Spontaneous Urticaria, Is Associated with High Disease Activity, Autoimmunity, and Poor Response to Treatment. *J. Allergy Clin. Immunol. Pract.* **2020**, *8*, 318–325.e5. [CrossRef]
128. Ertaş, R.; Hawro, T.; Altrichter, S.; Özyurt, K.; Erol, K.; Ertaş, K.; Maurer, M. Antinuclear antibodies are common and linked to poor response to omalizumab treatment in patients with CSU. *Allergy* **2020**, *75*, 468–470. [CrossRef]
129. Palacios, T.; Stillman, L.; Borish, L.; Lawrence, M. Lack of basophil CD203c-upregulating activity as an immunological marker to predict response to treatment with omalizumab in patients with symptomatic chronic urticaria. *J. Allergy Clin. Immunol. Pract.* **2016**, *4*, 529–530. [CrossRef]
130. Maronese, C.A.; Ferrucci, S.M.; Moltrasio, C.; Lorini, M.; Carbonelli, V.; Asero, R.; Marzano, A.V.; Cugno, M. IgG and IgE Autoantibodies to IgE Receptors in Chronic Spontaneous Urticaria and Their Role in the Response to Omalizumab. *J. Clin. Med.* **2023**, *12*, 378. [CrossRef]
131. Cakmak, M.E. Comparison of the Patients with Chronic Urticaria Who Responded and Did Not Respond to Omalizumab Treatment: A Single-Center Retrospective Study. *Int. Arch. Allergy Immunol.* **2022**, *183*, 1209–1215. [CrossRef]
132. Asero, R.; Marzano, A.V.; Cugno, M. Unresponsiveness to Omalizumab in Chronic Spontaneous Urticaria. *Curr. Treat. Options Allergy* **2020**, *7*, 135–141. [CrossRef]
133. Calzari, P.; Chiei Gallo, A.; Barei, F.; Bono, E.; Cugno, M.; Marzano, A.V.; Ferrucci, S.M. Omalizumab for the Treatment of Chronic Spontaneous Urticaria in Adults and Adolescents: An Eight-Year Real-Life Experience. *J. Clin. Med.* **2024**, *13*, 5610. [CrossRef] [PubMed]
134. Lowe, P.J.; Georgiou, P.; Canvin, J. Revision of omalizumab dosing table for dosing every 4 instead of 2 weeks for specific ranges of bodyweight and baseline IgE. *Regul. Toxicol. Pharmacol.* **2015**, *71*, 68–77. [CrossRef] [PubMed]
135. Normansell, R.; Walker, S.; Milan, S.J.; Walters, E.H.; Nair, P. Omalizumab for asthma in adults and children. *Cochrane Database Syst. Rev.* **2014**, *2014*, CD003559. [CrossRef]
136. Tharp, M.D.; Bernstein, J.A.; Kavati, A.; Ortiz, B.; MacDonald, K.; Denhaerynck, K.; Abraham, I.; Lee, C.S. Benefits and Harms of Omalizumab Treatment in Adolescent and Adult Patients with Chronic Idiopathic (Spontaneous) Urticaria: A Meta-analysis of "Real-world" Evidence. *JAMA Dermatol.* **2019**, *155*, 29–38. [CrossRef]
137. Di Bona, D.; Fiorino, I.; Taurino, M.; Frisenda, F.; Minenna, E.; Pasculli, C.; Kourtis, G.; Rucco, A.S.; Nico, A.; Albanesi, M.; et al. Long-term "real-life" safety of omalizumab in patients with severe uncontrolled asthma: A nine-year study. *Respir. Med.* **2017**, *130*, 55–60. [CrossRef]
138. Harrison, R.G.; MacRae, M.; Karsh, J.; Santucci, S.; Yang, W.H. Anaphylaxis and serum sickness in patients receiving omalizumab: Reviewing the data in light of clinical experience. *Ann. Allergy Asthma Immunol.* **2015**, *115*, 77–78. [CrossRef]
139. Gülsen, A.; Wedi, B.; Jappe, U. Hypersensitivity reactions to biologics (part I): Allergy as an important differential diagnosis in complex immune-derived adverse events. *Allergo J. Int.* **2020**, *29*, 32–61. [CrossRef]
140. Li, L.; Wang, Z.; Cui, L.; Xu, Y.; Guan, K.; Zhao, B. Anaphylactic risk related to omalizumab, benralizumab, reslizumab, mepolizumab, and dupilumab. *Clin. Transl. Allergy* **2021**, *11*, e12038. [CrossRef]
141. Casale, T.B.; Gimenez-Arnau, A.M.; Bernstein, J.A.; Holden, M.; Zuberbier, T.; Maurer, M. Omalizumab for Patients with Chronic Spontaneous Urticaria: A Narrative Review of Current Status. *Dermatol. Ther.* **2023**, *13*, 2573–2588. [CrossRef]
142. Soegiharto, R.; Alizadeh Aghdam, M.; Sørensen, J.A.; van Lindonk, E.; Bulut Demir, F.; Porras, N.M.; Matsuo, Y.; Kiefer, L.; Knulst, A.C.; Maurer, M.; et al. Multinational Drug Survival Study of Omalizumab in Patients with Chronic Urticaria and Potential Predictors for Discontinuation. *JAMA Dermatol.* **2024**, *160*, 927–935. [CrossRef] [PubMed]
143. Gasser, P.; Tarchevskaya, S.S.; Guntern, P.; Brigger, D.; Ruppli, R.; Zbären, N.; Kleinboelting, S.; Heusser, C.; Jardetzky, T.S.; Eggel, A. The mechanistic and functional profile of the therapeutic anti-IgE antibody ligelizumab differs from omalizumab. *Nat. Commun.* **2020**, *11*, 165. [CrossRef] [PubMed]
144. Maurer, M.; Ensina, L.F.; Gimenez-Arnau, A.M.; Sussman, G.; Hide, M.; Saini, S.; Grattan, C.; Fomina, D.; Rigopoulos, D.; Berard, F.; et al. Efficacy and safety of ligelizumab in adults and adolescents with chronic spontaneous urticaria: Results of two phase 3 randomised controlled trials. *Lancet* **2024**, *403*, 147–159. [CrossRef] [PubMed]

145. Harris, J.M.; Cabanski, C.R.; Scheerens, H.; Samineni, D.; Bradley, M.S.; Cochran, C.; Staubach, P.; Metz, M.; Sussman, G.; Maurer, M. A randomized trial of quilizumab in adults with refractory chronic spontaneous urticaria. *J. Allergy Clin. Immunol.* **2016**, *138*, 1730–1732. [CrossRef]
146. Lee, J.K.; Simpson, R.S. Dupilumab as a novel therapy for difficult to treat chronic spontaneous urticaria. *J. Allergy Clin. Immunol. Pract.* **2019**, *7*, 1659–1661.e1. [CrossRef]
147. Errichetti, E.; Stinco, G. Recalcitrant chronic urticaria treated with dupilumab: Report of two instances refractory to H1-antihistamines, omalizumab and cyclosporine and brief literature review. *Dermatol. Therapy.* **2021**, *34*, e14821. [CrossRef]
148. Sun, Y.; Lin, S.Y.; Lan, C.E. Dupilumab as a rescue therapy for a chronic urticaria patient who showed secondary failure to omalizumab. *Kaohsiung J. Med. Sci.* **2022**, *38*, 610–611. [CrossRef]
149. Puxkandl, V.; Hoetzenecker, W.; Altrichter, S. Case report: Severe chronic spontaneous urticaria successfully treated with omalizumab and dupilumab. *Allergol. Select.* **2023**, *7*, 17–19. [CrossRef]
150. Sirufo, M.M.; Catalogna, A.; Raggiunti, M.; De Pietro, F.; Ginaldi, L.; De Martinis, M. Cholinergic Urticaria, an Effective and Safe "Off Label" Use of Dupilumab: A Case Report with Literature Review. *Clin. Cosmet. Investig. Dermatol.* **2022**, *15*, 253–260. [CrossRef]
151. Marchal, V.; Reguiai, Z. Efficacity of dupilumab in severe idiopathic cold urticaria: A case report. *J. Dermatol. Treat.* **2023**, *34*, 2182620. [CrossRef]
152. Ferrucci, S.; Benzecry, V.; Berti, E.; Asero, R. Rapid disappearance of both severe atopic dermatitis and cold urticaria following dupilumab treatment. *Clin. Exp. Dermatol.* **2020**, *45*, 345–346. [CrossRef] [PubMed]
153. Zhu, C.; Fok, J.S.; Lin, L.; Su, H.; Maurer, M. Complete response to dupilumab in a patient with chronic spontaneous urticaria who did not tolerate omalizumab. *JAAD Case Rep.* **2022**, *32*, 109–112. [CrossRef] [PubMed]
154. Goodman, B.; Jariwala, S. Dupilumab as a novel therapy to treat adrenergic urticaria. *Ann. Allergy Asthma Immunol.* **2021**, *126*, 205–206. [CrossRef] [PubMed]
155. Holm, J.G.; Sørensen, J.A.; Thomsen, S.F. Concurrent use of omalizumab and dupilumab in a 47-year-old woman with chronic spontaneous urticaria and atopic dermatitis. *Int. J. Dermatol.* **2022**, *61*, e173–e174. [CrossRef]
156. Föhr, J.; Herbst, M.; Jahn, S. Treatment of simultaneously occurring urticaria and atopic dermatitis with dupilumab. *Hautarzt* **2021**, *72*, 249–251. [CrossRef]
157. Valtellini, L.; Barei, F.; Zussino, M.; Marzano, A.V.; Ferrucci, S.M. Dupilumab: A new frontier for chronic urticaria. A case series and review of the literature. *Int. J. Dermatol.* **2024**, *63*, 399–401. [CrossRef]
158. Feldborg, S.E.B.; Thomsen, S.F.; Vestergaard, C. Treatment refractory chronic spontaneous urticaria may benefit from treatment with dupilumab: A case series of eight patients. *J. Eur. Acad. Dermatol. Venereol.* **2024**, *38*, e877–e879. [CrossRef]
159. Altrichter, S.; Frischbutter, S.; Fok, J.S.; Kolkhir, P.; Jiao, Q.; Skov, P.S.; Metz, M.; Church, M.K.; Maurer, M. The role of eosinophils in chronic spontaneous urticaria. *J. Allergy Clin. Immunol.* **2020**, *145*, 1510–1516. [CrossRef]
160. Abadeh, A.; Lee, J.K. Long-term follow-up of patients treated with dupilumab for chronic spontaneous urticaria: A case report. *SAGE Open Med. Case Rep.* **2022**, *10*, 2050313X221117702. [CrossRef]
161. Bernstein, J.A.; Singh, U.; Rao, M.B.; Berendts, K.; Zhang, X.; Mutasim, D. Benralizumab for Chronic Spontaneous Urticaria. *N. Engl. J. Med.* **2020**, *383*, 1389–1391. [CrossRef]
162. Magen, E.; Komarova, I.; Magen, I.; Phirtskhalava, S. Case of benralizumab-induced exacerbations of chronic spontaneous urticaria. *Clin. Case Rep.* **2022**, *10*, e05930. [CrossRef] [PubMed]
163. Menzies-Gow, A.; Corren, J.; Bourdin, A.; Chupp, G.; Israel, E.; Wechsler, M.E.; Brightling, C.E.; Griffiths, J.M.; Hellqvist, Å.; Bowen, K.; et al. Tezepelumab in Adults and Adolescents with Severe, Uncontrolled Asthma. *N. Engl. J. Med.* **2021**, *384*, 1800–1809. [CrossRef] [PubMed]
164. Kay, A.B.; Clark, P.; Maurer, M.; Ying, S. Elevations in T-helper-2-initiating cytokines (interleukin-33, interleukin-25 and thymic stromal lymphopoietin) in lesional skin from chronic spontaneous ('idiopathic') urticaria. *Br. J. Dermatol.* **2015**, *172*, 1294–1302. [CrossRef]
165. Shtessel, M.; Limjunyawong, N.; Oliver, E.T.; Chichester, K.; Gao, L.; Dong, X.; Saini, S.S. MRGPRX2 Activation Causes Increased Skin Reactivity in Patients with Chronic Spontaneous Urticaria. *J. Investig. Dermatol.* **2021**, *141*, 678–681.e2. [CrossRef]
166. McNeil, B.D.; Pundir, P.; Meeker, S.; Han, L.; Undem, B.J.; Kulka, M.; Dong, X. Identification of a mast-cell-specific receptor crucial for pseudo-allergic drug reactions. *Nature* **2015**, *519*, 237–241. [CrossRef]
167. Ogasawara, H.; Noguchi, M. Therapeutic Potential of MRGPRX2 Inhibitors on Mast Cells. *Cells* **2021**, *10*, 2906. [CrossRef]
168. Lerner, L.; Babina, M.; Zuberbier, T.; Stevanovic, K. Beyond Allergies-Updates on The Role of Mas-Related G-Protein-Coupled Receptor X2 in Chronic Urticaria and Atopic Dermatitis. *Cells* **2024**, *13*, 220. [CrossRef]
169. Lao, K.; Mak, H.W.F.; Chiang, V.; Kumar, M.; Chow, B.K.C.; Li, P.H. Mas-Related G-Protein Coupled Receptor-X2 and Chemokine (C-C Motif) Ligand 2 Correlate with Disease Activity Among Treatment-Naïve Chinese Patients with Chronic Spontaneous Urticaria. *Clin. Exp. Allergy* **2024**. *ahead of print*. [CrossRef]
170. Kumar, M.; Duraisamy, K.; Annapureddy, R.R.; Chan, C.B.; Chow, B.K. Novel small molecule MRGPRX2 antagonists inhibit a murine model of allergic reaction. *J. Allergy Clin. Immunol.* **2023**, *151*, 1110–1122. [CrossRef]
171. Wollam, J.; Solomon, M.; Villescaz, C.; Lanier, M.; Evans, S.; Bacon, C.; Freeman, D.; Vasquez, A.; Vest, A.; Napora, J.; et al. Inhibition of mast cell degranulation by novel small molecule MRGPRX2 antagonists. *J. Allergy Clin. Immunol.* **2024**, *154*, 1033–1043. [CrossRef]

172. Ferrer, M.; Nakazawa, K.; Kaplan, A.P. Complement dependence of histamine release in chronic urticaria. *J. Allergy Clin. Immunol.* **1999**, *104*, 169–172. [CrossRef] [PubMed]
173. Kolkhir, P.; Giménez-Arnau, A.M.; Kulthanan, K.; Peter, J.; Metz, M.; Maurer, M. Urticaria. *Nat. Rev. Dis. Primers.* **2022**, *8*, 61. [CrossRef] [PubMed]
174. Altrichter, S.; Staubach, P.; Pasha, M.; Singh, B.; Chang, A.T.; Bernstein, J.A.; Rasmussen, H.S.; Siebenhaar, F.; Maurer, M. An open-label, proof-of-concept study of lirentelimab for antihistamine-resistant chronic spontaneous and inducible urticaria. *J. Allergy Clin. Immunol.* **2022**, *149*, 1683–1690.e7. [CrossRef]
175. Muñoz, M.; Kocatürk, E.; Maurer, M.; Kolkhir, P. Emerging Therapeutics in Chronic Urticaria. *Immunol. Allergy Clin. N. Am.* **2024**, *44*, 517–528. [CrossRef]
176. Valent, P.; Akin, C.; Hartmann, K.; Nilsson, G.; Reiter, A.; Hermine, O.; Sotlar, K.; Sperr, W.R.; Escribano, L.; George, T.I.; et al. Mast cells as a unique hematopoietic lineage and cell system: From Paul Ehrlich's visions to precision medicine concepts. *Theranostics* **2020**, *10*, 10743–10768. [CrossRef]
177. Davis, M.I.; Hunt, J.P.; Herrgard, S.; Ciceri, P.; Wodicka, L.M.; Pallares, G.; Hocker, M.; Treiber, D.K.; Zarrinkar, P.P. Comprehensive analysis of kinase inhibitor selectivity. *Nat. Biotechnol.* **2011**, *29*, 1046–1051. [CrossRef]
178. Alvarado, D.; Maurer, M.; Gedrich, R.; Seibel, S.B.; Murphy, M.B.; Crew, L.; Goldstein, J.; Crocker, A.; Vitale, L.A.; Morani, P.A.; et al. Anti-KIT monoclonal antibody CDX-0159 induces profound and durable mast cell suppression in a healthy volunteer study. *Allergy* **2022**, *77*, 2393–2403. [CrossRef]
179. Grimbaldeston, M.A.; Chen, C.-C.; Piliponsky, A.M.; Tsai, M.; Tam, S.-Y.; Galli, S.J. Mast cell-deficient W-sash c-kit mutant Kit W-sh/W-sh mice as a model for investigating mast cell biology in vivo. *Am. J. Pathol.* **2005**, *167*, 835–848. [CrossRef]
180. Cerny-Reiterer, S.; Rabenhorst, A.; Stefanzl, G.; Herndlhofer, S.; Hoermann, G.; Müllauer, L.; Baumgartner, S.; Beham-Schmid, C.; Sperr, W.R.; Mannhalter, C.; et al. Long-term treatment with imatinib results in profound mast cell deficiency in Ph+ chronic myeloid leukemia. *Oncotarget* **2014**, *6*, 3071–3084. [CrossRef]
181. Hata, D.; Kawakami, Y.; Inagaki, N.; Lantz, C.S.; Kitamura, T.; Khan, W.N.; Maeda-Yamamoto, M.; Miura, T.; Han, W.; Hartman, S.E.; et al. Involvement of Bruton's tyrosine kinase in FcepsilonRI-dependent mast cell degranulation and cytokine production. *J. Exp. Med.* **1998**, *187*, 1235–1247. [CrossRef]
182. Shen, P.; Wang, Y.; Jia, X.; Xu, P.; Qin, L.; Feng, X.; Li, Z.; Qiu, Z. Dual-target Janus kinase (JAK) inhibitors: Comprehensive review on the JAK-based strategies for treating solid or hematological malignancies and immune-related diseases. *Eur. J. Med. Chem.* **2022**, *239*, 114551. [CrossRef] [PubMed]
183. Zarrin, A.A.; Bao, K.; Lupardus, P.; Vucic, D. Kinase inhibition in autoimmunity and inflammation. *Nat. Rev. Drug Discov.* **2021**, *20*, 39–63. [CrossRef] [PubMed]
184. Gu, D.; Tang, H.; Wu, J.; Li, J.; Miao, Y. Targeting Bruton tyrosine kinase using non-covalent inhibitors in B cell malignancies. *J. Hematol. Oncol.* **2021**, *14*, 40. [CrossRef] [PubMed]
185. Estupiñán, H.Y.; Berglöf, A.; Zain, R.; Smith, C.I.E. Comparative Analysis of BTK Inhibitors and Mechanisms Underlying Adverse Effects. *Front. Cell Dev. Biol.* **2021**, *9*, 630942. [CrossRef]
186. Gabizon, R.; London, N. A Fast and Clean BTK Inhibitor. *J. Med. Chem.* **2020**, *63*, 5100–5101. [CrossRef]
187. Metz, M.; Sussman, G.; Gagnon, R.; Staubach, P.; Tanus, T.; Yang, W.H.; Lim, J.J.; Clarke, H.J.; Galanter, J.; Chinn, L.W.; et al. Fenebrutinib in H1 antihistamine-refractory chronic spontaneous urticaria: A randomized phase 2 trial. *Nat. Med.* **2021**, *27*, 1961–1969. [CrossRef]
188. Cohen, S.; Tuckwell, K.; Katsumoto, T.R.; Zhao, R.; Galanter, J.; Lee, C.; Rae, J.; Toth, B.; Ramamoorthi, N.; Hackney, J.A.; et al. Fenebrutinib versus Placebo or Adalimumab in Rheumatoid Arthritis: A Randomized, Double-Blind, Phase II Trial (ANDES Study). *Arthritis Rheumatol.* **2020**, *72*, 1435–1446. [CrossRef]
189. Isenberg, D.; Furie, R.; Jones, N.S.; Guibord, P.; Galanter, J.; Lee, C.; McGregor, A.; Toth, B.; Rae, J.; Hwang, O.; et al. Efficacy, Safety, and Pharmacodynamic Effects of the Bruton's Tyrosine Kinase Inhibitor Fenebrutinib (GDC-0853) in Systemic Lupus Erythematosus: Results of a Phase II, Randomized, Double-Blind, Placebo-Controlled Trial. *Arthritis Rheumatol.* **2021**, *73*, 1835–1846. [CrossRef]
190. Asero, R.; Ferrucci, S.; Tedeschi, A.; Cugno, M. Biologics for chronic spontaneous urticaria: Toward a personalized treatment. *Expert. Rev. Clin. Immunol.* **2022**, *18*, 1297–1305. [CrossRef]
191. Murakami, J.; Senoo, Y.; Tanimoto, T. Rilzabrutinib in Immune Thrombocytopenia. *N. Engl. J. Med.* **2022**, *386*, 2537–2538.
192. Damsky, W.; King, B.A. JAK inhibitors in dermatology: The promise of a new drug class. *J. Am. Acad. Dermatol.* **2017**, *76*, 736–744. [CrossRef] [PubMed]
193. Mansouri, P.; Mozafari, N.; Chalangari, R.; Martits-Chalangari, K. Efficacy of oral tofacitinib in refractory chronic spontaneous urticaria and urticarial vasculitis. *Dermatol. Ther.* **2022**, *35*, e15932. [CrossRef] [PubMed]
194. Fukunaga, A.; Ito, M.; Nishigori, C. Efficacy of Oral Ruxolitinib in a Patient with Refractory Chronic Spontaneous Urticaria. *Acta Derm. Venereol.* **2018**, *98*, 904–905. [CrossRef] [PubMed]
195. Auphan, N.; DiDonato, J.A.; Rosette, C.; Helmberg, A.; Karin, M. Immunosuppression by glucocorticoids: Inhibition of NF-kappa B activity through induction of I kappa B synthesis. *Science* **1995**, *270*, 286–290. [CrossRef]
196. Almawi, W.Y.; Beyhum, H.N.; Rahme, A.A.; Rieder, M.J. Regulation of cytokine and cytokine receptor expression by glucocorticoids. *J. Leukoc. Biol.* **1996**, *60*, 563–572. [CrossRef]
197. Cain, D.W.; Cidlowski, J.A. Immune regulation by glucocorticoids. *Nat. Rev. Immunol.* **2017**, *17*, 233–247. [CrossRef]

198. Brazzini, B.; Pimpinelli, N. New and established topical corticosteroids in dermatology: Clinical pharmacology and therapeutic use. *Am. J. Clin. Dermatol.* **2002**, *3*, 47–58. [CrossRef]
199. Rhen, T.; Cidlowski, J.A. Antiinflammatory action of glucocorticoids—New mechanisms for old drugs. *N. Engl. J. Med.* **2005**, *353*, 1711–1723. [CrossRef]
200. Asero, R.; Tedeschi, A. Usefulness of a short course of oral prednisone in antihistamine-resistant chronic urticaria: A retrospective analysis. *J. Investig. Allergol. Clin. Immunol.* **2010**, *20*, 386–390.
201. Zuberbier, T.; Iffländer, J.; Semmler, C.; Henz, B.M. Acute urticaria: Clinical aspects and therapeutic responsiveness. *Acta Derm. Venereol.* **1996**, *76*, 295–297. [CrossRef]
202. Yen, H.; Yen, H.; Huang, C.H.; Huang, I.H.; Hung, W.K.; Su, H.J.; Tai, C.C.; Haw, W.W.Y.; Flohr, C.; You, Z.Z.N.; et al. Systematic Review and Critical Appraisal of Urticaria Clinical Practice Guidelines: A Global Guidelines in Dermatology Mapping Project (GUIDEMAP). *J. Allergy Clin. Immunol. Pract.* **2023**, *11*, 3213–3220.e11. [CrossRef] [PubMed]
203. Chu, X.; Wang, J.; Ologundudu, L.; Brignardello-Petersen, R.; Guyatt, G.H.; Oykhman, P.; Bernstein, J.A.; Saini, S.S.; Beck, L.A.; Waserman, S.; et al. Efficacy and Safety of Systemic Corticosteroids for Urticaria: A Systematic Review and Meta-Analysis of Randomized Clinical Trials. *J. Allergy Clin. Immunol. Pract.* **2024**, *12*, 1879–1889.e8. [CrossRef] [PubMed]
204. Augey, F.; Guillot-Pouget, I.; Gunera-Saad, N.; Berard, F.; Nicolas, J.F. Impact of corticosteroid withdrawal in chronic urticaria: A prospective study of 17 patients. *Ann. Dermatol. Venereol.* **2008**, *135*, 21–25. [CrossRef] [PubMed]
205. Augey, F.; Nosbaum, A.; Ben-Said, B.; Bérard, F.; Nicolas, J.F. Chronic urticaria and corticodependence: Corticosteroids have no role in the treatment of urticaria. *Ann. Dermatol. Venereol.* **2011**, *138*, 3–4. [CrossRef] [PubMed]
206. Lee, H.; Myoung, H.; Kim, S.M. Review of two immunosuppressants: Tacrolimus and cyclosporine. *J. Korean Assoc. Oral. Maxillofac. Surg.* **2023**, *49*, 311–323. [CrossRef]
207. Grattan, C.E.; O'Donnell, B.F.; Francis, D.M.; Niimi, N.; Barlow, R.J.; Seed, P.T.; Kobza Black, A.; Greaves, M.W. Randomized double-blind study of cyclosporin in chronic "idiopathic" urticaria. *Br. J. Dermatol.* **2000**, *143*, 365–372. [CrossRef]
208. Di Leo, E.; Nettis, E.; Aloia, A.; Moschetta, M.; Carbonara, M.; Dammacco, F.; Vacca, A. Cyclosporin-A efficacy in chronic idiopathic urticaria. *Int. J. Immunopathol. Pharmacol.* **2011**, *24*, 195–200. [CrossRef]
209. Loria, M.P.; Dambra, P.P.; D'Oronzio, L.; Nettis, E.; Pannofino, A.; Cavallo, E.; Ferrannini, A.; Tursi, A. Cyclosporin A in patients affected by chronic idiopathic urticaria: A therapeutic alternative. *Immunopharmacol. Immunotoxicol.* **2001**, *23*, 205–213. [CrossRef]
210. Kulthanan, K.; Chaweekulrat, P.; Komoltri, C.; Hunnangkul, S.; Tuchinda, P.; Chularojanamontri, L.; Maurer, M. Cyclosporine for Chronic Spontaneous Urticaria: A Meta-Analysis and Systematic Review. *J. Allergy Clin. Immunol. Pract.* **2018**, *6*, 586–599. [CrossRef]
211. LaCava, A.F.; Fadugba, O.O. Cyclosporine for omalizumab-refractory chronic urticaria: A report of five cases. *Allergy Asthma Clin. Immunol.* **2023**, *19*, 78. [CrossRef]
212. Mateu-Arrom, L.; Giménez-Arnau, A.M.; Expósito-Serrano, V.; Bonfill-Ortí, M.; Serra-Baldrich, E.; Yélamos, O.; Spertino, J. Cyclosporine for the treatment of chronic spontaneous urticaria refractory to antihistamines and omalizumab: A case series. *Int. J. Dermatol.* **2024**. *ahead of print*. [CrossRef] [PubMed]
213. Vena, G.A.; Cassano, N.; Colombo, D.; Peruzzi, E.; Pigatto, P. Neo-I-30 Study Group. Cyclosporine in chronic idiopathic urticaria: A double-blind, randomized, placebo-controlled trial. *J. Am. Acad. Dermatol.* **2006**, *55*, 705–709. [CrossRef] [PubMed]
214. Tapia, C.; Nessel, T.A.; Zito, P.M. Cyclosporine. In *StatPearls [Internet]*; StatPearls Publishing: Treasure Island, FL, USA, 2024.
215. Kocatürk, E.; Başkan, E.B.; Küçük, Ö.S.; Özdemir, M.; Örnek, S.; Can, P.K.; Haşal, E.; Engin, B.; Atakan, N.; Alpsoy, E. Omalizumab versus cyclosporin-A for the treatment of chronic spontaneous urticaria: Can we define better-responding endotypes? *An. Bras. Dermatol.* **2022**, *97*, 592–600. [CrossRef]
216. Maoz-Segal, R.; Levy, T.; Haj-Yahia, S.; Offengenden, I.; Iancovich-Kidon, M.; Agmon-Levin, N. Combination therapy with omalizumab and an immune-suppressive agent for resistant chronic spontaneous rrticaria—A real-life experience. *World Allergy Organ J.* **2020**, *13*, 100448. [CrossRef] [PubMed]
217. Pizzorno, G.; Diasio, R.B.; Cheng, Y.C. Purine Analogs. In *Holland-Frei Cancer Medicine [Internet]*, 6th ed.; BC Decker: Hamilton, ON, Canada, 2003.
218. Tal, Y.; Toker, O.; Agmon-Levin, N.; Shalit, M. Azathioprine as a therapeutic alternative for refractory chronic urticaria. *Int. J. Dermatol.* **2015**, *54*, 367–369. [CrossRef]
219. Ghoshal, L.; Bhanja, D.C.; Das, S.; Das, S.; Roy, A.K. Azathioprine in autologous serum skin test positive chronic urticaria: A case-control study in a tertiary care hospital of eastern India. *Indian Dermatol. Online J.* **2015**, *6*, 185–188. [CrossRef]
220. Pathania, Y.S.; Bishnoi, A.; Parsad, D.; Kumar, A.; Kumaran, M.S. Comparing azathioprine with cyclosporine in the treatment of antihistamine refractory chronic spontaneous urticaria: A randomized prospective active-controlled non-inferiority study. *World Allergy Organ J.* **2019**, *12*, 100033. [CrossRef]
221. Cronstein, B.N.; Aune, T.M. Methotrexate and its mechanisms of action in inflammatory arthritis. *Nat. Rev. Rheumatol.* **2020**, *16*, 145–154. [CrossRef]
222. Sandhu, J.; Kumar, A.; Gupta, S.K. The therapeutic role of methotrexate in chronic urticaria: A systematic review. *Indian. J. Dermatol. Venereol. Leprol.* **2022**, *88*, 313–321. [CrossRef]
223. Sharma, V.K.; Singh, S.; Ramam, M.; Kumawat, M.; Kumar, R. A randomized placebo-controlled double-blind pilot study of methotrexate in the treatment of H1 antihistamine-resistant chronic spontaneous urticaria. *Indian. J. Dermatol. Venereol. Leprol.* **2014**, *80*, 122–128. [CrossRef]
224. Unsel, M. Safety of Methotrexate in Chronic Urticaria Unresponsive to Omalizumab. *Iran. J. Allergy Asthma Immunol.* **2021**, *20*, 500–504. [CrossRef]

225. Garbayo-Salmons, P.; Butt, S.; Dawe, R.S. Methotrexate combined with omalizumab for difficult to treat urticaria: A further step-up treatment? *Clin. Exp. Dermatol.* **2021**, *46*, 350–351. [CrossRef] [PubMed]
226. Shea, B.; Swinden, M.V.; Ghogomu, E.T.; Ortiz, Z.; Katchamart, W.; Rader, T.; Bombardier, C.; Wells, G.A.; Tugwell, P. Folic acid and folinic acid for reducing side effects in patients receiving methotrexate for rheumatoid arthritis. *J. Rheumatol.* **2014**, *41*, 1049–1060. [CrossRef] [PubMed]
227. Cassano, N.; D'Argento, V.; Filotico, R.; Vena, G.A. Low-dose dapsone in chronic idiopathic urticaria: Preliminary results of an open study. *Acta Derm. Venereol.* **2005**, *85*, 254–255. [CrossRef] [PubMed]
228. Noda, S.; Asano, Y.; Sato, S. Long-term complete resolution of severe chronic idiopathic urticaria after dapsone treatment. *J. Dermatol.* **2012**, *39*, 496–497. [CrossRef]
229. Liang, S.E.; Hoffmann, R.; Peterson, E.; Soter, N.A. Use of Dapsone in the Treatment of Chronic Idiopathic and Autoimmune Urticaria. *JAMA Dermatol.* **2019**, *155*, 90–95. [CrossRef]
230. Engin, B.; Ozdemir, M. Prospective randomized non-blinded clinical trial on the use of dapsone plus antihistamine vs. antihistamine in patients with chronic idiopathic urticaria. *J. Eur. Acad. Dermatol. Venereol.* **2008**, *22*, 481–486. [CrossRef]
231. Morgan, M.; Cooke, A.; Rogers, L.; Adams-Huet, B.; Khan, D.A. Double-blind placebo-controlled trial of dapsone in antihistamine refractory chronic idiopathic urticaria. *J. Allergy Clin. Immunol. Pract.* **2014**, *2*, 601–606. [CrossRef]
232. Kurien, G.; Jamil, R.T.; Preuss, C.V. Dapsone. In *StatPearls [Internet]*; StatPearls Publishing: Treasure Island, FL, USA, 2024.
233. Schrezenmeier, E.; Dörner, T. Mechanisms of action of hydroxychloroquine and chloroquine: Implications for rheumatology. *Nat. Rev. Rheumatol.* **2020**, *16*, 155–166. [CrossRef]
234. Boonpiyathad, T.; Sangasapaviliya, A. Hydroxychloroquine in the treatment of anti-histamine refractory chronic spontaneous urticaria, randomized single-blinded placebo-controlled trial and an open label comparison study. *Eur. Ann. Allergy Clin. Immunol.* **2017**, *49*, 220–224. [CrossRef]
235. Khan, N.; Epstein, T.E.; DuBuske, I.; Strobel, M.; Bernstein, D.I. Effectiveness of Hydroxychloroquine and Omalizumab in Chronic Spontaneous Urticaria: A Real-World Study. *J. Allergy Clin. Immunol. Pract.* **2022**, *10*, 3300–3305. [CrossRef] [PubMed]
236. Allison, A.C. Mechanisms of action of mycophenolate mofetil. *Lupus* **2005**, *14* (Suppl. S1), S2–S8. [CrossRef] [PubMed]
237. Shahar, E.; Bergman, R.; Guttman-Yassky, E.; Pollack, S. Treatment of severe chronic idiopathic urticaria with oral mycophenolate mofetil in patients not responding to antihistamines and/or corticosteroids. *Int. J. Dermatol.* **2006**, *45*, 1224–1227. [CrossRef]
238. Zimmerman, A.B.; Berger, E.M.; Elmariah, S.B.; Soter, N.A. The use of mycophenolate mofetil for the treatment of autoimmune and chronic idiopathic urticaria: Experience in 19 patients. *J. Am. Acad. Dermatol.* **2012**, *66*, 767–770. [CrossRef]
239. Behrend, M. Adverse gastrointestinal effects of mycophenolate mofetil: Aetiology, incidence and management. *Drug Saf.* **2001**, *24*, 645–663. [CrossRef]
240. Steinweg, S.A.; Gaspari, A.A. Rituximab for the Treatment of Recalcitrant Chronic Autoimmune Urticaria. *J. Drugs Dermatol.* **2015**, *14*, 1387.
241. Chakravarty, S.D.; Yee, A.F.; Paget, S.A. Rituximab successfully treats refractory chronic autoimmune urticaria caused by IgE receptor autoantibodies. *J. Allergy Clin. Immunol.* **2011**, *128*, 1354–1355. [CrossRef]
242. Arkwright, P.D. Anti-CD20 or anti-IgE therapy for severe chronic autoimmune urticaria. *J. Allergy Clin. Immunol.* **2009**, *123*, 510–511, author reply 511. [CrossRef]
243. Combalia, A.; Losno, R.A.; Prieto-González, S.; Mascaró, J.M. Rituximab in Refractory Chronic Spontaneous Urticaria: An Encouraging Therapeutic Approach. *Ski. Skin. Pharmacol. Physiol.* **2018**, *31*, 184–187. [CrossRef]
244. Mallipeddi, R.; Grattan, C.E.H. Lack of response of severe steroid-dependent chronic urticaria to rituximab. *Clin. Exp. Dermatol.* **2007**, *32*, 333–334. [CrossRef]
245. Rovesti, M.; Pierobon, E.; Vaschieri, C.; Genovese, G.; Marzano, A.V.; Lotti, T.; Satolli, F.; Feliciani, C. Case of a severe vulgaris and foliaceus pemphigus in a young patient treated with rituximab, with subsequent development of chronic urticaria. *Dermatol. Ther.* **2020**, *33*, e13665. [CrossRef] [PubMed]
246. Asero, R.; Tedeschi, A.; Cugno, M. Heparin and tranexamic Acid therapy may be effective in treatment-resistant chronic urticaria with elevated d-dimer: A pilot study. *Int. Arch. Allergy Immunol.* **2010**, *152*, 384–389. [CrossRef] [PubMed]
247. Dabas, G.; Thakur, V.; Bishnoi, A.; Parsad, D.; Kumar, A.; Kumaran, M.S. Causal Relationship between D-Dimers and Disease Status in Chronic Spontaneous Urticaria and Adjuvant Effect of Oral Tranexamic Acid. *Indian Dermatol. Online J.* **2021**, *12*, 726–730. [CrossRef] [PubMed]
248. Dunn, C.J.; Goa, K.L. Tranexamic acid: A review of its use in surgery and other indications. *Drugs* **1999**, *57*, 1005–1032. [CrossRef]

pharmaceuticals

MDPI

Review

Novel Approaches to Allergen Immunotherapy for Respiratory Allergies

Mongkol Lao-Araya

Division of Allergy and Clinical Immunology, Department of Pediatrics, Faculty of Medicine, Chiang Mai University, Chiang Mai 50200, Thailand; laoaraya@gmail.com

Abstract: Allergen immunotherapy (AIT) remains the cornerstone for managing respiratory allergies, offering long-term symptom relief, disease modification, and prevention of disease progression. While novel approaches like intralymphatic and epicutaneous immunotherapy and the combination of allergens with adjuvants show promise, traditional methods remain effective and safe. Hypoallergenic T-cell peptide vaccines and recombinant allergens require further research to confirm their clinical benefits. Passive immunotherapy, while demonstrating effectiveness in specific cases, needs exploration of its long-term efficacy and broader applicability. Combining AIT with biologics may enhance safety and treatment outcomes. Despite emerging innovations, allergen-specific immunotherapy with natural allergen extracts remains the primary disease-modifying treatment, offering long-term symptom relief and prevention of disease progression. Continued research is essential to refine and optimize allergen immunotherapy strategies, providing patients with more effective and personalized treatment options.

Keywords: allergy; allergen immunotherapy; allergic rhinitis; modified allergen; biologics; adjuvant

1. Introduction

Allergen immunotherapy (AIT), a therapeutic approach rooted in the concept of immunization, has evolved significantly since its inception. Its origins can be traced back to Edward Jenner's pioneering smallpox vaccine in 1796, demonstrating the therapeutic potential of inducing immunity. The modern understanding of allergic disease emerged in the late 19th century with Blackley's observations linking pollen exposure to hay fever symptoms [1,2]. The therapeutic application of AIT for hay fever was first introduced by Noon and Freeman in 1911, marking the beginning of a century-long journey of research and development [3]. While early studies laid the groundwork, rigorous clinical trials with well-characterized allergen extracts did not emerge until the 1980s, establishing the dose-dependent therapeutic effect of AIT [2,4–7].

Over the past century, AIT has undergone significant advancements. Despite its initial discovery over 110 years ago, AIT remains the standard therapy for allergic rhinitis (AR) and asthma [1,2]. Its proven efficacy in reducing symptoms and improving quality of life has earned the recommendation of numerous medical organizations [8–10]. AIT offers a unique disease-modifying approach, inducing long-term allergen tolerance and reducing allergic inflammation [11]. This is achieved by administering increasing doses of allergens via subcutaneous (SCIT) or sublingual (SLIT) routes.

While AIT offers substantial benefits, traditional treatment regimens can be lengthy and associated with adverse reactions. The need for prolonged administration, often spanning three years or more, can deter patients. Additionally, the risk of adverse reactions, particularly during dose escalation, can lead to treatment discontinuation [12]. Furthermore, AIT's effectiveness varies across different allergens and patient populations [13].

To address these limitations, ongoing research focuses on optimizing AIT delivery methods, treatment procedures, and patient adherence, particularly in pediatric populations. Novel approaches, such as allergen component therapy, hypoallergenic immunotherapy, new delivery routes, and the combination of allergens with adjuvants or biologics, hold promise in enhancing the efficacy and safety of AIT [2,14–18]. These innovations are expanding the therapeutic landscape for AIT, offering hope for individuals with respiratory allergies (Figure 1).

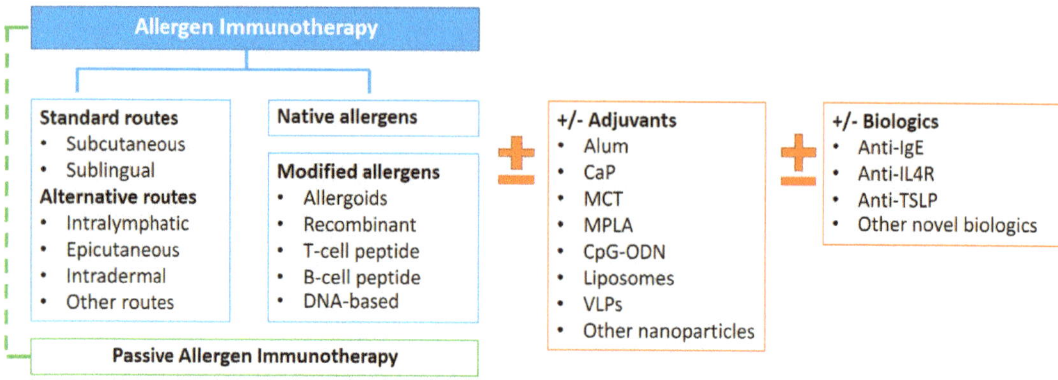

Figure 1. Approaches of allergen immunotherapy for respiratory allergies.

This review will explore the latest advancements in AIT, encompassing improvements in allergen extracts, delivery methods, and treatment strategies. By highlighting these innovations, we aim to provide insights into the future of AIT and its potential to enhance the lives of individuals with respiratory allergies.

2. Mechanisms of AIT (Table 1)

The allergic response is a multifaceted process involving the interaction of various immune cells, mediators, and cytokines. It begins when antigen-presenting cells (APCs), such as dendritic cells (DCs), recognize an allergen. These APCs, activated by epithelial-derived cytokines and those from type 2 innate lymphoid cells (ILC2) [19] and basophils, present the allergen to naive T cells, guiding their differentiation into T-helper 2 (TH2) cells. TH2 and follicular T-helper (Tfh) cells play a pivotal role in driving the allergic response by producing IL-4 and IL-13. These cytokines promote IgE production by B cells, enhancing the allergic inflammatory environment. In individuals with allergies, repeated exposure to low-dose allergens through a compromised epithelial barrier can lead to increased sIgE levels and subsequent allergic reactions [20–22].

While research on AIT mechanisms has primarily focused on aeroallergens, studies suggest that high-dose allergen exposure can play a pivotal role in restoring the epithelial barrier and inducing a shift from allergic TH2 inflammation to a more tolerant TH1 response [23]. This shift involves the generation of suppressive regulatory immune cells and a decrease in pro-allergic cytokines (IL-4, IL-5, IL-9, and IL-13). The reduction in allergic inflammation is accompanied by a decrease in mast cells, basophils, and eosinophils, key cells involved in allergic reactions. Additionally, there is an increase in allergen-specific T regulatory (Treg) cells [24,25], T follicular regulatory (Tfr) cells [26], and B regulatory (Breg) cells, which can help suppress the allergic immune response [22,23].

Furthermore, AIT is effective in inducing dendritic cell-derived regulatory cells (DCregs) [27] and innate lymphoid cell-derived regulatory cells (ILCregs) [28–30]. These regulatory cells produce cytokines like TGF-β, IL-12, IL-27, and IL-10, which can suppress allergic responses [24,31]. AIT is also associated with the generation of Treg cell subsets, which can further suppress TH2 and Tfh-cell responses, leading to a shift towards TH1 cells [32].

Initial immunotherapy may lead to a temporary increase in sIgE levels. However, over time, the immune response shifts towards a tolerogenic state. Breg cells, stimulated by cytokines like IL-10 and IL-35, play a crucial role in this process. These cells promote the production of blocking antibodies, including IgG1, IgG4, IgA1, and IgA2, which can bind to allergens and prevent them from triggering allergic responses [33]. These blocking antibodies are found both in the bloodstream and in mucosal secretions. For SCIT, IgG4 is the primary blocking antibody, while for SLIT, IgA1 and IgA2 are more prominent in both nasal and systemic compartments [23,34–36].

In summary, the mechanisms of immunotherapy involve a complex interplay of innate and adaptive immune cells, cytokines, and antibodies, ultimately leading to a shift towards a more tolerant immune response and reduced allergic symptoms [23,37].

Table 1. A summary of the main mechanisms and proven clinical benefits of allergen immunotherapy.

Mechanism of AIT
• Restoration of epithelial cell integrity • Decrease in allergen-dependent mast cell/basophil degranulation • Reduction in type 2 immune responses • Regulation of T-cell responses: suppression of TH2 and immune deviation toward a TH1 response, reduction of circulating Tfh cells • Modulation of ILCs: reduction of circulating ILC2s, induction of IL-10+ regulatory ILC2s • Induction of regulatory response: induction of Treg and Breg cells • Stimulation of allergen-specific blocking antibody production, including IgG1, IgG2, IgG4, and IgA, in both systemic and mucosal immune responses • Induction of tolerogenic cytokines: IL-10, IL-12, IL-27, IL-35 and TGF-β
Proven clinical benefits of AIT in allergic rhinoconjunctivitis +/− asthma
• Reduced symptoms and medication use • Improved quality of life • The benefits can last for many years, even after treatment is stopped. • Reduced risk of developing asthma in children with AR • Prevent subsequent allergic sensitization

3. Conventional AIT: SCIT and SLIT

SCIT and SLIT have been used as standard treatments for respiratory allergies for decades [10]. SCIT involves administering allergen extracts in gradually increasing doses over several weeks or months, followed by a maintenance phase of monthly injections for 3 to 5 years. While SCIT is generally safe, it carries a risk of systemic allergic reactions (up to 22%), including anaphylaxis [8,10,38–40]. However, the risk can be minimized with appropriate patient selection, adequate facilities, well-trained staff, and availability of emergency treatment [8,10]. The efficacy of SCIT varies depending on the allergen and the specific product used. Meta-analyses have demonstrated that SCIT is approximately 30% more effective than placebo in treating seasonal and perennial allergic rhinitis, [41] exceeding the World Allergy Organization's defined minimally clinically important difference of 20% [42].

While SCIT has been shown to be as effective as or more effective than pharmacotherapy in extrapolated pooled analyses, there are few direct comparisons between the two [43,44]. In practice, adherence and persistence with SCIT can be challenging, with studies showing that less than 50% of users completed the recommended 3 years of treatment [12,45].

In recent years, SLIT has emerged as a well-validated alternative to SCIT. Several large randomized controlled trials have confirmed the efficacy of SLIT tablets for patients with house dust mite (HDM), [46–48] grass pollen, [49] ragweed, [50] and Japanese cedar [51,52] pollen allergic rhinitis, including those with mild to moderately severe controlled HDM-induced allergic asthma [53,54].

SLIT involves taking tablets or drops sublingually daily for 3 years or starting 2 to 4 months before the allergy season in patients with seasonal AR [55]. After initial supervision and a 30-min observation period, SLIT can be self-administered, making it convenient for patients. Home administration and scheduled follow-up visits contribute to improved adherence with SLIT. Compared to SCIT, SLIT is generally safer. While SLIT is associated with local side effects like oropharyngeal itching and swelling, these are typically self-limiting and resolve within 1 to 2 weeks. Systemic side effects are rare, making SLIT a safer alternative to SCIT [38,56,57].

Both SCIT and SLIT have been shown to be effective for both seasonal and perennial allergies [41]. Indirect meta-analyses suggest that SLIT is at least as effective as current pharmacotherapy, although head-to-head controlled studies are needed for definitive confirmation [44,58]. A recent direct comparison using nasal allergen challenge found that SCIT was more effective than SLIT in the first year of treatment. However, the two treatments were equally effective in the second year [36]. Due to the heterogeneity between studies, treatment decisions should be based on the evidence available for specific products and individual patient factors [57,59,60].

4. Alternative Routes (Table 2)

4.1. Intralymphatic Immunotherapy

Intralymphatic immunotherapy (ILIT) is a targeted immunotherapy approach that involves injecting allergen extracts directly into lymph nodes, usually in the groin, under ultrasound guidance [61]. An ILIT injection of recombinant allergens (phospholipase A2 and Fel d 1) has demonstrated a significant increase in IgG levels compared to SCIT, achieving a 10-fold increase in just two weeks at a 100-fold lower dose [62,63]. This direct approach targets the immune system, potentially enhancing allergen presentation to T cells and avoiding direct mast cell activation [18,64].

A randomized open-label trial compared a 3-dose ILIT regimen administered over 2 months to a 3-year SCIT regimen in patients with grass pollen allergy, finding that ILIT achieved a persistent effect over 3 years with fewer side effects and significantly improved compliance [61]. While ILIT resulted in slightly less medication use and similar symptom score improvements, the low compliance rate in the SCIT group and the open-label nature of the study make it challenging to draw definitive conclusions.

Several studies have shown the efficacy of ILIT for grass and tree pollen allergy, although not all studies have confirmed its effectiveness [61,65,66]. A small-scale study showed that three intralymphatic injections of a recombinant cat Fel d 1 allergen, fused with a translocation sequence and a human invariant chain fragment, were effective in protecting against nasal challenge with whole cat allergen extract [62].

Overall, ILIT offers potential advantages in terms of reduced side effects, improved compliance, and shorter treatment duration [61,67]. However, it requires specialist skills, experience, and ultrasound guidance for injections, making it more technically demanding than traditional routes. Individual products, doses, and timing of injections still need to be optimized [64]. Further research is needed to confirm its efficacy and safety for various allergens and patient populations.

Table 2. Routes of allergen immunotherapy administration.

Routes of AIT	Advantages	Drawbacks
Subcutaneous (SCIT)	• Proven efficacy and safety • Standard applications in respiratory and venom AIT	• Repeated injections • Healthcare unit dependency • Long duration of treatment • Risk of severe hypersensitivity reactions

Table 2. *Cont.*

Routes of AIT	Advantages	Drawbacks
Sublingual (SLIT)	• Proven efficacy and safety • Standard applications in respiratory AIT • No injections • Less healthcare unit dependency • Home application • Lower risk of severe hypersensitivity reactions	• Need for daily self-applications which may affect the adherence • Higher allergen dose
Intralymphatic (ILIT)	• Applicability in respiratory and venom allergens • Reduced number of injections • Reduced treatment duration • Reduced allergen dosage use • Early clinical studies revealed promising results	• Requirement of experienced HCP for injections under ultrasound guidance • Risk for side effects due to allergens injected into lymph nodes • Further clinical study needed
Epicutaneous (EPIT)	• Applicability in food and respiratory allergens • Good safety profile • Early clinical studies revealed promising results	• Risk of local adverse reactions • Further clinical study needed
Intradermal (IDIT)	• May reduce allergen dosage use	• No clinical efficacy proven

4.2. Epicutaneous Immunotherapy

Epicutaneous immunotherapy (EPIT) involves applying allergen patches to the skin for several hours, aiming to increase local antigen presentation while preventing systemic allergen absorption. By removing the top layer of skin with adhesive tape, keratinocytes can be activated, increasing allergen exposure and potentially stimulating DC responses. This needle-free approach can improve patient compliance, especially in children [68,69].

A placebo-controlled randomized trial applied grass pollen extract in petroleum to the skin, stripped with adhesive tape, weekly for 6 months pre-seasonally in 48 participants. The study observed a 48% improvement in seasonal symptom scores in the first year compared to a 10% improvement in the placebo group. However, there were no significant differences in combined treatment and medication scores. Two further randomized controlled trials achieved similar results [70]. While higher doses were effective, they also led to high rates of local irritation, eczema, and occasional systemic allergic side effects, limiting their clinical utility compared to currently available SCIT [17,71].

A placebo-controlled randomized trial applied grass pollen extract to the skin, prepared with adhesive tape, weekly for 6 months pre-seasonally in 48 participants. The study observed a significant improvement in seasonal symptom scores in the treatment group compared to the placebo group [70]. However, while higher doses were effective, they also led to increased local skin reactions and systemic side effects, limiting their clinical utility. Two further randomized controlled trials yielded similar results. While EPIT has shown promise, its efficacy and safety profile still need to be optimized to compete with established SCIT [17,71].

4.3. Intradermal Immunotherapy

Intradermal allergen administration may increase the immune response and decrease the required allergen dose due to the presence of DCs in the intradermal area [17,71]. Early studies suggested that repeated low-dose intradermal injections could suppress late allergic responses and induce allergen-specific IgG antibodies [17,72]. However, a phase 2b trial of pre-seasonal low-dose intradermal grass pollen allergen failed to demonstrate significant clinical improvement. In fact, nasal symptoms worsened, and a heightened TH2 response was observed at the injection site [73]. These findings suggest that intradermal allergen administration may have paradoxical effects, potentially inducing both sensitization and tolerance. Therefore, this approach is not currently recommended for allergen immunotherapy.

5. Adjuvants (Table 3)

An adjuvant is a substance that enhances the immune response to a vaccine. By physically or chemically interacting with antigens, adjuvants can modify the pharmacological and immunological effects of allergen vaccines. They can modulate allergen delivery, act as a depot, stimulate immune responses, and steer the immune response towards either tolerance or a TH1-biased response. Additionally, adjuvants can help reduce the risk of anaphylactic reactions and unwanted side effects [14,17,18,74].

Traditionally, adjuvants have been classified into first-generation (aluminum hydroxide, microcrystalline tyrosine [MCT], and calcium phosphate) and second-generation (Monophosphoryl Lipid A [MPLA], Toll-like receptor [TLR] agonists) categories. Other promising adjuvants include liposomes and virus-like particles (VLP) [14]. The adjuvants currently approved for use in humans (aluminum hydroxide, calcium phosphate, MCT, and MPLA) [18] offer several advantages for improving AIT. These include prolonging antigen exposure at the injection site and stimulating the production of allergen-specific IgG antibodies.

Table 3. Adjuvants in allergen immunotherapy.

Adjuvants	Approved for Clinical Use [18]	Mechanism of Action
Aluminum hydroxide (alum)	EU (1937)	• Allergen depot • Inhibits TH2 and enhances TH1 responses • Low biodegradability, may lead to adverse reactions
Calcium Phosphate (CaP)	EU (1980)	• Allergen depot • Natural component • High biodegradability
Microcrystalline tyrosine (MCT)	EU (1970)	• Biodegradable depot adjuvant • Inhibits TH2 and enhances TH1 responses
Monophosphoryl Lipid A (MPLA)	EU (1999)	• TLR-4 agonist • Stimulates TH1 response • Works synergistically with MCT
CpG-Oligodesoxy-nucleotides	No	• TLR-9 agonist • Stimulates TH1 response • Combined in VLP as 'allergen-independent TH1 simulant' • Conflicting results in Phase 3 clinical trial
Nanoparticles: lipophilic liposomes, virus-like particles (VLPs) and other particles from synthetic and natural polymers	No	• Encapsulation of allergen • Allowing uptake into APCs without IgE binding • Activation of innate immunity without T cell help • Limited data in clinical trials

5.1. Alum and Calcium Phosphate

Aluminum salts (alum) have been used as a vaccine adjuvant since 1926 [75] and remain one of the most widely used adjuvants in human vaccines [74]. While alum-based allergen extracts are licensed for SCIT in Europe, they are not approved for use in the United States. Alum functions by adsorbing the allergen and triggering both innate and adaptive immune responses, including inflammasome activation and T-cell activation, which can enhance antibody responses. Although alum can increase TH2 responses in mouse models during sensitization, in humans, it has been shown to inhibit established allergic TH2 responses and promote TH1 responses, both in vitro and in vivo [14,74].

Alum-based allergy extracts have a long history of safe and effective use in Europe. While alum is well-tolerated, it can induce acute and chronic inflammation at the injection site due to its low biodegradability. Although there is a theoretical risk of aluminum accumulation and systemic side effects, this has not been observed in humans [74,76].

Calcium phosphate, a natural component of the body, is another depot adjuvant with better biodegradability and biocompatibility than alum [14]. Although calcium phosphate-adjuvanted AIT products were once available in the European market, they are no longer available for reasons that remain unclear [74].

5.2. Microcrystalline Tyrosine (MCT)

MCT, the crystalline form of the non-essential amino acid L-tyrosine, is a promising adjuvant for AIT [14,74]. While less commonly used than alum, MCT has demonstrated safety and efficacy in humans. It is a biodegradable depot adjuvant with a short half-life of 48 h. Since its initial report in the 1980s, MCT has been shown to enhance the induction of IgG antibodies when used with allergenic molecules. Unlike aluminum, which can accumulate at injection sites in murine models of AIT and is associated with granuloma formation, MCT is rapidly released and metabolized, reducing the risk of long-term accumulation [77,78].

MCT, a non-toxic adjuvant except in individuals with tyrosine metabolism disorders, [14] is currently patented for immunotherapy. It is integrated into glutaraldehyde allergoids to alleviate allergic symptoms and reduce reliance on relief medications [79].

5.3. Toll-like Receptors (TLRs)

Toll-like receptors (TLRs), a class of pattern-recognition receptors, are primarily expressed on APCs. Upon recognition of specific pathogen-associated molecular patterns (PAMPs), they initiate both innate and adaptive immune responses [14,17,74].

Monophosphoryl lipid A (MPL), a TLR4 agonist derived from the lipopolysaccharide of *Salmonella minnesota*, stimulates the production of IFN-γ and IL-12 but does not promote IL-5 synthesis [74]. MPL has shown promise as an adjuvant for AIT. In a study of grass pollen allergy, pre-seasonal injections with MPL-containing allergoids led to a significant reduction in symptoms compared to placebo, with effects lasting up to 5 years after discontinuation [80,81].

MCT-adjuvanted allergen vaccines, which may include native or modified (allergoid) allergens, are often combined with MPL, as exemplified by Pollinex®Quattro, an allergen therapeutic available for the treatment of seasonal allergic rhinoconjunctivitis. Combining allergens with MPL and MCT may address some of the major drawbacks of traditional AIT, including long treatment durations, poor patient adherence, and adverse effects [82–85]. While Pollinex®Quattro is currently available in Germany, sufficient clinical human data supporting marketing authorization in other European states have not been reported [74].

Cytosine-phosphodiester-guanine (CpG) motifs, conserved PAMPs-bacterial DNA sequences, are recognized by TLR-9, a receptor primarily expressed on B cells and plasmacytoid dendritic cells (pDCs). Activation of TLR-9 stimulates the innate immune response in a TH1-type fashion [18,74]. A phase 2 trial demonstrated that combining CpG motifs with the ragweed allergen Amb a 1 suppressed seasonal symptoms in ragweed allergy patients [86]. However, these results were not replicated in a larger phase 3 trial [17]. While TLR-9 agonists show potential as adjuvants for AIT, additional research is needed to fully elucidate the mechanisms of action of these adjuvants and optimize their clinical application.

5.4. Liposomes and Virus-like Particles (VLPs)

Polymeric biodegradable nanoparticles, including polyesters, polysaccharides, polyamides, liposomes, and virus-like particles (VLPs), offer promising strategies for encapsulating allergens or proteins and delivering them to APCs without IgE binding. While many of these delivery systems are still under development, they have shown potential for inducing TH1-biased immune responses in preclinical studies [14,17,74].

Liposomes, spherical or vesicular structures composed of lipids, can effectively package and deliver water-soluble antigens to target cells. Studies have demonstrated that liposome-encapsulated allergens can induce higher levels of allergen-specific IgG while reducing IgE production in mice [87]. Liposomes may also enhance lymph node allergen delivery, potentially improving the efficacy of AIT [64].

VLPs, derived from viral capsids, can activate the immune system through innate pathways, bypassing the need for T-cell help. VLPs are efficiently taken up by APCs, resulting in the activation of cytotoxic T cells and the complement system. VLPs can be used in various ways for AIT, including as standalone VLPs with or without embedded adjuvants, as solutions mixed with allergens, or with allergens encapsulated within the VLPs. These different approaches offer flexibility in designing AIT regimens and may have varying effects on the immune response. Conjugating allergens with VLPs can enhance their uptake into the lymphatic system, potentially minimizing the risk of mast cell degranulation [2,16,74].

VLPs have demonstrated promising results in preclinical studies. A phase 2 trial involving patients with HDM allergy found that combining VLPs with a cytosine-phosphodiester-guanine TLR-9 agonist (CβG10) and allergen encapsulation (CYT003) resulted in similar symptom improvements compared to the adjuvant alone [88,89]. Encouraged by these findings, larger placebo-controlled trials were conducted. A double-blind, randomized trial involving 299 HDM allergy patients found that QβG10, a VLP-based therapy administered without additional allergen, reduced symptom scores in a dose-dependent manner [90]. Additionally, a higher dose of QβG10 was associated with a greater number of patients achieving increased allergen tolerance [90]. These results suggest that VLP-based therapies, even without the addition of allergens, may have therapeutic benefits in allergic diseases [16,74].

However, subsequent trials yielded mixed results. A study in asthmatic patients undergoing steroid withdrawal found that QβG10 reduced asthma-related symptom scores and increased the number of patients with well-controlled asthma [88]. However, a larger phase IIb trial in patients with persistent moderate-to-severe allergic asthma did not demonstrate significant differences between QβG10 and placebo [91].

Nanoparticle-based delivery systems offer potential advantages for AIT by improving allergen delivery, modulating immune responses, and potentially reducing side effects. However, further research is necessary to evaluate their safety and efficacy in clinical trials.

6. Modified Allergens (Table 4)

Modifying allergens to alter their tertiary protein structure or target non-IgE-reactive epitopes can help preserve or enhance their ability to induce immune responses while minimizing allergic reactions, promoting tolerogenic outcomes.

Table 4. Modified allergens and novel approaches in allergen immunotherapy.

Modified Allergens	Advantages	Drawbacks
• Allergoids	Reduced allergenicity, improved safety profiles, shorter up-dosing phase	Limited efficacy data compared to conventional allergen extracts
• Recombinant allergens	Personalized AIT, almost unlimited supply, may improve safety and efficacy	Limited efficacy and safety advantages compared to conventional extracts, reported late-phase adverse allergic reactions
• T-cell peptides	Retained T-cell epitope stimulation, reduced IgE binding, may improve safety and efficacy	Potential for late-phase adverse responses, similar side effects to SCIT, failure to demonstrate clinical efficacy in phase 3 trials
• B-cell peptides	Induce protective humoral antibody responses without stimulating IgE production, demonstrated increases in blocking IgG1 and IgG4 antibodies in phase 2 trial	Limited clinical data, did not reach statistical significance in primary analysis of combined seasonal symptom medication scores

Table 4. *Cont.*

Modified Allergens	Advantages	Drawbacks
• DNA-based vaccine	Induce TH1 and Treg cell responses while downregulating TH2 cell responses in preclinical studies	Concern of theoretical risks of plasmid DNA integration into the human genome and development of anti-DNA antibodies, failure to demonstrate clinical efficacy in phase 3 trials
Passive immunotherapy (monoclonal antibodies)	Protection against nasal allergen challenge for almost 3 months after 1 dose injection	No long-term clinical efficacy shown
AIT combined with biologics	Enhanced efficacy and safety, potential for long-term allergen tolerance	High cost, further research needed to evaluate long-term benefits

6.1. Allergoids

Allergoids are chemically modified allergens produced through polymerization with glutaraldehyde or formaldehyde or monomerization with carbamylation. These modifications aim to alter the tertiary protein structure, reducing the ability of allergens to cross-link IgE while preserving shorter linear T-cell epitopes, thereby retaining immunogenicity. This approach allows for higher doses to be administered during a shorter-term accumulation phase, potentially improving treatment efficiency and reducing the risk of side effects [14,18,92].

Several allergoids have demonstrated efficacy in placebo-controlled trials for various allergens, including ragweed [92,93], grass [94–96], tree pollen [97–99], and mite [100–104] allergy. A phase 3 trial of a formaldehyde-treated, alum-adsorbed 6-grass pollen mix showed a significant 26.6% reduction in combined seasonal symptom medication scores after one year compared to placebo. Although some participants experienced mild to moderate late systemic reactions, no serious adverse events, such as anaphylaxis, were reported [105].

Carbamylation, a chemical modification of the lysine groups, has been used to develop low molecular weight allergoids that can be easily absorbed by the mucosa. A sublingual allergoid produced using this method reduced the need for antihistamines during the pollination season and maintained its clinical benefits for at least two years [106,107]. Another example is the HDM-monomeric allergoid SLIT, which has shown promise in improving rhinitis severity and reducing drug intake in phase II research [102,104]. These findings suggest that allergoids may offer a viable treatment option for respiratory allergies, with potential advantages over traditional allergen extracts.

Head-to-head comparisons between allergoids and conventional allergen extracts are limited, making it difficult to directly assess their relative efficacy. Quantification of modified allergens can be complex, leading to batch-to-batch variation and hindering comparisons of hypoallergenic effects between allergoids and whole allergens, both in vitro and in vivo [17,108].

6.2. Recombinant Allergens

Molecular diagnostics and therapeutics have significantly advanced the field of allergy medicine, enabling the identification of individual allergic components. This has paved the way for more precise allergy diagnosis and treatment, including the potential for personalized "tailor-made" allergen immunotherapy [109–111].

Molecular diagnosis also helps assess the clinical relevance of allergen sensitization profiles, particularly in cases of cross-reactivity between pollens and certain foods or different pollen types. By differentiating between true significant sensitization and pan-allergen sensitization, clinicians can select the most appropriate allergens for inclusion in immunotherapy, optimizing treatment outcomes for patients with complex sensitization profiles [109–111].

The potential of recombinant allergens to improve the safety and efficacy of AIT has been explored. The first cloning of allergen cDNAs was attempted in the late 1980s, and the first clinical trial using recombinant hypoallergens was conducted in the early 2000s [16,112,113].

A phase 2 trial showed that a mixture of six-grass pollen recombinant allergens was effective in treating seasonal allergic rhinitis. This treatment was associated with increases in allergen-specific IgG but not specific IgE, unlike whole allergen extract immunotherapy [114]. A phase 3 randomized controlled trial of recombinant birch allergen Bet v 1 demonstrated a 50% improvement in medication and symptom scores in patients with seasonal allergic rhinitis. While effective, it did not show significant differences in efficacy or side effects compared to natural protein or whole Bet v 1 extract [115].

Recombinant allergens offer several advantages, including standardization, genetic modification to deliver specific IgE-binding and T-cell epitopes, and an almost unlimited supply of purified allergen [14,16]. However, there are also potential disadvantages. One limitation of recombinant proteins is that they expose patients to only one or a few allergen molecules, unlike natural extracts that contain multiple allergens. While targeting a single allergen component may be effective for some patients, those sensitized to multiple components may benefit less from this approach. Additionally, recombinant allergens were initially thought to be safer due to their potential to stimulate only T or B cells, avoiding mast cell activation and related adverse events. However, clinical trials have reported adverse allergic reactions, including anaphylaxis, even hours after administration [16,112].

Despite showing promise in phase 2 trials, recombinant vaccines and hypoallergenic variants have not yet demonstrated significant improvements in efficacy or safety compared to current standardized allergen extracts. Further research is necessary to fully assess their potential benefits and address their limitations. With increasing knowledge of individual sensitization profiles and the role of major allergen epitopes, recombinant approaches may become more significant in the future of AIT [16].

6.3. T-Cell Peptides

T-cell epitopes are short, linear sequences of amino acids recognized by T-cell receptors. Unlike whole allergens, which can trigger IgE-mediated allergic reactions, T-cell epitopes do not induce IgE-mediated responses. When presented without co-stimulation, peptides can induce T-cell unresponsiveness (anergy) to the whole allergen. Additionally, peptides may induce tolerance by eliminating pathogenic allergen-specific T cells or altering the dominant T-cell phenotype towards Treg cells [116–118].

While peptide-based vaccines may have limited impact on humoral antibody responses compared to whole allergen immunotherapy, they offer potential advantages in terms of safety and the ability to modulate T-cell responses. However, it is important to note that while minimizing the risk of IgE-mediated anaphylaxis, peptide-based therapies may still induce T-cell-dependent late-phase asthmatic responses [118].

Several phase 2 studies have evaluated the efficacy of T-cell peptide immunotherapy. Initial studies on T-cell peptide immunotherapy showed promise, with a clinical trial demonstrating reduced rhinoconjunctivitis symptoms in cat-allergic patients treated with a mixture of seven Fel d 1 peptides [119]. However, larger phase 3 field trials involving Fel d 1-derived T-cell peptides (ClinicalTrials.gov, NCT01620762) failed to demonstrate efficacy, leading to the discontinuation of further development for these peptides. These setbacks may be attributed to factors such as a high placebo response in the control group and the inclusion of cat owners who might already have some degree of tolerance due to ongoing exposure to the allergen [2].

Contiguous overlapping peptides are longer sequences of amino acids that encompass a broader range of T-cell epitopes while disrupting IgE epitopes. This approach aims to target T-cell responses without triggering allergic reactions. A phase 2b dose-finding study of birch pollen contiguous overlapping peptides demonstrated a modest but statistically significant treatment effect (7%) over placebo at the highest dose [120,121].

Hydrolyzing whole allergens into medium-chain length peptides can reduce their allergenicity while preserving their ability to induce T- and B-cell responses. This approach may offer a broader range of epitopes compared to synthetic allergen sources [118].

A large clinical trial found that hydrolyzed rye grass allergen peptides administered in a short-term pre-seasonal regimen resulted in a significant reduction in allergy symptoms compared to placebo. The side effects associated with this approach were similar to those observed with conventional SCIT, suggesting that the primary benefit lies in the shortened treatment course [122,123].

6.4. B-Cell Peptides

B-cell peptide immunotherapy aims to induce protective humoral antibody responses without stimulating IgE production. One approach involves developing non-IgE-reactive peptides and conjugating them with a carrier protein unrelated to the allergen. This strategy exploits alternative T-helper responses, facilitated by the carrier protein, to induce protective allergen-specific IgG responses while preventing IgE stimulation [17,124].

A placebo-controlled field study involving 181 participants evaluated a mixture of recombinant non-IgE-reactive linear peptides (BM32) derived from grass pollen allergens, fused to a carrier protein (Pre-S protein). The study showed increased levels of allergen-specific IgG1 and IgG4 antibodies with minimal changes in IgE levels. While the primary analysis of combined seasonal symptom medication scores did not reach statistical significance, improvements were observed in asthma symptom scores and quality of life [125–127]. The results of phase 3 trials are eagerly awaited to further evaluate the efficacy and safety of this B-cell peptide immunotherapy approach.

6.5. DNA-Based Vaccine

DNA-based vaccines have shown promise in mouse models of allergy, inducing preferential TH1 and Treg cell responses while downregulating TH2 cell responses. The repeated use of DNA-based vaccines in humans has raised concerns, including the theoretical risk of plasmid DNA integration into the human genome, the development of anti-DNA antibodies, and the potential for long-term allergen persistence, which could lead to severe allergic reactions [2,16].

A clinical study evaluated a DNA-based vaccine targeting Cry j 2, a major allergen of Japanese cedar pollen allergy. The vaccine incorporated lysosomal-associated membrane protein 1 (LAMP1), a protein that directs the plasmid to the lysosomal compartment, reducing the risk of allergen release and anaphylaxis. After four intramuscular injections, 10 out of 12 participants showed a reduced immediate skin test response to Cry j 2 at 4 months. However, the study did not assess other clinical outcomes [128].

Another approach has involved combining allergens with bacterial DNA sequences containing CpG motifs, which are recognized by TLR-9, a receptor predominantly expressed on human B cells and dendritic cells. A phase 2 trial using a ragweed allergen (Amb a 1) covalently linked to a B-type CpG-containing oligodeoxynucleotide (ODN) showed promising results in ragweed pollen-induced hay fever [86]. However, these findings were not confirmed in a larger phase 3 trial, leading to the discontinuation of this approach [2].

Given their remarkable effectiveness against SARS-CoV-2 during the COVID-19 pandemic, mRNA-based vaccines have garnered significant interest for their potential applications in various medical fields, including allergic diseases [2,16]. Preclinical studies have demonstrated their ability to induce type 1 immune deviation and suppress allergic inflammation in mouse models of allergy [129].

7. Passive Immunotherapy

In 1935, Cooke et al. demonstrated that passive transfer of serum from ragweed immunotherapy patients could confer localized protection against ragweed skin prick test reactions in passively sensitized individuals [130]. This passive transfer of immunity was attributed to the transfer of blocking antibodies.

Subsequent studies in cat allergy patients have further validated this concept [131]. A single subcutaneous injection of a mixture of two recombinant anti-Fel d 1 antibodies conferred protection against nasal challenge with whole cat allergen extract for nearly 3 months, accompanied by a reduction in nasal fluid TH2-type cytokines and an increase in serum and nasal IgE-blocking activity [132].

A similar approach has been used to treat seasonal birch pollen allergy, where a cocktail of three monoclonal antibodies targeting the major birch allergen Bet v 1 effectively inhibited the clinical response to birch pollen nasal challenge for at least 2 months [133].

These findings suggest that passive immunotherapy, utilizing monoclonal antibodies targeting specific allergens, may offer a potential treatment option for allergic diseases, particularly for short-term protection or as a bridge therapy during periods of allergen exposure.

8. AIT Combination with Biologics

The combination of AIT with biologics, such as monoclonal antibodies targeting specific immune pathways, has emerged as a promising strategy for improving the management of allergic diseases. By combining the disease-modifying effects of AIT with the targeted therapeutic actions of biologics, this approach aims to enhance efficacy and safety while addressing specific challenges associated with AIT [134].

Omalizumab, a humanized monoclonal antibody, targets IgE, preventing it from binding to its receptors and triggering allergic reactions. It is currently approved for the treatment of moderate to severe asthma, chronic rhinosinusitis with nasal polyps, and chronic spontaneous urticaria. When used concurrently with AIT, omalizumab can lessen AIT-associated side effects, increasing tolerability. This allows patients to receive higher doses of allergen more quickly, making AIT suitable for higher-risk patients with asthma and enabling the use of rush protocols [135]. The combination of AIT with omalizumab has demonstrated efficacy in various allergens, including birch, grass, ragweed, perennial allergens, cat, dog, and HDM. Studies have shown a significant reduction in symptom scores, up to 48% less than SCIT alone, with a decrease in rescue medication use during seasonal exposure [136,137].

While the combination of grass pollen subcutaneous immunotherapy and dupilumab, an anti-IL-4 receptor antibody, reduced circulating IL-4-expressing TH2 cells, it did not significantly alter the magnitude or duration of allergen-induced late skin responses compared to allergen immunotherapy alone [138]. A clinical trial (NCT04502966) is currently evaluating the combination of grass pollen allergen with dupilumab, targeting both IL-4-dependent and IL-13-dependent pathways, in the context of inhalant immunotherapy [134].

Tezepelumab, a humanized monoclonal antibody targeting thymic stromal lymphopoietin (TSLP), has demonstrated promise in reducing eosinophilic inflammation, airway hyperresponsiveness, and asthma exacerbations. Additionally, it decreases serum IL-5, IL-13, and total IgE, suggesting potential synergy with AIT. A recent clinical trial investigated the combination of cat dander SCIT with tezepelumab. The study found that tezepelumab combined with SCIT was more effective than SCIT alone at reducing nasal response to cat allergen challenge after 52 weeks. This suppression persisted even one year after stopping treatment, suggesting a potential long-term benefit [139]. These findings suggest that tezepelumab may enhance the effectiveness of AIT by promoting long-term allergen tolerance [134].

Combining AIT with biologics has shown promise in improving short-term efficacy, enhancing safety, and improving patient tolerance during dose escalation. However, further research is needed to assess the long-term benefits and cost-effectiveness of these combination therapies.

9. Conclusions

AIT, including SLIT and SCIT, remains a safe and effective treatment for respiratory allergies. While novel approaches, such as the use of adjuvants, recombinant allergens, and biologics, show promise, their clinical efficacy and safety profiles still require further investigation.

Key findings and future directions include:

- Traditional AIT: SCIT and SLIT continue to be the primary options for AIT, offering long-term symptom relief and the potential to prevent progression to asthma;
- Novel Approaches: While modified allergens combined with novel adjuvants have shown promise in preclinical and early phase clinical trials, their superiority over traditional AIT has not been definitively established;
- Personalized Immunotherapy: The development of personalized allergen immunotherapy based on individual sensitization profiles and the identification of specific epitopes, recombinant allergen, offers potential for improved efficacy and safety;
- Combination Therapies: Combining AIT with biologics may enhance safety, treatment outcomes and address specific challenges associated with AIT;
- Passive Immunotherapy: Recent studies suggest that passive immunotherapy using monoclonal antibodies may offer a viable option for short-term protection against allergic symptoms.

Overall, while AIT remains a valuable treatment option for respiratory allergies, ongoing research is essential to further refine existing approaches and develop novel strategies that can improve efficacy, safety, and patient outcomes.

Funding: This research received no external funding.

Data Availability Statement: The datasets generated during the current study are available from the corresponding author upon reasonable request.

Conflicts of Interest: M.L. has received honoraria for scientific lectures from Abbott, A. Menarini, AstraZeneca, GSK, Takeda, Viatris, Organon, Sanofi, Novartis, and research supports from Amgen.

Abbreviations

AIT	allergen immunotherapy
APC	antigen-presenting cell
AR	allergic rhinitis
Breg	B regulatory cell
CpG	Cytosine-phosphodiester-guanine
DC	dendritic cell
DCreg	dendritic cell-derived regulatory cell
EPIT	epicutaneous immunotherapy
HCP	health care personnel
HDM	house dust mite
Ig	Immunoglobulin
IDIT	Intradermal Immunotherapy
IL	interleukin
ILC2	type 2 innate lymphoid cell
ILCreg	innate lymphoid cell-derived regulatory cell
ILIT	Intralymphatic immunotherapy
LAMP1	lysosomal-associated membrane protein 1
MCT	microcrystalline tyrosine
MPLA	Monophosphoryl lipid A
ODN	oligodeoxynucleotide
pDC	plasmacytoid dendritic cell
SCIT	subcutaneous immunotherapy
SLIT	sublingual immunotherapy
Tfh	T-helper cell
Tfr	T follicular regulatory cell
TGF	transforming growth factor
TH1	T-helper 1 cell
TH2	T-helper 2 cell

TLR	Toll-like receptor
Treg	T regulatory cells
TSLP	thymic stromal lymphopoietin
VLP	virus-like particle

References

1. Gutermuth, J.; Grosber, M.; Pfaar, O.; Bergmann, K.C.; Ring, J. 111 years of allergen-immunotherapy: A long and successful history of the only available disease-modifier in allergic diseases. *Allergol. Select* **2022**, *6*, 248–258. [CrossRef] [PubMed]
2. Durham, S.R.; Shamji, M.H. Allergen immunotherapy: Past, present and future. *Nat. Rev. Immunol.* **2023**, *23*, 317–328. [CrossRef] [PubMed]
3. Noon, L. Prophylactic inoculation against hay fever (historical document). *Ann. Allergy* **1955**, *13*, 713–716. [PubMed]
4. Frankland, A.W.; Augustin, R. Prophylaxis of summer hay-fever and asthma: A controlled trial comparing crude grass-pollen extracts with the isolated main protein component. *Lancet* **1954**, *266*, 1055–1057. [CrossRef] [PubMed]
5. Lowell, F.C.; Franklin, W. A double-blind study of the effectiveness and specificity of injection therapy in ragweed hay fever. *N. Engl. J. Med.* **1965**, *273*, 675–679. [CrossRef]
6. Norman, P.S.; Lichtenstein, L.M. The clinical and immunologic specificity of immunotherapy. *J. Allergy Clin. Immunol.* **1978**, *61*, 370–377. [CrossRef]
7. Hunt, K.J.; Valentine, M.D.; Sobotka, A.K.; Benton, A.W.; Amodio, F.J.; Lichtenstein, L.M. A controlled trial of immunotherapy in insect hypersensitivity. *N. Engl. J. Med.* **1978**, *299*, 157–161. [CrossRef]
8. Cox, L.; Nelson, H.; Lockey, R.; Calabria, C.; Chacko, T.; Finegold, I.; Nelson, M.; Weber, R.; Bernstein, D.I.; Blessing-Moore, J.; et al. Allergen immunotherapy: A practice parameter third update. *J. Allergy Clin. Immunol.* **2011**, *127*, S1–S55. [CrossRef]
9. Agache, I.; Lau, S.; Akdis, C.A.; Smolinska, S.; Bonini, M.; Cavkaytar, O.; Flood, B.; Gajdanowicz, P.; Izuhara, K.; Kalayci, O.; et al. EAACI Guidelines on Allergen Immunotherapy: House dust mite-driven allergic asthma. *Allergy* **2019**, *74*, 855–873. [CrossRef]
10. Roberts, G.; Pfaar, O.; Akdis, C.A.; Ansotegui, I.J.; Durham, S.R.; Gerth van Wijk, R.; Halken, S.; Larenas-Linnemann, D.; Pawankar, R.; Pitsios, C.; et al. EAACI Guidelines on Allergen Immunotherapy: Allergic rhinoconjunctivitis. *Allergy* **2018**, *73*, 765–798. [CrossRef]
11. Arshad, H.; Lack, G.; Durham, S.R.; Penagos, M.; Larenas-Linnemann, D.; Halken, S. Prevention Is Better than Cure: Impact of Allergen Immunotherapy on the Progression of Airway Disease. *J. Allergy Clin. Immunol. Pract.* **2024**, *12*, 45–56. [CrossRef] [PubMed]
12. Larenas-Linnemann, D. Long-term adherence strategies for allergen immunotherapy. *Allergy Asthma Proc.* **2022**, *43*, 299–304. [CrossRef] [PubMed]
13. Bonertz, A.; Roberts, G.C.; Hoefnagel, M.; Timon, M.; Slater, J.E.; Rabin, R.L.; Bridgewater, J.; Pini, C.; Pfaar, O.; Akdis, C.; et al. Challenges in the implementation of EAACI guidelines on allergen immunotherapy: A global perspective on the regulation of allergen products. *Allergy* **2018**, *73*, 64–76. [CrossRef] [PubMed]
14. Pavon-Romero, G.F.; Parra-Vargas, M.I.; Ramirez-Jimenez, F.; Melgoza-Ruiz, E.; Serrano-Perez, N.H.; Teran, L.M. Allergen Immunotherapy: Current and Future Trends. *Cells* **2022**, *11*, 212. [CrossRef] [PubMed]
15. Zemelka-Wiacek, M.; Agache, I.; Akdis, C.A.; Akdis, M.; Casale, T.B.; Dramburg, S.; Jahnz-Rozyk, K.; Kosowska, A.; Matricardi, P.M.; Pfaar, O.; et al. Hot topics in allergen immunotherapy, 2023: Current status and future perspective. *Allergy* **2024**, *79*, 823–842. [CrossRef]
16. Pfaar, O.; Portnoy, J.; Nolte, H.; Chaker, A.M.; Luna-Pech, J.A.; Patterson, A.; Pandya, A.; Larenas-Linnemann, D. Future Directions of Allergen Immunotherapy for Allergic Rhinitis: Experts' Perspective. *J. Allergy Clin. Immunol. Pract.* **2024**, *12*, 32–44. [CrossRef]
17. Gunawardana, N.C.; Durham, S.R. New approaches to allergen immunotherapy. *Ann. Allergy Asthma Immunol.* **2018**, *121*, 293–305. [CrossRef]
18. Sosic, L.; Paolucci, M.; Flory, S.; Jebbawi, F.; Kundig, T.M.; Johansen, P. Allergen immunotherapy: Progress and future outlook. *Expert. Rev. Clin. Immunol.* **2023**, *19*, 745–769. [CrossRef]
19. Licona-Limon, P.; Kim, L.K.; Palm, N.W.; Flavell, R.A. TH2, allergy and group 2 innate lymphoid cells. *Nat. Immunol.* **2013**, *14*, 536–542. [CrossRef]
20. Rondon, C.; Campo, P.; Togias, A.; Fokkens, W.J.; Durham, S.R.; Powe, D.G.; Mullol, J.; Blanca, M. Local allergic rhinitis: Concept, pathophysiology, and management. *J. Allergy Clin. Immunol.* **2012**, *129*, 1460–1467. [CrossRef]
21. Rosenwasser, L.J. Current understanding of the pathophysiology of allergic rhinitis. *Immunol. Allergy Clin. N. Am.* **2011**, *31*, 433–439. [CrossRef] [PubMed]
22. Shamji, M.H.; Durham, S.R. Mechanisms of allergen immunotherapy for inhaled allergens and predictive biomarkers. *J. Allergy Clin. Immunol.* **2017**, *140*, 1485–1498. [CrossRef] [PubMed]
23. Layhadi, J.A.; Lalioti, A.; Palmer, E.; van Zelm, M.C.; Wambre, E.; Shamji, M.H. Mechanisms and Predictive Biomarkers of Allergen Immunotherapy in the Clinic. *J. Allergy Clin. Immunol. Pract.* **2024**, *12*, 59–66. [CrossRef] [PubMed]
24. Ling, E.M.; Smith, T.; Nguyen, X.D.; Pridgeon, C.; Dallman, M.; Arbery, J.; Carr, V.A.; Robinson, D.S. Relation of CD4+CD25+ regulatory T-cell suppression of allergen-driven T-cell activation to atopic status and expression of allergic disease. *Lancet* **2004**, *363*, 608–615. [CrossRef] [PubMed]

25. Boonpiyathad, T.; Sozener, Z.C.; Akdis, M.; Akdis, C.A. The role of Treg cell subsets in allergic disease. *Asian Pac. J. Allergy Immunol.* **2020**, *38*, 139–149. [CrossRef]
26. Sharif, H.; Acharya, S.; Dhondalay, G.K.R.; Varricchi, G.; Krasner-Macleod, S.; Laisuan, W.; Switzer, A.; Lenormand, M.; Kashe, E.; Parkin, R.V.; et al. Altered chromatin landscape in circulating T follicular helper and regulatory cells following grass pollen subcutaneous and sublingual immunotherapy. *J. Allergy Clin. Immunol.* **2021**, *147*, 663–676. [CrossRef]
27. Zimmer, A.; Bouley, J.; Le Mignon, M.; Pliquet, E.; Horiot, S.; Turfkruyer, M.; Baron-Bodo, V.; Horak, F.; Nony, E.; Louise, A.; et al. A regulatory dendritic cell signature correlates with the clinical efficacy of allergen-specific sublingual immunotherapy. *J. Allergy Clin. Immunol.* **2012**, *129*, 1020–1030. [CrossRef]
28. Golebski, K.; Layhadi, J.A.; Sahiner, U.; Steveling-Klein, E.H.; Lenormand, M.M.; Li, R.C.Y.; Bal, S.M.; Heesters, B.A.; Vila-Nadal, G.; Hunewald, O.; et al. Induction of IL-10-producing type 2 innate lymphoid cells by allergen immunotherapy is associated with clinical response. *Immunity* **2021**, *54*, 291–307.e7. [CrossRef]
29. Lao-Araya, M.; Steveling, E.; Scadding, G.W.; Durham, S.R.; Shamji, M.H. Seasonal increases in peripheral innate lymphoid type 2 cells are inhibited by subcutaneous grass pollen immunotherapy. *J. Allergy Clin. Immunol.* **2014**, *134*, 1193–1195.e4. [CrossRef]
30. Boonpiyathad, T.; Tantilipikorn, P.; Ruxrungtham, K.; Pradubpongsa, P.; Mitthamsiri, W.; Piedvache, A.; Thantiworasit, P.; Sirivichayakul, S.; Jacquet, A.; Suratannon, N.; et al. IL-10-producing innate lymphoid cells increased in patients with house dust mite allergic rhinitis following immunotherapy. *J. Allergy Clin. Immunol.* **2021**, *147*, 1507–1510.e8. [CrossRef]
31. Bohle, B.; Kinaciyan, T.; Gerstmayr, M.; Radakovics, A.; Jahn-Schmid, B.; Ebner, C. Sublingual immunotherapy induces IL-10-producing T regulatory cells, allergen-specific T-cell tolerance, and immune deviation. *J. Allergy Clin. Immunol.* **2007**, *120*, 707–713. [CrossRef] [PubMed]
32. Gueguen, C.; Bouley, J.; Moussu, H.; Luce, S.; Duchateau, M.; Chamot-Rooke, J.; Pallardy, M.; Lombardi, V.; Nony, E.; Baron-Bodo, V.; et al. Changes in markers associated with dendritic cells driving the differentiation of either TH2 cells or regulatory T cells correlate with clinical benefit during allergen immunotherapy. *J. Allergy Clin. Immunol.* **2016**, *137*, 545–558. [CrossRef] [PubMed]
33. Boonpiyathad, T.; van de Veen, W.; Wirz, O.; Sokolowska, M.; Ruckert, B.; Tan, G.; Sangasapaviliya, A.; Pradubpongsa, P.; Fuengthong, R.; Thantiworasit, P.; et al. Role of Der p 1-specific B cells in immune tolerance during 2 years of house dust mite-specific immunotherapy. *J. Allergy Clin. Immunol.* **2019**, *143*, 1077–1086.e10. [CrossRef] [PubMed]
34. Shamji, M.H.; Larson, D.; Eifan, A.; Scadding, G.W.; Qin, T.; Lawson, K.; Sever, M.L.; Macfarlane, E.; Layhadi, J.A.; Wurtzen, P.A.; et al. Differential induction of allergen-specific IgA responses following timothy grass subcutaneous and sublingual immunotherapy. *J. Allergy Clin. Immunol.* **2021**, *148*, 1061–1071.e11. [CrossRef] [PubMed]
35. Shamji, M.H.; Kappen, J.; Abubakar-Waziri, H.; Zhang, J.; Steveling, E.; Watchman, S.; Kouser, L.; Eifan, A.; Switzer, A.; Varricchi, G.; et al. Nasal allergen-neutralizing IgG(4) antibodies block IgE-mediated responses: Novel biomarker of subcutaneous grass pollen immunotherapy. *J. Allergy Clin. Immunol.* **2019**, *143*, 1067–1076. [CrossRef]
36. Scadding, G.W.; Calderon, M.A.; Shamji, M.H.; Eifan, A.O.; Penagos, M.; Dumitru, F.; Sever, M.L.; Bahnson, H.T.; Lawson, K.; Harris, K.M.; et al. Effect of 2 Years of Treatment With Sublingual Grass Pollen Immunotherapy on Nasal Response to Allergen Challenge at 3 Years Among Patients With Moderate to Severe Seasonal Allergic Rhinitis: The GRASS Randomized Clinical Trial. *JAMA* **2017**, *317*, 615–625. [CrossRef]
37. Boonpiyathad, T.; Lao-Araya, M.; Chiewchalermsri, C.; Sangkanjanavanich, S.; Morita, H. Allergic Rhinitis: What Do We Know About Allergen-Specific Immunotherapy? *Front. Allergy* **2021**, *2*, 747323. [CrossRef]
38. Calderon, M.A.; Vidal, C.; Rodriguez Del Rio, P.; Just, J.; Pfaar, O.; Tabar, A.I., Sanchez-Machin, I.; Bubel, P.; Borja, J.; Eberle, P.; et al. European Survey on Adverse Systemic Reactions in Allergen Immunotherapy (EASSI): A real-life clinical assessment. *Allergy* **2017**, *72*, 462–472. [CrossRef]
39. Asllani, J.; Mitsias, D.; Konstantinou, G.; Priftanji, A.; Hoxha, M.; Sinani, G.; Christoff, G.; Zlatko, D.; Makris, M.; Aggelidis, X.; et al. The Allergen Immunotherapy Adverse Events Registry: Setup & methodology of a European Academy of Allergy and Clinical Immunology taskforce project. *Clin. Transl. Allergy* **2023**, *13*, e12266. [CrossRef]
40. Bernstein, D.I.; Epstein, T.E.G. Safety of allergen immunotherapy in North America from 2008-2017: Lessons learned from the ACAAI/AAAAI National Surveillance Study of adverse reactions to allergen immunotherapy. *Allergy Asthma Proc.* **2020**, *41*, 108–111. [CrossRef]
41. Dhami, S.; Nurmatov, U.; Arasi, S.; Khan, T.; Asaria, M.; Zaman, H.; Agarwal, A.; Netuveli, G.; Roberts, G.; Pfaar, O.; et al. Allergen immunotherapy for allergic rhinoconjunctivitis: A systematic review and meta-analysis. *Allergy* **2017**, *72*, 1597–1631. [CrossRef] [PubMed]
42. Canonica, G.W.; Baena-Cagnani, C.E.; Bousquet, J.; Bousquet, P.J.; Lockey, R.F.; Malling, H.J.; Passalacqua, G.; Potter, P.; Valovirta, E. Recommendations for standardization of clinical trials with Allergen Specific Immunotherapy for respiratory allergy. A statement of a World Allergy Organization (WAO) taskforce. *Allergy* **2007**, *62*, 317–324. [CrossRef] [PubMed]
43. Durham, S.R.; Penagos, M. Sublingual or subcutaneous immunotherapy for allergic rhinitis? *J. Allergy Clin. Immunol.* **2016**, *137*, 339–349.e0. [CrossRef] [PubMed]
44. Penagos, M.; Durham, S.R. Allergen immunotherapy for long-term tolerance and prevention. *J. Allergy Clin. Immunol.* **2022**, *149*, 802–811. [CrossRef]
45. Conroy, E.R.; Banzon, T.M.; Simoneau, T.; Phipatanakul, W.; van Boven, J.F.M.; Larenas-Linnemann, D. An Overview of Adherence-What It Is and Why It Is Important. *J. Allergy Clin. Immunol. Pract.* 2024, *in press*. [CrossRef]

46. Kulalert, P.; Phinyo, P.; Lao-Araya, M. Efficacy and safety of house dust mite sublingual immunotherapy tablets in allergic rhinitis: A systematic review and meta-analysis. *World Allergy Organ. J.* **2022**, *15*, 100691. [CrossRef]
47. Bergmann, K.C.; Demoly, P.; Worm, M.; Fokkens, W.J.; Carrillo, T.; Tabar, A.I.; Nguyen, H.; Montagut, A.; Zeldin, R.K. Efficacy and safety of sublingual tablets of house dust mite allergen extracts in adults with allergic rhinitis. *J. Allergy Clin. Immunol.* **2014**, *133*, 1608–1614.e6. [CrossRef]
48. Demoly, P.; Corren, J.; Creticos, P.; De Blay, F.; Gevaert, P.; Hellings, P.; Kowal, K.; Le Gall, M.; Nenasheva, N.; Passalacqua, G.; et al. A 300 IR sublingual tablet is an effective, safe treatment for house dust mite-induced allergic rhinitis: An international, double-blind, placebo-controlled, randomized phase III clinical trial. *J. Allergy Clin. Immunol.* **2021**, *147*, 1020–1030.e10. [CrossRef]
49. Durham, S.R.; Emminger, W.; Kapp, A.; de Monchy, J.G.; Rak, S.; Scadding, G.K.; Wurtzen, P.A.; Andersen, J.S.; Tholstrup, B.; Riis, B.; et al. SQ-standardized sublingual grass immunotherapy: Confirmation of disease modification 2 years after 3 years of treatment in a randomized trial. *J. Allergy Clin. Immunol.* **2012**, *129*, 717–725.e5. [CrossRef]
50. Creticos, P.S.; Maloney, J.; Bernstein, D.I.; Casale, T.; Kaur, A.; Fisher, R.; Liu, N.; Murphy, K.; Nekam, K.; Nolte, H. Randomized controlled trial of a ragweed allergy immunotherapy tablet in North American and European adults. *J. Allergy Clin. Immunol.* **2013**, *131*, 1342–1349e6. [CrossRef]
51. Yonekura, S.; Gotoh, M.; Kaneko, S.; Maekawa, Y.; Okubo, K.; Okamoto, Y. Disease-Modifying Effect of Japanese Cedar Pollen Sublingual Immunotherapy Tablets. *J. Allergy Clin. Immunol. Pract.* **2021**, *9*, 4103–4116.e4. [CrossRef] [PubMed]
52. Okamoto, Y.; Okubo, K.; Yonekura, S.; Hashiguchi, K.; Goto, M.; Otsuka, T.; Murata, T.; Nakao, Y.; Kanazawa, C.; Nagakura, H.; et al. Efficacy and safety of sublingual immunotherapy for two seasons in patients with Japanese cedar pollinosis. *Int. Arch. Allergy Immunol.* **2015**, *166*, 177–188. [CrossRef] [PubMed]
53. Virchow, J.C.; Backer, V.; Kuna, P.; Prieto, L.; Nolte, H.; Villesen, H.H.; Ljorring, C.; Riis, B.; de Blay, F. Efficacy of a House Dust Mite Sublingual Allergen Immunotherapy Tablet in Adults With Allergic Asthma: A Randomized Clinical Trial. *JAMA* **2016**, *315*, 1715–1725. [CrossRef] [PubMed]
54. Mosbech, H.; Deckelmann, R.; de Blay, F.; Pastorello, E.A.; Trebas-Pietras, E.; Andres, L.P.; Malcus, I.; Ljorring, C.; Canonica, G.W. Standardized quality (SQ) house dust mite sublingual immunotherapy tablet (ALK) reduces inhaled corticosteroid use while maintaining asthma control: A randomized, double-blind, placebo-controlled trial. *J. Allergy Clin. Immunol.* **2014**, *134*, 568–575.e7. [CrossRef] [PubMed]
55. Horak, F.; Jaeger, S.; Worm, M.; Melac, M.; Didier, A. Implementation of pre-seasonal sublingual immunotherapy with a five-grass pollen tablet during optimal dosage assessment. *Clin. Exp. Allergy* **2009**, *39*, 394–400. [CrossRef]
56. Greenhawt, M.; Oppenheimer, J.; Nelson, M.; Nelson, H.; Lockey, R.; Lieberman, P.; Nowak-Wegrzyn, A.; Peters, A.; Collins, C.; Bernstein, D.I.; et al. Sublingual immunotherapy: A focused allergen immunotherapy practice parameter update. *Ann. Allergy Asthma Immunol.* **2017**, *118*, 276–282.e2. [CrossRef]
57. Lao-Araya, M.; Sompornrattanaphan, M.; Kanjanawasee, D.; Tantilipikorn, P.; Allergy Asthma and Immunology Association of Thailand (AAIAT) interesting group on immunotherapy. Allergen immunotherapy for respiratory allergies in clinical practice: A comprehensive review. *Asian Pac. J. Allergy Immunol.* **2022**, *40*, 283–294. [CrossRef]
58. Durham, S.R.; Creticos, P.S.; Nelson, H.S.; Li, Z.; Kaur, A.; Meltzer, E.O.; Nolte, H. Treatment effect of sublingual immunotherapy tablets and pharmacotherapies for seasonal and perennial allergic rhinitis: Pooled analyses. *J. Allergy Clin. Immunol.* **2016**, *138*, 1081–1088.e4. [CrossRef]
59. Kennedy, J.L.; Robinson, D.; Christophel, J.; Borish, L.; Payne, S. Decision-making analysis for allergen immunotherapy versus nasal steroids in the treatment of nasal steroid-responsive allergic rhinitis. *Am. J. Rhinol. Allergy* **2014**, *28*, 59–64. [CrossRef]
60. Settipane, R.A.; Bukstein, D.A. Allergen immunotherapy and shared decision-making. *Allergy Asthma Proc.* **2022**, *43*, 350–355. [CrossRef]
61. Senti, G.; Prinz Vavricka, B.M.; Erdmann, I.; Diaz, M.I.; Markus, R.; McCormack, S.J.; Simard, J.J.; Wuthrich, B.; Crameri, R.; Graf, N.; et al. Intralymphatic allergen administration renders specific immunotherapy faster and safer: A randomized controlled trial. *Proc. Natl. Acad. Sci. USA* **2008**, *105*, 17908–17912. [CrossRef]
62. Senti, G.; Crameri, R.; Kuster, D.; Johansen, P.; Martinez-Gomez, J.M.; Graf, N.; Steiner, M.; Hothorn, L.A.; Gronlund, H.; Tivig, C.; et al. Intralymphatic immunotherapy for cat allergy induces tolerance after only 3 injections. *J. Allergy Clin. Immunol.* **2012**, *129*, 1290–1296. [CrossRef] [PubMed]
63. Chabot, A.; Senti, G.; Erdmann, I.; Prinz, B.M.; Wuthrich, B.; Sosic, L.; Kundig, T.M.; Johansen, P. Intralymphatic Immunotherapy (ILIT) With Bee Venom Allergens: A Clinical Proof-of-Concept Study and the Very First ILIT in Humans. *Front. Allergy* **2022**, *3*, 832010. [CrossRef] [PubMed]
64. Senti, G.; Freiburghaus, A.U.; Larenas-Linnemann, D.; Hoffmann, H.J.; Patterson, A.M.; Klimek, L.; Di Bona, D.; Pfaar, O.; Ahlbeck, L.; Akdis, M.; et al. Intralymphatic Immunotherapy: Update and Unmet Needs. *Int. Arch. Allergy Immunol.* **2019**, *178*, 141–149. [CrossRef] [PubMed]
65. Konradsen, J.R.; Grundstrom, J.; Hellkvist, L.; Tran, T.A.T.; Andersson, N.; Gafvelin, G.; Kiewiet, M.B.G.; Hamsten, C.; Tang, J.; Parkin, R.V.; et al. Intralymphatic immunotherapy in pollen-allergic young adults with rhinoconjunctivitis and mild asthma: A randomized trial. *J. Allergy Clin. Immunol.* **2020**, *145*, 1005–1007.e7. [CrossRef] [PubMed]
66. Skaarup, S.H.; Schmid, J.M.; Skjold, T.; Graumann, O.; Hoffmann, H.J. Intralymphatic immunotherapy improves grass pollen allergic rhinoconjunctivitis: A 3-year randomized placebo-controlled trial. *J. Allergy Clin. Immunol.* **2021**, *147*, 1011–1019 [CrossRef]

67. Hoang, M.P.; Seresirikachorn, K.; Chitsuthipakorn, W.; Snidvongs, K. Intralymphatic immunotherapy for allergic rhinoconjunctivitis: A systematic review and meta-analysis. *Rhinology* **2021**, *59*, 236–244. [CrossRef]
68. Senti, G.; von Moos, S.; Kundig, T.M. Epicutaneous allergen administration: Is this the future of allergen-specific immunotherapy? *Allergy* **2011**, *66*, 798–809. [CrossRef]
69. Senti, G.; Graf, N.; Haug, S.; Ruedi, N.; von Moos, S.; Sonderegger, T.; Johansen, P.; Kundig, T.M. Epicutaneous allergen administration as a novel method of allergen-specific immunotherapy. *J. Allergy Clin. Immunol.* **2009**, *124*, 997–1002. [CrossRef]
70. Senti, G.; von Moos, S.; Tay, F.; Graf, N.; Johansen, P.; Kundig, T.M. Determinants of efficacy and safety in epicutaneous allergen immunotherapy: Summary of three clinical trials. *Allergy* **2015**, *70*, 707–710. [CrossRef]
71. Senti, G.; Kundig, T.M. Novel Delivery Routes for Allergy Immunotherapy: Intralymphatic, Epicutaneous, and Intradermal. *Immunol. Allergy Clin. N. Am.* **2016**, *36*, 25–37. [CrossRef] [PubMed]
72. Rotiroti, G.; Shamji, M.; Durham, S.R.; Till, S.J. Repeated low-dose intradermal allergen injection suppresses allergen-induced cutaneous late responses. *J. Allergy Clin. Immunol.* **2012**, *130*, 918–924.e1. [CrossRef] [PubMed]
73. Slovick, A.; Douiri, A.; Muir, R.; Guerra, A.; Tsioulos, K.; Hay, E.; Lam, E.P.S.; Kelly, J.; Peacock, J.L.; Ying, S.; et al. Intradermal grass pollen immunotherapy increases T(H)2 and IgE responses and worsens respiratory allergic symptoms. *J. Allergy Clin. Immunol.* **2017**, *139*, 1830–1839.e13. [CrossRef] [PubMed]
74. Lin, Y.J.; Zimmermann, J.; Schulke, S. Novel adjuvants in allergen-specific immunotherapy: Where do we stand? *Front. Immunol.* **2024**, *15*, 1348305. [CrossRef] [PubMed]
75. Norman, P.S.; Lichtenstein, L.M. Comparisons of alum-precipitated and unprecipitated aqueous ragweed pollen extracts in the treatment of hay fever. *J. Allergy Clin. Immunol.* **1978**, *61*, 384–389. [CrossRef]
76. Principi, N.; Esposito, S. Aluminum in vaccines: Does it create a safety problem? *Vaccine* **2018**, *36*, 5825–5831. [CrossRef]
77. Baldrick, P.; Richardson, D.; Wheeler, A.W. Review of L-tyrosine confirming its safe human use as an adjuvant. *J. Appl. Toxicol.* **2002**, *22*, 333–344. [CrossRef]
78. Wheeler, A.W.; Moran, D.M.; Robins, B.E.; Driscoll, A. l-Tyrosine as an immunological adjuvant. *Int. Arch. Allergy Appl. Immunol.* **1982**, *69*, 113–119. [CrossRef]
79. Becker, S.; Zieglmayer, P.; Canto, G.; Fassio, F.; Yong, P.; Acikel, C.; Raskopf, E.; Steveling-Klein, E.H.; Allekotte, S.; Mosges, R. A meta-analysis on allergen-specific immunotherapy using MCT((R)) (MicroCrystalline Tyrosine)-adsorbed allergoids in pollen allergic patients suffering from allergic rhinoconjunctivitis. *Clin. Transl. Allergy* **2021**, *11*, e12037. [CrossRef]
80. Mothes, N.; Heinzkill, M.; Drachenberg, K.J.; Sperr, W.R.; Krauth, M.T.; Majlesi, Y.; Semper, H.; Valent, P.; Niederberger, V.; Kraft, D.; et al. Allergen-specific immunotherapy with a monophosphoryl lipid A-adjuvanted vaccine: Reduced seasonally boosted immunoglobulin E production and inhibition of basophil histamine release by therapy-induced blocking antibodies. *Clin. Exp. Allergy* **2003**, *33*, 1198–1208. [CrossRef]
81. Drachenberg, K.J.; Wheeler, A.W.; Stuebner, P.; Horak, F. A well-tolerated grass pollen-specific allergy vaccine containing a novel adjuvant, monophosphoryl lipid A, reduces allergic symptoms after only four preseasonal injections. *Allergy* **2001**, *56*, 498–505. [CrossRef] [PubMed]
82. Bell, A.J.; Heath, M.D.; Hewings, S.J.; Skinner, M.A. The adsorption of allergoids and 3-O-desacyl-4′-monophosphoryl lipid A (MPL(R)) to microcrystalline tyrosine (MCT) in formulations for use in allergy immunotherapy. *J. Inorg. Biochem.* **2015**, *152*, 147–153. [CrossRef] [PubMed]
83. Jutek, M.; Bachert, C. Ultra-short-course seasonal allergy vaccine (Pollinex Quattro): Viewpoints. *Drugs* **2006**, *66*, 939–940. [CrossRef] [PubMed]
84. Rosewich, M.; Lee, D.; Zielen, S. Pollinex Quattro: An innovative four injections immunotherapy in allergic rhinitis. *Hum. Vaccin. Immunother.* **2013**, *9*, 1523–1531. [CrossRef]
85. Worm, M.; Higenbottam, T.; Pfaar, O.; Mosges, R.; Aberer, W.; Gunawardena, K.; Wessiepe, D.; Lee, D.; Kramer, M.F.; Skinner, M.; et al. Randomized controlled trials define shape of dose response for Pollinex Quattro Birch allergoid immunotherapy. *Allergy* **2018**, *73*, 1812–1822. [CrossRef]
86. Creticos, P.S.; Schroeder, J.T.; Hamilton, R.G.; Balcer-Whaley, S.L.; Khattignavong, A.P.; Lindblad, R.; Li, H.; Coffman, R.; Seyfert, V.; Eiden, J.J.; et al. Immunotherapy with a ragweed-toll-like receptor 9 agonist vaccine for allergic rhinitis. *N. Engl. J. Med.* **2006**, *355*, 1445–1455. [CrossRef]
87. Kawakita, A.; Shirasaki, H.; Yasutomi, M.; Tokuriki, S.; Mayumi, M.; Naiki, H.; Ohshima, Y. Immunotherapy with oligomannose-coated liposomes ameliorates allergic symptoms in a murine food allergy model. *Allergy* **2012**, *67*, 371–379. [CrossRef]
88. Beeh, K.M.; Kanniess, F.; Wagner, F.; Schilder, C.; Naudts, I.; Hammann-Haenni, A.; Willers, J.; Stocker, H.; Mueller, P.; Bachmann, M.F.; et al. The novel TLR-9 agonist QbG10 shows clinical efficacy in persistent allergic asthma. *J. Allergy Clin. Immunol.* **2013**, *131*, 866–874. [CrossRef]
89. Senti, G.; Johansen, P.; Haug, S.; Bull, C.; Gottschaller, C.; Muller, P.; Pfister, T.; Maurer, P.; Bachmann, M.F.; Graf, N.; et al. Use of A-type CpG oligodeoxynucleotides as an adjuvant in allergen-specific immunotherapy in humans: A phase I/IIa clinical trial. *Clin. Exp. Allergy* **2009**, *39*, 562–570. [CrossRef]
90. Klimek, L.; Willers, J.; Hammann-Haenni, A.; Pfaar, O.; Stocker, H.; Mueller, P.; Renner, W.A.; Bachmann, M.F. Assessment of clinical efficacy of CYT003-QbG10 in patients with allergic rhinoconjunctivitis: A phase IIb study. *Clin. Exp. Allergy* **2011**, *41*, 1305–1312. [CrossRef]

91. Casale, T.B.; Cole, J.; Beck, E.; Vogelmeier, C.F.; Willers, J.; Lassen, C.; Hammann-Haenni, A.; Trokan, L.; Saudan, P.; Wechsler, M.E. CYT003, a TLR9 agonist, in persistent allergic asthma—a randomized placebo-controlled Phase 2b study. *Allergy* **2015**, *70*, 1160–1168. [CrossRef] [PubMed]
92. Marsh, D.G.; Lichtenstein, L.M.; Campbell, D.H. Studies on "allergoids" prepared from naturally occurring allergens. I. Assay of allergenicity and antigenicity of formalinized rye group I component. *Immunology* **1970**, *18*, 705–722. [PubMed]
93. Norman, P.S.; Lichtenstein, L.M.; Kagey-Sobotka, A.; Marsh, D.G. Controlled evaluation of allergoid in the immunotherapy of ragweed hay fever. *J. Allergy Clin. Immunol.* **1982**, *70*, 248–260. [CrossRef] [PubMed]
94. Bousquet, J.; Braquemond, P.; Feinberg, J.; Guerin, B.; Maasch, H.; Michel, F.B. Specific IgE response before and after rush immunotherapy with a standardized allergen or allergoid in grass pollen allergy. *Ann. Allergy* **1986**, *56*, 456–459.
95. Bozek, A.; Cudak, A.; Walter Canonica, G. Long-term efficacy of injected allergen immunotherapy for treatment of grass pollen allergy in elderly patients with allergic rhinitis. *Allergy Asthma Proc.* **2020**, *41*, 271–277. [CrossRef]
96. Bousquet, J.; Hejjaoui, A.; Soussana, M.; Michel, F.B. Double-blind, placebo-controlled immunotherapy with mixed grass-pollen allergoids. IV. Comparison of the safety and efficacy of two dosages of a high-molecular-weight allergoid. *J. Allergy Clin. Immunol.* **1990**, *85*, 490–497. [CrossRef]
97. Worm, M.; Rak, S.; Samolinski, B.; Antila, J.; Hoiby, A.S.; Kruse, B.; Lipiec, A.; Rudert, M.; Valovirta, E. Efficacy and safety of birch pollen allergoid subcutaneous immunotherapy: A 2-year double-blind, placebo-controlled, randomized trial plus 1-year open-label extension. *Clin. Exp. Allergy* **2019**, *49*, 516–525. [CrossRef]
98. Lund, L.; Henmar, H.; Wurtzen, P.A.; Lund, G.; Hjortskov, N.; Larsen, J.N. Comparison of allergenicity and immunogenicity of an intact allergen vaccine and commercially available allergoid products for birch pollen immunotherapy. *Clin. Exp. Allergy* **2007**, *37*, 564–571. [CrossRef]
99. Klimek, L.; Dormann, D.; Jarman, E.R.; Cromwell, O.; Riechelmann, H.; Reske-Kunz, A.B. Short-term preseasonal birch pollen allergoid immunotherapy influences symptoms, specific nasal provocation and cytokine levels in nasal secretions, but not peripheral T-cell responses, in patients with allergic rhinitis. *Clin. Exp. Allergy* **1999**, *29*, 1326–1335. [CrossRef]
100. Klimek, L.; Fox, G.C.; Thum-Oltmer, S. SCIT with a high-dose house dust mite allergoid is well tolerated: Safety data from pooled clinical trials and more than 10 years of daily practice analyzed in different subgroups. *Allergo J. Int.* **2018**, *27*, 131–139. [CrossRef]
101. Jutel, M.; Bruggenjurgen, B.; Richter, H.; Vogelberg, C. Real-world evidence of subcutaneous allergoid immunotherapy in house dust mite-induced allergic rhinitis and asthma. *Allergy* **2020**, *75*, 2050–2058. [CrossRef] [PubMed]
102. Passalacqua, G.; Albano, M.; Fregonese, L.; Riccio, A.; Pronzato, C.; Mela, G.S.; Canonica, G.W. Randomised controlled trial of local allergoid immunotherapy on allergic inflammation in mite-induced rhinoconjunctivitis. *Lancet* **1998**, *351*, 629–632. [CrossRef] [PubMed]
103. Gallego, M.T.; Iraola, V.; Himly, M.; Robinson, D.S.; Badiola, C.; Garcia-Robaina, J.C.; Briza, P.; Carnes, J. Depigmented and polymerised house dust mite allergoid: Allergen content, induction of IgG4 and clinical response. *Int. Arch. Allergy Immunol.* **2010**, *153*, 61–69. [CrossRef] [PubMed]
104. Di Gioacchino, M.; Cavallucci, E.; Ballone, E.; Cervone, M.; Di Rocco, P.; Piunti, E.; Filardo, G.S.; Turi, M.C.; Mangifesta, R.; Quecchia, C.; et al. Dose-dependent clinical and immunological efficacy of sublingual immunotherapy with mite monomeric allergoid. *Int. J. Immunopathol. Pharmacol.* **2012**, *25*, 671–679. [CrossRef] [PubMed]
105. Corrigan, C.J.; Kettner, J.; Doemer, C.; Cromwell, O.; Narkus, A.; Study, G. Efficacy and safety of preseasonal-specific immunotherapy with an aluminium-adsorbed six-grass pollen allergoid. *Allergy* **2005**, *60*, 801–807. [CrossRef] [PubMed]
106. Agostinis, F.; Foglia, C.; Bruno, M.E.; Falagiani, P. Efficacy, safety and tolerability of sublingual monomeric allergoid in tablets given without up-dosing to pediatric patients with allergic rhinitis and/or asthma due to grass pollen. *Eur. Ann. Allergy Clin. Immunol.* **2009**, *41*, 177–180.
107. Mosges, R.; Ritter, B.; Kayoko, G.; Allekotte, S. Carbamylated monomeric allergoids as a therapeutic option for sublingual immunotherapy of dust mite- and grass pollen-induced allergic rhinoconjunctivitis: A systematic review of published trials with a meta-analysis of treatment using Lais(R) tablets. *Acta Dermatovenerol. Alp. Pannonica Adriat.* **2010**, *19*, 3–10.
108. Klimek, L.; Pfaar, O.; Bousquet, J.; Senti, G.; Kundig, T. Allergen immunotherapy in allergic rhinitis: Current use and future trends. *Expert. Rev. Clin. Immunol.* **2017**, *13*, 897–906. [CrossRef]
109. Barber, D.; Diaz-Perales, A.; Escribese, M.M.; Kleine-Tebbe, J.; Matricardi, P.M.; Ollert, M.; Santos, A.F.; Sastre, J. Molecular allergology and its impact in specific allergy diagnosis and therapy. *Allergy* **2021**, *76*, 3642–3658. [CrossRef]
110. Dramburg, S.; Hilger, C.; Santos, A.F.; de Las Vecillas, L.; Aalberse, R.C.; Acevedo, N.; Aglas, L.; Altmann, F.; Arruda, K.L.; Asero, R.; et al. EAACI Molecular Allergology User's Guide 2.0. *Pediatr. Allergy Immunol.* **2023**, *34* (Suppl. S28), e13854. [CrossRef]
111. Gonzalez-Perez, R.; Poza-Guedes, P.; Pineda, F.; Sanchez-Machin, I. Advocacy of Precision Allergy Molecular Diagnosis in Decision Making for the Eligibility of Customized Allergen Immunotherapy. *Curr. Issues Mol. Biol.* **2023**, *45*, 9976–9984. [CrossRef] [PubMed]
112. Valenta, R.; Campana, R.; Focke-Tejkl, M.; Niederberger, V. Vaccine development for allergen-specific immunotherapy based on recombinant allergens and synthetic allergen peptides: Lessons from the past and novel mechanisms of action for the future. *J. Allergy Clin. Immunol.* **2016**, *137*, 351–357. [CrossRef] [PubMed]
113. Valenta, R.; Linhart, B.; Swoboda, I.; Niederberger, V. Recombinant allergens for allergen-specific immunotherapy: 10 years anniversary of immunotherapy with recombinant allergens. *Allergy* **2011**, *66*, 775–783. [CrossRef] [PubMed]

114. Jutel, M.; Jaeger, L.; Suck, R.; Meyer, H.; Fiebig, H.; Cromwell, O. Allergen-specific immunotherapy with recombinant grass pollen allergens. *J. Allergy Clin. Immunol.* **2005**, *116*, 608–613. [CrossRef] [PubMed]
115. Pauli, G.; Larsen, T.H.; Rak, S.; Horak, F.; Pastorello, E.; Valenta, R.; Purohit, A.; Arvidsson, M.; Kavina, A.; Schroeder, J.W.; et al. Efficacy of recombinant birch pollen vaccine for the treatment of birch-allergic rhinoconjunctivitis. *J. Allergy Clin. Immunol.* **2008**, *122*, 951–960. [CrossRef]
116. Larche, M. Immunotherapy with allergen peptides. *Allergy Asthma Clin. Immunol.* **2007**, *3*, 53–59. [CrossRef]
117. Moldaver, D.; Larche, M. Immunotherapy with peptides. *Allergy* **2011**, *66*, 784–791. [CrossRef]
118. Wraith, D.C.; Krishna, M.T. Peptide allergen-specific immunotherapy for allergic airway diseases-State of the art. *Clin. Exp. Allergy* **2021**, *51*, 751–769. [CrossRef]
119. Patel, D.; Couroux, P.; Hickey, P.; Salapatek, A.M.; Laidler, P.; Larche, M.; Hafner, R.P. Fel d 1-derived peptide antigen desensitization shows a persistent treatment effect 1 year after the start of dosing: A randomized, placebo-controlled study. *J. Allergy Clin. Immunol.* **2013**, *131*, 103–109.e7. [CrossRef]
120. Oldfield, W.L.; Larche, M.; Kay, A.B. Effect of T-cell peptides derived from Fel d 1 on allergic reactions and cytokine production in patients sensitive to cats: A randomised controlled trial. *Lancet* **2002**, *360*, 47–53. [CrossRef]
121. Kettner, A.; DellaCorte, G.; de Blay, F.; Jacobsen, L.; Jutel, M.; Worm, M.; Charlon, V.; Simonsen, K.; Reymond, C.; Spertini, F. Benefit of Bet v 1 contiguous overlapping peptide immunotherapy persists during first follow-up season. *J. Allergy Clin. Immunol.* **2018**, *142*, 678–680.e7. [CrossRef] [PubMed]
122. Sharif, H.; Singh, I.; Kouser, L.; Mosges, R.; Bonny, M.A.; Karamani, A.; Parkin, R.V.; Bovy, N.; Kishore, U.; Robb, A.; et al. Immunologic mechanisms of a short-course of Lolium perenne peptide immunotherapy: A randomized, double-blind, placebo-controlled trial. *J. Allergy Clin. Immunol.* **2019**, *144*, 738–749. [CrossRef] [PubMed]
123. Mosges, R.; Kasche, E.M.; Raskopf, E.; Singh, J.; Sohlich, L.; Astvatsatourov, A.; Shah-Hosseini, K.; Pirotton, S.; Haazen, L.; Durham, S.R.; et al. A randomized, double-blind, placebo-controlled, dose-finding trial with Lolium perenne peptide immunotherapy. *Allergy* **2018**, *73*, 896–904. [CrossRef] [PubMed]
124. Narayanan, M.; Freidl, R.; Focke-Tejkl, M.; Baranyi, U.; Wekerle, T.; Valenta, R.; Linhart, B. A B Cell Epitope Peptide Derived from the Major Grass Pollen Allergen Phl p 1 Boosts Allergen-Specific Secondary Antibody Responses without Allergen-Specific T Cell Help. *J. Immunol.* **2017**, *198*, 1685–1695. [CrossRef]
125. Niederberger, V.; Neubauer, A.; Gevaert, P.; Zidarn, M.; Worm, M.; Aberer, W.; Malling, H.J.; Pfaar, O.; Klimek, L.; Pfutzner, W.; et al. Safety and efficacy of immunotherapy with the recombinant B-cell epitope-based grass pollen vaccine BM32. *J. Allergy Clin. Immunol.* **2018**, *142*, 497–509.e9. [CrossRef]
126. Rauber, M.M.; Mobs, C.; Campana, R.; Henning, R.; Schulze-Dasbeck, M.; Greene, B.; Focke-Tejkl, M.; Weber, M.; Valenta, R.; Pfutzner, W. Allergen immunotherapy with the hypoallergenic B-cell epitope-based vaccine BM32 modifies IL-10- and IL-5-secreting T cells. *Allergy* **2020**, *75*, 450–453. [CrossRef]
127. Eckl-Dorna, J.; Weber, M.; Stanek, V.; Linhart, B.; Ristl, R.; Waltl, E.E.; Villazala Merino, S.; Hummel, A.; Focke-Tejkl, M.; Froeschel, R.; et al. Two years of treatment with the recombinant grass pollen allergy vaccine BM32 induces a continuously increasing allergen-specific IgG(4) response. *EBioMedicine* **2019**, *50*, 421–432. [CrossRef]
128. Su, Y.; Romeu-Bonilla, E.; Anagnostou, A.; Fitz-Patrick, D.; Hearl, W.; Heiland, T. Safety and long-term immunological effects of CryJ2-LAMP plasmid vaccine in Japanese red cedar atopic subjects: A phase I study. *Hum. Vaccin. Immunother.* **2017**, *13*, 2804–2813. [CrossRef]
129. Roesler, E.; Weiss, R.; Weinberger, E.E.; Fruehwirth, A.; Stoecklinger, A.; Mostbock, S.; Ferreira, F.; Thalhamer, J.; Scheiblhofer, S. Immunize and disappear-safety-optimized mRNA vaccination with a panel of 29 allergens. *J. Allergy Clin. Immunol.* **2009**, *124*, 1070–1077.e11. [CrossRef]
130. Cooke, R.A.; Barnard, J.H.; Hebald, S.; Stull, A. Serological Evidence of Immunity with Coexisting Sensitization in a Type of Human Allergy (Hay Fever). *J. Exp. Med.* **1935**, *62*, 733–750. [CrossRef]
131. Orengo, J.M.; Radin, A.R.; Kamat, V.; Badithe, A.; Ben, L.H.; Bennett, B.L.; Zhong, S.; Birchard, D.; Limnander, A.; Rafique, A.; et al. Treating cat allergy with monoclonal IgG antibodies that bind allergen and prevent IgE engagement. *Nat. Commun.* **2018**, *9*, 1421. [CrossRef] [PubMed]
132. Shamji, M.H.; Singh, I.; Layhadi, J.A.; Ito, C.; Karamani, A.; Kouser, L.; Sharif, H.; Tang, J.; Handijiev, S.; Parkin, R.V.; et al. Passive Prophylactic Administration with a Single Dose of Anti-Fel d 1 Monoclonal Antibodies REGN1908-1909 in Cat Allergen-induced Allergic Rhinitis: A Randomized, Double-Blind, Placebo-controlled Clinical Trial. *Am. J. Respir. Crit. Care Med.* **2021**, *204*, 23–33. [CrossRef] [PubMed]
133. Gevaert, P.; De Craemer, J.; De Ruyck, N.; Rottey, S.; de Hoon, J.; Hellings, P.W.; Volckaert, B.; Lesneuck, K.; Orengo, J.M.; Atanasio, A.; et al. Novel antibody cocktail targeting Bet v 1 rapidly and sustainably treats birch allergy symptoms in a phase 1 study. *J. Allergy Clin. Immunol.* **2022**, *149*, 189–199. [CrossRef] [PubMed]
134. Olivieri, B.; Gunaydin, F.E.; Corren, J.; Senna, G.; Durham, S.R. The combination of allergen immunotherapy and biologics for inhalant allergies: Exploring the synergy. *Ann. Allergy Asthma Immunol.* 2024, *in press*. [CrossRef] [PubMed]
135. Casale, T.B.; Busse, W.W.; Kline, J.N.; Ballas, Z.K.; Moss, M.H.; Townley, R.G.; Mokhtarani, M.; Seyfert-Margolis, V.; Asare, A.; Bateman, K.; et al. Omalizumab pretreatment decreases acute reactions after rush immunotherapy for ragweed-induced seasonal allergic rhinitis. *J. Allergy Clin. Immunol.* **2006**, *117*, 134–140. [CrossRef]
136. Dantzer, J.A.; Wood, R.A. The use of omalizumab in allergen immunotherapy. *Clin. Exp. Allergy* **2018**, *48*, 232–240. [CrossRef]

137. De Filippo, M.; Votto, M.; Caminiti, L.; Carella, F.; Castro, G.; Landi, M.; Olcese, R.; Panasiti, I.; Vernich, M.; Barberi, S.; et al. Omalizumab and allergen immunotherapy for respiratory allergies: A mini-review from the Allergen-Immunotherapy Committee of the Italian Society of Pediatric Allergy and Immunology (SIAIP). *Allergol. Immunopathol.* **2022**, *50*, 47–52. [CrossRef]
138. Corren, J.; Saini, S.S.; Gagnon, R.; Moss, M.H.; Sussman, G.; Jacobs, J.; Laws, E.; Chung, E.S.; Constant, T.; Sun, Y.; et al. Short-Term Subcutaneous Allergy Immunotherapy and Dupilumab are Well Tolerated in Allergic Rhinitis: A Randomized Trial. *J. Asthma Allergy* **2021**, *14*, 1045–1063. [CrossRef]
139. Corren, J.; Larson, D.; Altman, M.C.; Segnitz, R.M.; Avila, P.C.; Greenberger, P.A.; Baroody, F.; Moss, M.H.; Nelson, H.; Burbank, A.J.; et al. Effects of combination treatment with tezepelumab and allergen immunotherapy on nasal responses to allergen: A randomized controlled trial. *J. Allergy Clin. Immunol.* **2023**, *151*, 192–201. [CrossRef]

pharmaceuticals

MDPI

Brief Report

Biologic Agents in Idiopathic Hypereosinophilic Syndrome †

Ourania Papaioannou, Fotios Sampsonas, Panagiota Tsiri, Vasilina Sotiropoulou, Ioannis Christopoulos, Dimitrios Komninos and Argyrios Tzouvelekis *

Department of Respiratory Medicine, University Hospital of Patras, 26504 Patras, Greece; ouraniapapaioannou@outlook.com (O.P.); fsampsonas@gmail.com (F.S.); tsiripanayiota@gmail.com (P.T.); v.swtiropoulou@gmail.com (V.S.); christopoulosi94@gmail.com (I.C.); komninos312@gmail.com (D.K.)

* Correspondence: atzouvelekis@upatras.gr or argyris.tzouvelekis@gmail.com

† This article is a revised and expanded version of a paper entitled 'Biologic Agents in Idiopathic Hypereosinophilic Syndrome: A 4-Year-Follow Up in a Case Series', which was presented at the ERS 2024, Vienna, Austria, 7–11 September 2024.

Abstract: Background: Hypereosinophilic syndrome (HES) is a heterogeneous group of rare disorders defined by the presence of marked eosinophilia resulting in end organ damage. The diagnostic approach is multidisciplinary and treatment goals include reductions in flares and eosinophils with minimal drug-related side effects. **Results:** Eleven patients (n = 11) with a diagnosis of idiopathic HES were included in the study [M/F: 6/5, median age: 54 (95% CI: 38.2 to 68.5), smokers/never smokers: 5/6]. Asthma was present in the majority of them (n = 8, 72.7%); four patients (n = 4, 36.4%) presented with eosinophilic pleural effusions, two patients (n = 2, 18.2%) with cardiac arrhythmias, and one with bilateral eyelid angioedema. Eight patients (72.7%) were treated with mepolizumab (300 mg/month) and three (27.3%) with benralizumab (30 mg/4 weeks). The median values of eosinophils at baseline and 12 months after initiation of biologic agent were 3000 (95% CI: 2172 to 11,365) K/μL and 50 (95% CI: 3 to 190) K/μL, respectively, p = 0.0002. All patients with concomitant asthma (n = 8) experienced elimination of asthma flares, asthma control (ACQ < 0.75), functional improvement (mean ΔFEV1: 857 ± 594 mL), and an 82% reduction in oral corticosteroids, p = 0.0001. **Materials and Methods:** Patients with highly characterized idiopathic HES treated with anti-eosinophilic agents between 1 October 2019 and 1 October 2023 were retrospectively included in the study. The aim of this study was to present clinical, laboratory, and functional features and outcomes in patients with thoroughly investigated idiopathic HES treated with biologic agents targeting eosinophils. **Conclusions:** Biologic agents in patients with idiopathic HES—following thorough diagnostic investigation—are both safe and effective, sparing the toxicity of immunosuppressive agents. Real-life data from larger registries are greatly anticipated.

Keywords: hypereosinophilic syndrome; biologic agents; eosinophils

1. Introduction

Hypereosinophilic syndrome (HES) is a heterogeneous group of rare disorders characterized by the presence of remarkable eosinophilia, resulting in end organ damage if treatment is not timely and appropriate [1,2]. In order to diagnose idiopathic HES, we need to exclude all primary and secondary causes of hypereosinophilia [3]. The current definition of HES requires persistent eosinophilia with a corresponding absolute eosinophil count of $>1.5 \times 10^9/L$ for a shorter period of 2 to 4 weeks (compared to the historical criterion of more than 6 months outlined by Chusid and colleagues in 1975), and concomitant tissue damage [4,5]. More specifically, the diagnostic criteria for idiopathic HES include sustained hypereosinophilia (eosinophil count $\geq 1.5 \times 10^9$/L) recorded more than once in a minimum time interval of two weeks, ≥10% eosinophilia, organ failure attributable to the eosinophilia or tissue infiltration by eosinophils, and exclusion of reactive eosinophilia, lymphocyte-variant HES, chronic eosinophilic leukemia, and other myeloid or lymphoid neoplasm [4]. According to the World Health Organization classification for eosinophilic disorders, the diagnosis of idiopathic HES may be in the context of working diagnosis until the final cause of eosinophilia is determined. It is important to mention that in the era of multiple molecular markers of neoplasia, the percentage of patients diagnosed with idiopathic HES decreased [6]. Despite the fact that the epidemiology of HES is not well characterized, the estimated prevalence of HES is up to 6.3 per 100,000 person-years globally [7].

Clinical manifestations are highly variable depending on specific organ involvement. The most common symptomatology involved in HES includes cutaneous (e.g., rash, urticaria, angioedema), pulmonary (e.g., shortness of breath, cough, pulmonary infiltrates, pleural effusion), gastrointestinal (e.g., abdominal pain, nausea, vomiting), constitutional (e.g., fever, fatigue), cardiovascular (e.g., myocardial ischemia, arrhythmias), and neurological (e.g., numbness, weakness, muscle atrophy) manifestations. Among the signs and symptoms recorded, the most common were weakness, fatigue, and cough in 25% of patients, followed by dyspnea, myalgias or angioedema, rash or fever, and rhinitis [8]. Persistent eosinophilia might potentially involve every organ. Skin manifestations were the most common, reported in 69% of patients, followed by respiratory (44%) and gastrointestinal (38%) manifestations. Cardiac disease related to underlying eosinophilic disease was eventually identified in 20% of patients. It is notable that endocardial damage can lead to mural thrombi, increased embolic risk, and restrictive cardiomyopathy [9].

The main pillars of diagnostic approach are the exclusion of secondary reactive causes of eosinophilia, assessing end organ damage based on signs and symptoms, and evaluation for primary clonal eosinophilia [3]. With regard to the secondary causes of eosinophilia, a multidisciplinary discussion with subspecialty experts seems crucial in order to exclude infections, such as parasitic (strongyloides, toxocara, schistosoma, echinococcus, entamoeba, cystoisospora, ascaris, hookworm, trichinella, paragonimus, clonorchis, filariasis), viral (human immunodeficiency virus), fungal (coccidiodes, histoplasma, cryptococcus, pneumocystis), mycobacterial (tuberculosis), and bacterial infections; allergies, such as asthma, allergic rhinitis, atopic dermatitis, and allergic bronchopulmonary aspergillosis; autoimmune causes, such as inflammatory bowel disease, celiac disease, eosinophilic granulomatosis with polyangiitis, rheumatoid arthritis, sarcoidosis, systemic sclerosis, Sjogren's syndrome, bullous pemphigoid, and immunoglobulin (IgG)4-related disease; medications, such as aspirin, nonsteroidal anti-inflammatory drugs, antimicrobials which can lead to drug rash with eosinophilia and systemic symptoms (DRESS) syndrome; malignancies, including solid tumors (lung, renal, colon) and Hodgkin and non-Hodgkin lymphoma; metabolic causes, such as adrenal insufficiency; immune deficiency, including hyper-IgE syndromes, Omenn syndrome, and Wiskott–Aldrich syndrome; and other more rare causes [3]. In order to investigate all aforementioned causes, the diagnostic algorithm includes travel history and parasite testing, including stool culture and antibodies for specific parasites (e.g., strongyloides), in the appropriate clinical context. Additional laboratory testing [e.g., IgE, troponin, autoimmune antibodies] and imaging tests (e.g., chest X-ray; electrocardiogram and cardiac echo; and chest, abdomen, and pelvis computed tomography) are guided by the patient's history, symptomatology, and findings on clinical examination. For eosinophilic lung diseases, pulmonary function tests, bronchoscopy, and serology testing [e.g., aspergillus-specific IgE to evaluate for allergic bronchopulmonary aspergillosis (ABPA)] may be performed [10]. Evaluation of blood and/or bone marrow is characterized by meticulous investigation through serum B12 level, serum tryptase level, serum IgE level, FIP1 like-1 platelet-derived growth factor α-fusion gene (FIP1L1::PDGFRA) fusion by fluorescence in situ hybridization (FISH), or reverse transcription–polymerase chain reaction (RT-PCR) (either on blood sample or bone marrow biopsy), BCR::ABL1 fusion by FISH or RT-PCR (either on blood sample or bone marrow biopsy), T-cell receptor gene rearrangement by PCR (either on blood sample or bone marrow biopsy), immunophenotyping (either on blood sample or bone marrow biopsy), next-generation sequencing myeloid gene panel (either on blood sample or bone marrow biopsy), dysplasia and blast percentage (either on blood sample or bone marrow biopsy), bone marrow fibrosis, immunohistochemistry for CD117 and CD25 if serum tryptase is elevated (bone marrow biopsy), and standard karyotyping (bone marrow biopsy) [3,6,11–14]. The general diagnostic approach is depicted in a flow chart (Figure 1).

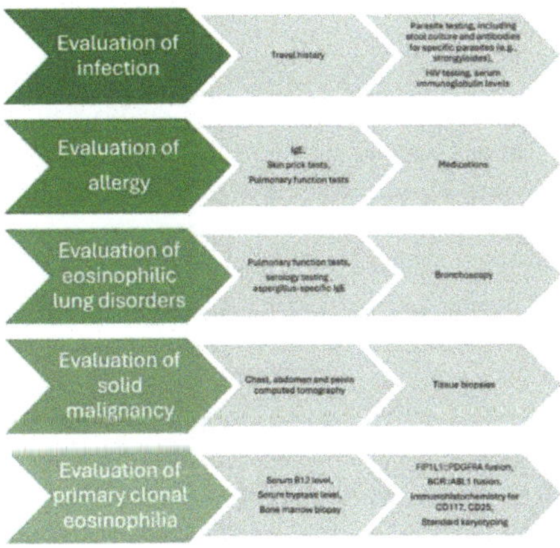

Figure 1. Flow chart of diagnostic approach in idiopathic HES.

It is very challenging to decipher to what extent sustained elevated blood or tissue eosinophils will lead to organ failure. The existing data are insufficient to support a specific eosinophil count for the initiation of treatment in the absence of organ disease. Based on the literature, an absolute eosinophil count of 1.5 to 2 $\times$ 10^9/L is the applied cut-off for initiating therapeutic modalities [3].

Traditional therapeutic options involve corticosteroids, characterized as first-line management unless FIP1L1/PDGFRA-positive; hydroxyurea, as a second-line therapeutic agent; vincristine, especially in children; other cytotoxic or immunomodulatory agents, such as rituximab; imatinib mesylate, as a first-line therapy for FIP1L1/PDGFRA-positive and myeloproliferative variants; and bone marrow transplants for FIP1L1/PDGFRA-positive and imatinib-resistant FIP1L1/PDGFRA-negative variants with disease progression despite standard of care therapies [15,16]. Over the past few years, extensive research efforts have dramatically improved our understanding of HES etiopathogenesis and led to actionable information for the diagnosis, prognosis, and therapeutic management of eosinophil disorders. In line with these, novel biologic agents, including mepolizumab, an anti-interleukin-(IL)5 monoclonal antibody, and benralizumab, a monoclonal antibody targeting IL-5 receptor alpha, have been shown to reduce disease flares and eosinophilic count and alleviate symptoms [5,17]. It is more than evident that the aforementioned beneficial role of IL-5-targeting monoclonal antibodies in the therapeutic management of HES stems from their mechanism of action. Mepolizumab directly binds to, and inactivates, circulating IL-5, while benralizumab, on the other hand, binds to the eosinophil cell membrane at the IL-5 receptor, preventing activation of the receptor, but simultaneously inducing apoptosis of the eosinophil by cross-binding with natural killer cells [18]. Mepolizumab was the first drug in over a decade to receive FDA approval for the treatment of HES without another identifiable non-blood-related cause [16,17,19]. More importantly, these targeted therapies not only present with noteworthy efficacy but also spare treatment-related toxicities. Nonetheless, real-life world evidence on both the safety and effectiveness of these agents is currently scarce and limited. To this end, we conducted a real-life study on biologic agents in patients with HES. The selection of specific biologic therapy was based on the physician's decision, taking into account concomitant severe asthma and the patient's preference.

2. Results

Eleven patients (n = 11) with a diagnosis of idiopathic HES were included in the study [M/F: 6/5, median age: 54 (95% CI: 38.2 to 68.5), smokers/never smokers: 5/6]. Asthma was present in the majority of them (n = 8, 72.7%); four patients (n = 4, 36.4%) presented with eosinophilic pleural effusions, two patients (n = 2, 18.2%) with cardiac arrhythmias, and one with bilateral eyelid angioedema. Eight patients (72.7%) were treated with mepolizumab (300 mg/month) and three (27.3%) with benralizumab (30 mg/4 weeks). The median values of eosinophils at baseline and 12 months after the initiation of biologic treatment were 3000 (95% CI: 2172 to 11,365) K/μL and 50 (95% CI: 3 to 190) K/μL, respectively, p = 0.0002. All patients with concomitant asthma (n = 8)—five of them were treated with mepolizumab (300 mg/month) and three of them were treated with benralizumab (30 mg/4 weeks)—experienced elimination of asthma flares, asthma control [Asthma Control Questionnaire (ACQ) < 0.75], and functional improvement (mean ΔFEV1: 857 ± 594 mL). No significant difference was observed between the two groups of applied biologic agents—mepolizumab and benralizumab—with regard to outcomes. HES flares had been defined as HES-attributable worsening of clinical symptomatology or blood eosinophil counts requiring an escalation in therapy. With regard to the longitudinal use of oral corticosteroids, we noticed that 82% of the patients achieved elimination (p = 0.0001), while the two patients that remained on maintenance oral corticosteroids achieved a reduction in dosing (Table 1, Figure 2). It is also remarkable that all patients improved in terms of forced expiratory volume in 1 s (FEV_1) and forced vital capacity (FVC) on the treatment, despite only one subset of them having been diagnosed with asthma. A diagnosis of asthma was not established in the other subgroup despite the functional improvement in spirometry. Importantly, none of our patients experienced any permanent organ damage and/or dysfunction attributable to tissue eosinophilia. No treatment-related adverse events were noticed. All patients were assessed through clinical examination, laboratory tests, vital signs, or electrocardiographic results for excluding major safety concerns such as hypereosinophilic flares, lymphocytopenia, renal failure, hepatitis, pneumonia, polyneuropathy, or cardiac arrhythmia, or adverse events such as headache, fatigue, peripheral edema, rash, or arthralgia. In addition, none of our patients experienced adverse events associated with the longitudinal use of oral corticosteroids.

Table 1. Characteristics of enrolled patients pre- and 12 months after initiation of biologic treatment (BT).

Characteristics	Pre-BT	Post BT
Oral corticosteroids: prednisone (longitudinal use)	11 (100%)–20 mg/d	2 (18%)–7.5 mg/d
Median value of eosinophils (K/μL) (95%CI)	3000 (2172 to 11,365)	50 (3 to 190)
HES flares	11 (100%)	0 (0%)
Asthma control (ACQ < 0.75)	0 * (0%)	8 * (100%)
ΔFEV1 ± SD	NA	857 ± 594 mL

* Asthma was present in 8 patients with HES.

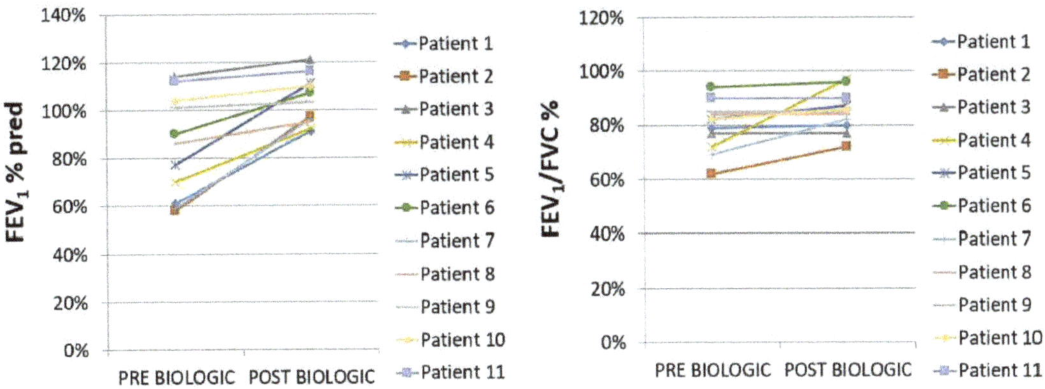

Figure 2. FEV1% pred and FEV1/FVC% tracings pre (baseline) vs. post (12 months after initiation of biologic agent) biologic treatment, $p = 0.04$ and $p = 0.14$, respectively.

3. Discussion

To our knowledge, this was one of the largest real-world studies including a considerable number of highly characterized patients with idiopathic HES treated with anti-eosinophilic biologic agents so far, considering disease rarity [20]. Based on a diagnostic algorithm of eosinophilic disorders, all patients enrolled in our cohort underwent mandatory first-line investigations, as well as further investigations according to patient history and clinical manifestations [6]. Infectious diseases, as well as drug-related hypereosinophilia, were ruled out. Subsequently, real-time quantitative PCR, or FISH and flow cytometry lymphocyte phenotyping, were performed in assessing FIP1L1-PDGFRA gene fusion, rare mutations and rearrangements, and clonal or aberrant T-cell populations in order to exclude clonal bone marrow disease [21]. Based on the fact that HES is a systemic disease and fully dependent on levels of eosinophils, including concomitant coagulation impairment, inflammation, and tissue damage, organ involvement was specifically addressed. The respiratory system, skin, gastrointestinal system, heart vessels, and nervous system were thoroughly assessed.

With regard to therapeutic management, we demonstrated that biologic agents in patients with idiopathic HES are both safe and effective, sparing the toxicity of immunosuppressive agents, including myelosuppression, opportunistic infections, malignancies, or further side effects of long-term corticosteroid use such as hypertension, diabetes mellitus, osteoporosis, myopathy, gastritis, and glaucoma. Our findings are in line with large-scale randomized controlled trials showing the superiority of mepolizumab compared to placebo in reducing disease flares and use of oral corticosteroids. We are also in accordance with a smaller phase 2 trial showing the efficacy of benralizumab in decreasing blood and tissue eosinophilia with no serious toxic effects in patients with severe, treatment-refractory hypereosinophilic syndrome [17,19]. It is important to know that in our country, Greece, mepolizumab is indicated for patients with HES other than asthma and benralizumab is administrated in patients with HES and concomitant severe asthma. Both of them are fully reimbursed following approval by national health committees.

Despite the exponential increase in our understanding of the therapeutic management of eosinophil disorders, the duration of administration of biologic agents targeting eosinophils is still puzzling, taking into account their high cost reimbursed by health systems. Data derived from the literature show that most patients are prone to a baseline level of blood eosinophils and increased risk of exacerbations following the cessation of biologic agents in the context of severe asthma treatment [22–24]. As a consequence, the sudden cessation of biologic treatment in patients with HES could lead to a loss of disease control. Recently, Soendergaard et al., in the OPTIMAL study, suggested that gradual down-titration of anti-IL-5 biologics in severe asthma could be a more appropriate approach to evaluate whether a reduction in or cessation of treatment could be possible, raising concerns for personalized dosing intervals in the future [25]. These data need further validation on a longitudinal basis. In addition, further caution should be applied for potential treatment cessation in disorders lying within the spectrum of hypereosinophilia, as excess eosinophilia requires continuous and more aggressive therapeutic (anti-eosinophilic and/or cytotoxic) approaches.

The number of patients included in our study could be a limitation, but idiopathic HES is a rare entity (10/1,000,000) with scarce real-life data in the literature, so our study could really contribute to this field. In particular, our data represent the largest real-life data on the management of highly characterized HES patients in Greece, and one of the largest published so far in Europe. Thus, we believe that our data add major and valuable knowledge on the effectiveness and safety of biologics in hypereosinophilic disorders in real-life clinical settings.

4. Materials and Methods

We recorded consecutive patients between 10 January 2019 and 1 January 2023 who presented in our Respiratory Department of the University Hospital of Patras, Greece, received a multidisciplinary diagnosis of idiopathic hypereosinophilic syndrome, and were treated with anti-eosinophilic biologic agents from diagnosis until the present. Diagnosis was based on clinical, laboratory, radiological, and histological examination. Secondary causes of eosinophilia, such as infections, particularly tissue-invasive parasites; allergy or atopy and hypersensitivity conditions; drug reactions; collagen–vascular disease (e.g., eosinophilic granulomatosis with polyangiitis, granulomatosis with polyangiitis, systemic lupus erythematosus, IgG4-related disease) pulmonary eosinophilic diseases (e.g., idiopathic acute or chronic eosinophilic pneumonia, allergic bronchopulmonary aspergillosis); allergic gastroenteritis (with associated peripheral eosinophilia); immune deficiency (e.g., hyper-IgE syndromes); and metabolic conditions such as adrenal insufficiency, were excluded, and an evaluation of primary bone marrow disorders was conducted. All patients had a negative immunological profile including *p*, c-ANCA, cyclic citrullinated peptides (CCPs), ANA and extractable nuclear antigen (ENA) panel, normal aspergillus-specific IgE, negative stool culture, normal examination of blood smear, normal serum B12, and tryptase, as well as negative FIP1L1-PDGFRA. A full-body computed tomography scan, pulmonary function testing, bronchoscopy, and hematological consult were included in the work-up of all patients. The diagnostic criteria used for idiopathic HES stem from the definition of the disorder and include hypereosinophilia (>1500 K/μL), related organ dysfunction, and exclusion of secondary causes of hypereosinophilia. Data collection and analysis was approved by the Institutional Review Board and the Local Ethics Committee (protocol number: 19281/05-JUL-2023). Data collection included demographics and history for previous administration of corticosteroids, exacerbations, and comorbidities. Informed consent was obtained from all individual participants included in the study.

5. Conclusions

In conclusion, following the exclusion of eosinophilia due to secondary causes, the diagnostic approach to primary eosinophilia necessitates a combination of a plethora of assessments. Our real-life clinical data support the effectiveness and safety of biologic agents in highly characterized idiopathic HES through the elimination of flares, a reduction in blood eosinophilia, and their steroid-sparing effects. Future real-world evidence from larger registries aiming to identify the safety and efficacy profiles of anti-eosinophilic biologic agents in HES is greatly anticipated.

Author Contributions: Conception: O.P. and A.T. Methodology: O.P. and A.T. Investigation: O.P., F.S., P.T., V.S., I.C. and D.K. Data analysis: O.P. and A.T. Writing of draft paper: O.P. and A.T. Supervision: A.T. Revision and approval of final paper: all authors. All authors have read and agreed to the published version of the manuscript.

Funding: The publication of this article has been financed by the University of Patras.

Institutional Review Board Statement: Data collection and analysis was approved by the Institutional Review Board and the Local Ethics Committee with protocol number: 19281/05-JUL-2023 on 5 July 2023.

Informed Consent Statement: Informed consent for publication was obtained from all individual participants included in this study.

Data Availability Statement: Data are available on request. O.P. and A.T. have full access to the data and are the guarantors for these data.

Acknowledgments: The authors thank the patients who participated in the study.

Conflicts of Interest: The authors declare no conflicts of interest.

References

1. Valent, P.; Klion, A.D.; Roufosse, F.; Simon, D.; Metzgeroth, G.; Leiferman, K.M.; Schwaab, J.; Butterfield, J.H.; Sperr, W.R.; Sotlar, K.; et al. Proposed refined diagnostic criteria and classification of eosinophil disorders and related syndromes. *Allergy* **2023**, *78*, 47–59. [CrossRef] [PubMed]
2. Valent, P.; Klion, A.D.; Horny, H.-P.; Roufosse, F.; Gotlib, J.; Weller, P.F.; Hellmann, A.; Metzgeroth, G.; Leiferman, K.M.; Arock, M., et al. Contemporary consensus proposal on criteria and classification of eosinophilic disorders and related syndromes. *J. Allergy Clin. Immunol.* **2012**, *130*, 607–612.e9. [CrossRef] [PubMed]
3. Shomali, W.; Gotlib, J. World Health Organization and International Consensus Classification of eosinophilic disorders: 2024 update on diagnosis, risk stratification, and management. *Am. J. Hematol.* **2024**, *99*, 946–968. [CrossRef] [PubMed]
4. Wang, S.A.; Orazi, A.; Gotlib, J.; Reiter, A.; Tzankov, A.; Hasserjian, R.P.; Arber, D.A.; Tefferi, A. The international consensus classification of eosinophilic disorders and systemic mastocytosis. *Am. J. Hematol.* **2023**, *98*, 1286–1306. [CrossRef]
5. Klion, A.D.; Bochner, B.S.; Gleich, G.J.; Nutman, T.B.; Rothenberg, M.E.; Simon, H.U.; Wechsler, M.E.; Weller, P.F.; The Hypereosinophilic Syndromes Working Group. Approaches to the treatment of hypereosinophilic syndromes: A workshop summary report. *J. Allergy Clin. Immunol.* **2006**, *117*, 1292–1302. [CrossRef]
6. Caminati, M.; Brussino, L.; Carlucci, M.; Carlucci, P.; Carpagnano, L.F.; Caruso, C.; Cosmi, L.; D'Amore, S.; Del Giacco, S.; Detoraki, A.; et al. Managing Patients with Hypereosinophilic Syndrome: A Statement from the Italian Society of Allergy, Asthma, and Clinical Immunology (SIAAIC). *Cells* **2024**, *13*, 1180. [CrossRef]
7. Crane, M.M.; Chang, C.M.; Kobayashi, M.G.; Weller, P.F. Incidence of myeloproliferative hypereosinophilic syndrome in the United States and an estimate of all hypereosinophilic syndrome incidence. *J. Allergy Clin. Immunol.* **2010**, *126*, 179–181. [CrossRef]
8. Weller, P.F.; Bubley, G.J. The idiopathic hypereosinophilic syndrome. *Blood* **1994**, *83*, 2759–2779. [CrossRef]
9. Gotlib, J.; Cools, J.; Malone, J.M.; Schrier, S.L., 3rd; Gilliland, D.G.; Coutre, S.E. The FIP1L1-PDGFRalpha fusion tyrosine kinase in hypereosinophilic syndrome and chronic eosinophilic leukemia: Implications for diagnosis, classification, and management. *Blood* **2004**, *103*, 2879–2891. [CrossRef]
10. Wardlaw, A.J.; Wharin, S.; Aung, H.; Shaffu, S.; Siddiqui, S. The causes of a peripheral blood eosinophilia in a secondary care setting. *Clin. Exp. Allergy* **2021**, *51*, 902–914. [CrossRef]
11. Klion, A.D.; Noel, P.; Akin, C.; Law, M.A.; Gilliland, D.G.; Cools, J.; Metcalfe, D.D.; Nutman, T.B. Elevated serum tryptase levels identify a subset of patients with a myeloproliferative variant of idiopathic hypereosinophilic syndrome associated with tissue fibrosis, poor prognosis, and imatinib responsiveness. *Blood* **2003**, *101*, 4660–4666. [PubMed]
12. Schwaab, J.; Jawhar, M.; Naumann, N.; Schmitt-Graeff, A.; Fabarius, A.; Horny, H.-P.; Cross, N.C.P.; Hofmann, W.-K.; Reiter, A.; Metzgeroth, G. Diagnostic challenges in the work up of hypereosinophilia: Pitfalls in bone marrow core biopsy interpretation. *Ann. Hematol.* **2016**, *95*, 557–562. [PubMed]

13. Metzgeroth, G.; Walz, C.; Score, J.; Siebert, R.; Schnittger, S.; Haferlach, C.; Popp, H.; Haferlach, T.; Erben, P.; Mix, J.; et al. Recurrent finding of the FIP1L1-PDGFRA fusion gene in eosinophilia-associated acute myeloid leukemia and lymphoblastic T-cell lymphoma. *Leukemia* **2007**, *21*, 1183–1188. [PubMed]
14. Caminati, M.; Carpagnano, L.F.; Alberti, C.; Amaddeo, F.; Bixio, R.; Caldart, F.; De Franceschi, L.; Del Giglio, M.; Festi, G.; Friso, S.; et al. Idiopathic hypereosinophilic syndromes and rare dysimmune conditions associated with hyper-eosinophilia in practice: An innovative multidisciplinary approach. *World Allergy Organ. J.* **2024**, *17*, 100928.
15. Curtis, C.; Ogbogu, P. Hypereosinophilic Syndrome. *Clin. Rev. Allergy Immunol.* **2016**, *50*, 240–251.
16. Steinfeld, J.; Rofousse, F.; Kahn, J.-E.; Gleich, G.; Rothenberg, M.; Wardlaw, A.; Kirby, S.Y.; Gilson, M.; Bentley, J.; Bradford, E.; et al. Efficacy and safety of mepolizumab in hypereosinophilic syndrome: A phase III, randomized, placebo-controlled trial. *J. Allergy Clin. Immunol.* **2020**, *146*, 1397–1405.
17. Kuang, F.L.; Legrand, F.; Makiya, M.; Ware, J.; Wetzler, L.; Brown, T.; Magee, T.; Piligian, B.; Yoon, P.; Ellis, J.H.; et al. Benralizumab for PDGFRA-Negative Hypereosinophilic Syndrome. *N. Engl. J. Med.* **2019**, *380*, 1336–1346. [CrossRef]
18. Langton, D.; Politis, J.; Collyer, T.; Khung, S.W.; Bardin, P. Benralizumab and mepolizumab treatment outcomes in two severe asthma clinics. *Respirology* **2023**, *28*, 1117–1125.
19. Steinfeld, J.; Gleich, G.; Roufosse, F.; Chupp, G.; Faguer, S.; Reiter, A.; Walz, B.; Bentley, J.; Bradford, E.; Yancey, S. Safety and Efficacy of Mepolizumab in Hypereosinophilic Syndrome: An Open-Label Extension Study. *J. Allergy Clin. Immunol. Pract.* **2021**, *9*, 4431–4440.e1.
20. Papaioannou, O.; Tsiri, P.; Sotiropoulou, V.; Christopoulos, I.; Komninos, D.; Koulousousa, E.; Theochari, E.; Tsirikos, G.; Sampsonas, F.; Tzouvelekis, A. Biologic agents in idiopathic hypereosinophilic syndrome: A 4-year-follow up in a case series. *Eur. Respir. J.* **2024**, *64* (Suppl. S68), PA1772.
21. Bacher, U.; Reiter, A.; Haferlach, T.; Mueller, L.; Schnittger, S.; Kern, W.; Schoch, C. A combination of cytomorphology, cytogenetic analysis, fluorescence in situ hybridization and reverse transcriptase polymerase chain reaction for establishing clonality in cases of persisting hypereosinophilia. *Haematologica* **2006**, *91*, 817–820. [PubMed]
22. Haldar, P.; Brightling, C.E.; Singapuri, A.; Hargadon, B.; Gupta, S.; Monteiro, W.; Bradding, P.; Green, R.H.; Wardlaw, A.J.; Ortega, H.; et al. Outcomes after cessation of mepolizumab therapy in severe eosinophilic asthma: A 12-month follow-up analysis. *J. Allergy Clin. Immunol.* **2014**, *133*, 921–923. [PubMed]
23. Ortega, H.; Lemiere, C.; Llanos, J.-P.; Forshag, M.; Price, R.; Albers, F.; Yancey, S.; Castro, M. Outcomes following mepolizumab treatment discontinuation: Real-world experience from an open-label trial. *Allergy Asthma Clin. Immunol.* **2019**, *15*, 37. [PubMed]
24. Moore, W.C.; Kornmann, O.; Humbert, M.; Poirier, C.; Bel, E.H.; Kaneko, N.; Smith, S.G.; Martin, N.; Gilson, M.J.; Price, R.G.; et al. Stopping versus continuing long-term mepolizumab treatment in severe eosinophilic asthma (COMET study). *Eur. Respir. J.* **2022**, *59*, 2100396.
25. Soendergaard, M.B.; Bjerrum, A.S.; Rasmussen, L.M.; Lock-Johansson, S.; Hilberg, O.; Hansen, S.; von Bulow, A.; Porsbjerg, C. Titration of anti-IL-5 biologics in severe asthma: An open-label randomised controlled trial (the OPTIMAL study). *Eur. Respir. J.* **2024**, *64*, 2400404.

pharmaceuticals MDPI

Article

Adjuvant Effect of *Lactobacillus paracasei* in Sublingual Immunotherapy of Asthmatic Mice

Dhafer Alwayli [1], Xiaoli Jiang [1], Jiaxu Liang [1], Syed Rafiq Hussain Shah [1], Atta Ullah [1], Mohammed F. Z. Abusidu [2] and Wen Shu [1,*]

1 Department of Pathogen Biology and Microecology, School of Basic Medical Sciences, Dalian Medical University, Dalian 116044, China; dhafer21@dmu.edu.cn (D.A.); xiaoly1109@163.com (X.J.); 18754663572@163.com (J.L.); syedrafiq223@gmail.com (S.R.H.S.); attaakhan902@gmail.com (A.U.)

2 Department of Biotechnology, School of Basic Medical Sciences, Dalian Medical University, Dalian 116044, China; mohammadabuseedo@gmail.com

* Correspondence: shuwen@dmu.edu.cn; Tel.: +86-136-2411-1836

Abstract: Background: Sublingual immunotherapy (SLIT) has shown promise in mitigating allergic asthma symptoms; nevertheless, its high dose and prolonged duration of treatment raise safety concerns. This study explored the potential of *Lactobacillus paracasei* (*L. paracasei*) to enhance the effectiveness of SLIT in a mouse model of allergic asthma. **Methods**: Allergic asthma was induced in Balb/c mice following sensitization and challenge with a house dust mite (HDM) allergen. Subsequently, the mice were subjected to SLIT (66 and 132 μg) either alone or in combination with *L. paracasei* supplementation. Asthma-associated parameters, including rubbing frequency, IgE level, cytokine profiles, and histological changes, were evaluated to assess treatment efficacy. **Results**: mice that received SLIT 132 μg combined with the probiotic (combined 132) demonstrated a significant reduction in allergic symptoms (rubbing). This treatment strategy led to a marked IgE and eosinophil level decrease in serum; an increase in anti-inflammatory cytokines like IFN-γ and IL-10; and a reduction in pro-inflammatory cytokines IL-17 and TNF-α. The combination therapy also mitigated lung inflammation and supported the restoration of the structural integrity of the colon, promoting the recovery of goblet cells and mucus secretion. Probiotic treatment alone also effectively reduced IgE levels, increased IFN-γ, and decreased levels of IL-17 and TNF-α. **Conclusions**: The adjuvant effect of *L. paracasei* in enhancing SLIT represents a promising approach for improving asthma treatment efficacy.

Keywords: allergic asthma; house dust mite; probiotic; sublingual immunotherapy

1. Introduction

Asthma is a complex and chronic lung condition affecting nearly 300 million people globally, with an additional 100 million cases increasing by 2025 [1]. Allergic asthma, the most common phenotype of the disease, is featured by chronic inflammation and airway hyperresponsiveness (AHR), which can remarkably impair life quality [1–3]. If severe, cases of allergic asthma can be fatal and besides its link to health problems, it also contributes to significant economic burdens, reducing productivity and impacting education and quality of work [3]. Key characteristics of allergic asthma involve persistent airway inflammation, AHR, and structural changes such as airway remodeling, which collectively contribute to airflow obstruction and worsen the symptom's severity [4,5].

The disturbed balance between various T-helper (Th) cell subtypes acts crucially in allergic asthma pathogenesis [6]. Specifically, a skewed Th2/Th1 balance is one of the key drivers of allergic asthma. Th2 cells produce cytokines such as IL-4, IL-5, and IL-13, which are pivotal in promoting IgE synthesis and subsequent histamine release (IL-4 and IL-13), eosinophilia (IL-5), and mucus oversecretion, airway hyperresponsiveness, and remodeling (IL-13). In contrast, Th1 cells typically act to counter-regulate Th2 responses through the production of IFN-γ. The Th2 pathway is overactivated in allergic asthma, whereas Th1-mediated responses are suppressed. This leads to persistent inflammation and worsened symptoms [7]. Furthermore, the development of allergic asthma is also influenced by the Th17/regulatory (Treg) imbalance. Th17 cells contribute to neutrophilic inflammation and remodeling through their production of IL-17. Increased levels of IL-17 have been linked to severe, steroid-resistant asthma. In contrast, Treg cells, which secrete anti-inflammatory cytokines like IL-10 and TGF-β, are in charge of preserving immunological tolerance and preventing excessive inflammatory responses. Treg cells are in charge of maintaining immune tolerance and averting overly inflammatory reactions because they emit anti-inflammatory cytokines including TGF-β and IL-10. A decrease in Treg cells or their malfunction exacerbates the inflammatory response, resulting in uncontrolled Th2 and Th17 activity and emphasizing the necessity of immunological balance-restoring treatment approaches [8].

Allergen immunotherapy (AIT) is one of the allergic asthma symptom modulators that involve gradually exposing patients to increasing doses of the offending allergen [9–11]. AIT can reduce allergic reactions through mechanisms that antagonize allergic asthma [12]. Among the various forms of AIT, sublingual immunotherapy (SLIT) has shown great potential in promoting tolerance to HDM in humans [13–15], and mice [16–19]. The primary mechanisms of SLIT involve the stimulation of allergen-specific IgG production by B cells and plasma cells. These IgG antibodies either compete with IgE for binding sites or prevent IgE cross-linking, thus inhibiting mast cell and basophil degranulation and the release of histamine [9–11,20,21]. Additionally, SLIT promotes the induction of tolerogenic dendritic cells (tDCs), which drive the production of Tregs and Bregs [22–26]. Despite the benefits, a SLIT high-dose and long-term treatment regimen (need 2–3 years) poses risks, including potential adverse reactions during treatment (particularly for children).

Probiotics have been demonstrated to play a substantial role in normalizing immune responses [27–29], though the exact mechanisms remain under investigation. Studies in murine models have shown that probiotics can trigger a shift from a Th2- to a Th1-dominant immune response, enrich T regulatory cells (Tregs), and restrict Th17 activity [30–32]. This immunomodulatory effect of probiotics has been associated with reducing allergic asthma in humans and mice [33,34]. Notably, *Bifidobacterium* and *Lactobacillus* augment short-chain fatty acids (SCFAs) like butyrate and acetate, which alleviate inflammation by enhancing Tregs and reducing the Th2-mediated allergic reactions [35,36]. While animal studies provide promising evidence of probiotics' role in reducing airway inflammation and potentially preventing allergic asthma, clinical trials in humans have produced mixed results [37,38]. The variability in results may be attributed to the use of different strains of probiotics across studies [39]. Because *L. paracasei* has been proven as safe in previous research [40–42], we used it in this study. Additionally, this strain has shown promising results and safety in earlier studies conducted in our lab utilizing OVA-sensitized rats and mice models. This study aims to explore the adjuvant effect of *L. paracasei* in SLIT of asthmatic mice. Overall, probiotics may rebalance immune response and reduce inflammation via IL-10 induction and SCFA production, which could complement SLIT by abolishing its side effects. Therefore, some synergistic effects are expected when probiotics are simultaneously administered during SLIT, and due to their favorable safety profile, probiotics could mitigate the side effects often associated with SLIT.

2. Results

2.1. Combined 132 Ameliorates Allergic Symptoms in Mice

Nasal scratching is largely associated with histamine release. In this experiment, we established an allergic asthma model in mice and evaluated the inhibitory effect of treatments on nasal itching by applying different treatments and counting the number of rubs in the different groups of mice within 15 min post-challenge on days 19, 21, and 24. HDM-induced allergic asthma mice displayed significantly increased frequencies of rubbing compared with control mice (Figure 1A–C; $p < 0.05$). As shown in Figure 1A–C, the number of rubs for allergic asthma mice given combined132 treatment was lower than the number for those not given treatment ($p < 0.01$, $p < 0.01$, and $p < 0.05$, respectively). These results suggested that combined 132 ameliorated the symptoms of rubbing in allergic asthma mice.

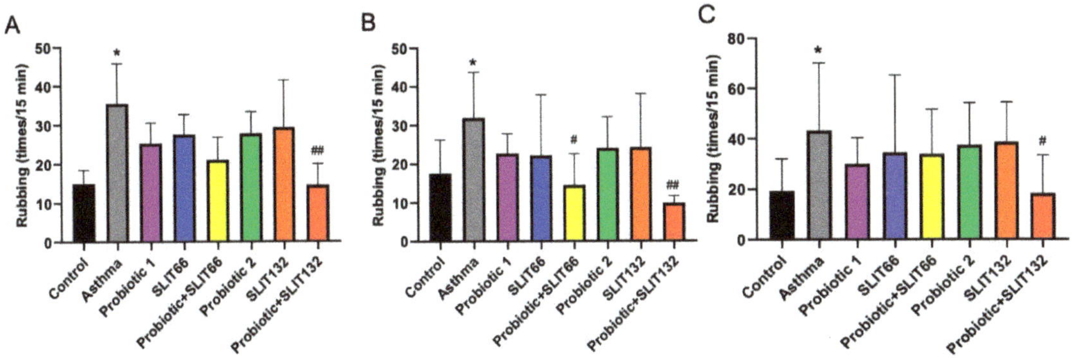

Figure 1. The effects of a probiotic, SLIT, and their combination on the frequency of nasal rubbing. Treatment with combined 132 demonstrated a significant decrease in the frequency of nasal rubbing on (**A**) day 19, (**B**) day 21, and (**C**) day 24 following an HDM challenge. * $p < 0.05$ vs. the control group; # $p < 0.05$ and ## $p < 0.01$ vs. the asthma group.

2.2. Changes in Serum IgE and Cytokine Levels After Treatment with SLIT and L. paracasei

To assess the effectiveness of the probiotic, SLIT, and their combination on HDM-induced allergic asthma in mice, various immune parameters, including serum IgE and cytokine levels (IL-4, IL-17, TNFα, IFN-γ, and IL-10), were detected using ELISA. As depicted in Figure 2A–I, HDM sensitization and subsequent challenge led to a significant elevation in the levels of IgE and IL-4, IL-17, and TNF-α when compared to the control group. On the other hand, the levels of IFN-γ and IL-10 were notably reduced in these HDM-exposed groups, indicating a clear immunological response consistent with HDM sensitization. After treatment application, IFN-γ levels showed a significant increase across all treatment groups (Figure 2B; $p < 0.0001$). IL-17 levels were significantly reduced following treatment, with the most notable reduction observed in the probiotic-only and combined groups (Figure 2E; $p < 0.0001$). The production of IL-10 was significantly elevated in the probiotic-only, SLIT 132, and combined 132 groups compared to the asthma group ($p < 0.001$) (Figure 2D). TNF-α levels also significantly decreased in both the probiotic-only and combined 132 groups ($p < 0.05$). IgE levels were markedly reduced following treatment with probiotic-only and combined 132 groups ($p < 0.05$). Although a downward trend in serum IL-4 levels was observed in the combined 132 group, the reduction was not statistically significant (Figure 2A).

2.3. Combined 132 Reduces Eosinophil and Neutrophil Levels in Mice Serum

Figure 2G,H show the total and differential inflammatory cells in serum for neutrophils and eosinophils. According to the results, there were no significant differences among the total cell counts in any of the treatment groups vs. asthma (Figure 2G). However, the evaluation of the differential cell counts for neutrophils and eosinophils revealed a percentual decrease in eosinophils and neutrophils in the combined 132 group compared to the asthma group (Figure 2H,I, $p < 0.001$ and $p = 0.05$, respectively).

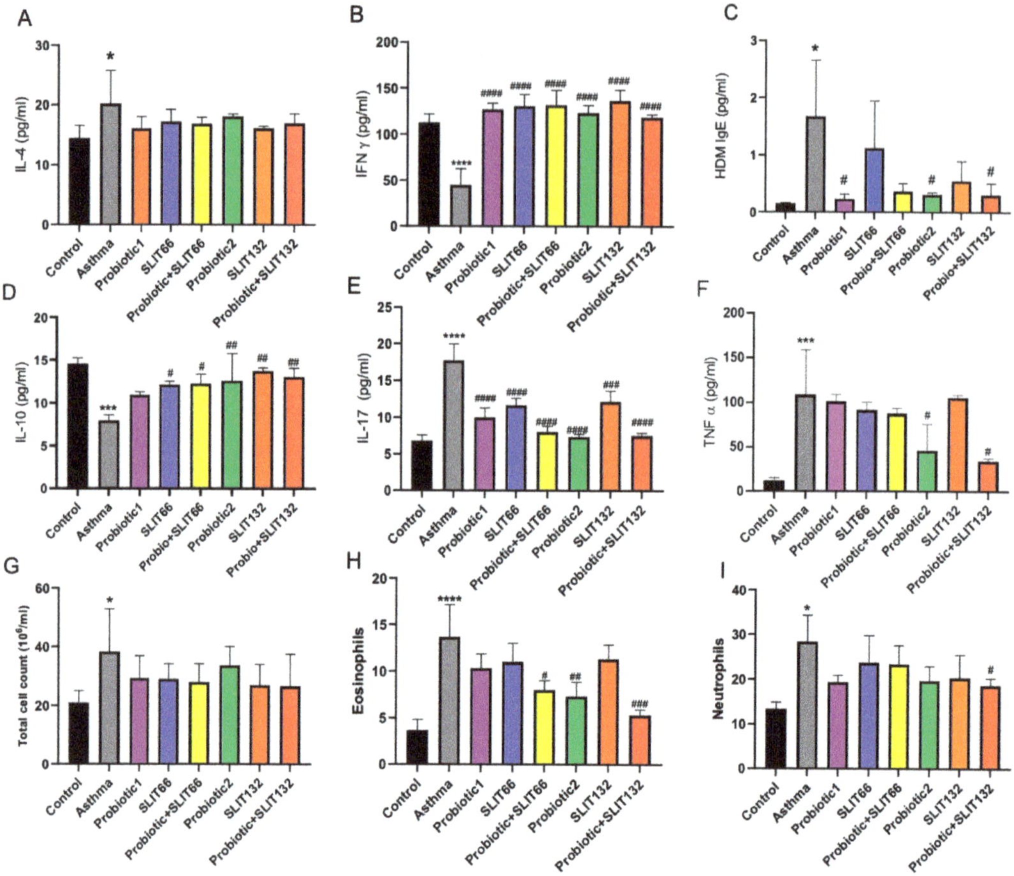

Figure 2. The effects of a probiotic, SLIT, and their combination on inflammatory cell count, IgE, and cytokine concentrations. Serum IgE and cytokines of asthmatic and treated mice of all groups were measured by ELISA. The concentrations of (**A**) pro-inflammatory cytokine IL-4, (**B**) Interferon gamma (IFN-γ), (**C**) HDM IgE, (**D**) IL-10, (**E**) IL-17, (**F**) tumor necrosis factor alpha (TNFα). The enumeration of inflammatory cells in blood, including (**G**) total blood cells, (**H**) eosinophils, and (**I**) neutrophils obtained from various groups. * $p < 0.05$, *** $p < 0.001$, and **** $p < 0.0001$ vs. the control group; # $p < 0.05$, ## $p < 0.01$, ### $p < 0.001$, and #### $p < 0.0001$ vs. the asthma group.

2.4. Combined 132 Mitigates Lung Damage and Reduces Airway Inflammation in HDM-Sensitized Mice

Histopathological assessments were conducted to further evaluate the degree of HDM-induced airway inflammation. Asthmatic mice displayed significant immune cell infiltration in lung tissues. As shown in Figure 3A, all treatments exhibited less lung inflammation and cell infiltration; however, treatment with combined 132 notably further improved outcomes. Inflammation in the lung tissue's peribronchial and perialveolar areas was graded using a subjective scale from 0 to 4. After treatment with combined 132, the inflammation score decreased significantly, approaching levels similar to those of the control group (Figure 3B, $p < 0.001$). To examine interstitial GC hyperplasia, we utilized PAS staining. The asthma group displayed a higher number of PAS-positive cells compared to the control group. However, treating asthmatic mice with combined 132 significantly reduced the area of PAS-stained and PAS-positive cells (Figure 3C,D, $p < 0.0001$).

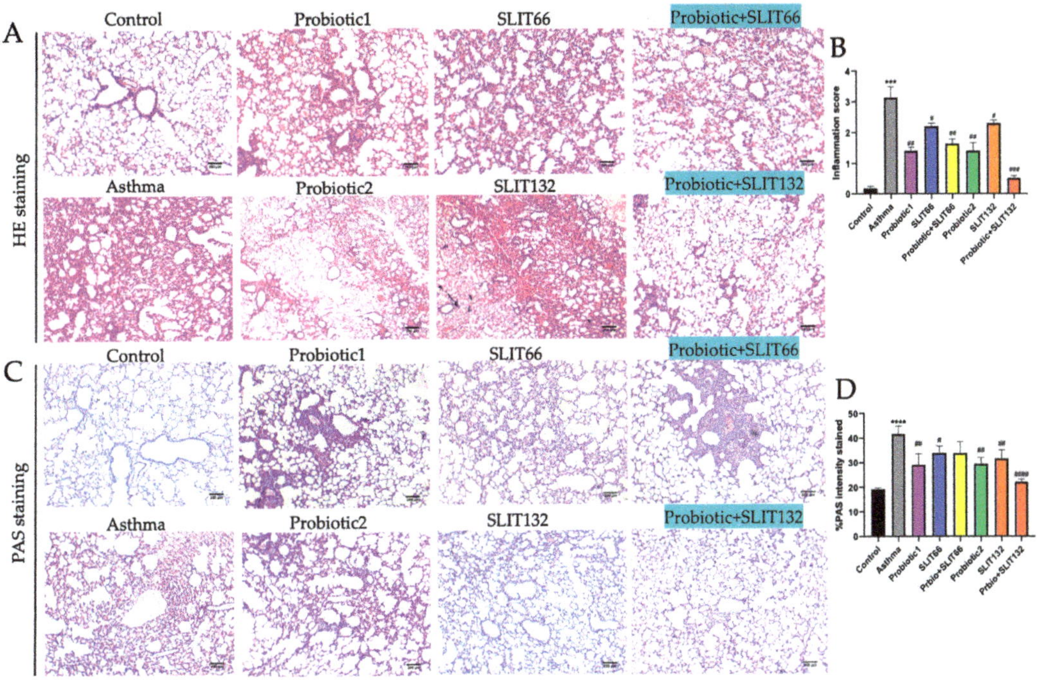

Figure 3. A probiotic, SLIT, and their combination improved asthma induced histopathological change in mice lungs. (**A**) H&E staining of mice lung tissues. Lung sections stained with H&E revealed infiltrations of inflammatory cells in HDM-sensitized and -challenged mice, contrasting with the control group where such aggregations were absent. Notably, treated mice exhibited distinctive features in this context. (**B**) Inflammation score. (**C**) PAS staining was applied to mouse lung sections following intranasal HDM exposure. (**D**) % PAS intensity of stained tissue. Scale bar = 200 μm; Magnification: 40×. *** $p < 0.001$ and **** $p < 0.0001$ vs. the control group; # $p < 0.05$, ## $p < 0.01$, ### $p < 0.001$, and #### $p < 0.0001$ vs. the asthma group.

2.5. Combined 132 Improves GCs' Number and Mucin Production in the Colon of HDM-Sensitized Mice

We here identified whether asthma in mice could lead to colon injury and possible improvement after treatment application. In the asthma group, mice exhibited apparent changes in the colon histostructure, with a damaged and unevenly arranged epithelium after staining with H&E. The mucosal space appeared to be ill defined, and the infiltration of inflammatory cells was observed (Figure 4A). To further assess the effect of asthma on goblet cells and mucin content within the colon, we conducted AB and PAS staining. This technique stains acidic mucins blue using AB and neutral mucins magenta with PAS. PAS and AB staining of the asthma lung revealed hallmarks of pathological features of allergic asthma, including a decrease in GCs' number, and intensity of acid mucin production (Figure 4B,E). The total mucin intensity and the number of GCs in colonic tissue sections were measured by ImageJ software (version 1.4.3.67) Figure 4C,D,F,G). However, GCs' number and mucin secretion were recovered after staining with PAS ($p < 0.001$ and $p < 0.0001$) and AB ($p < 0.0001$ and $p < 0.01$), and inflammatory infiltration was reduced following treatment, particularly with combined 132.

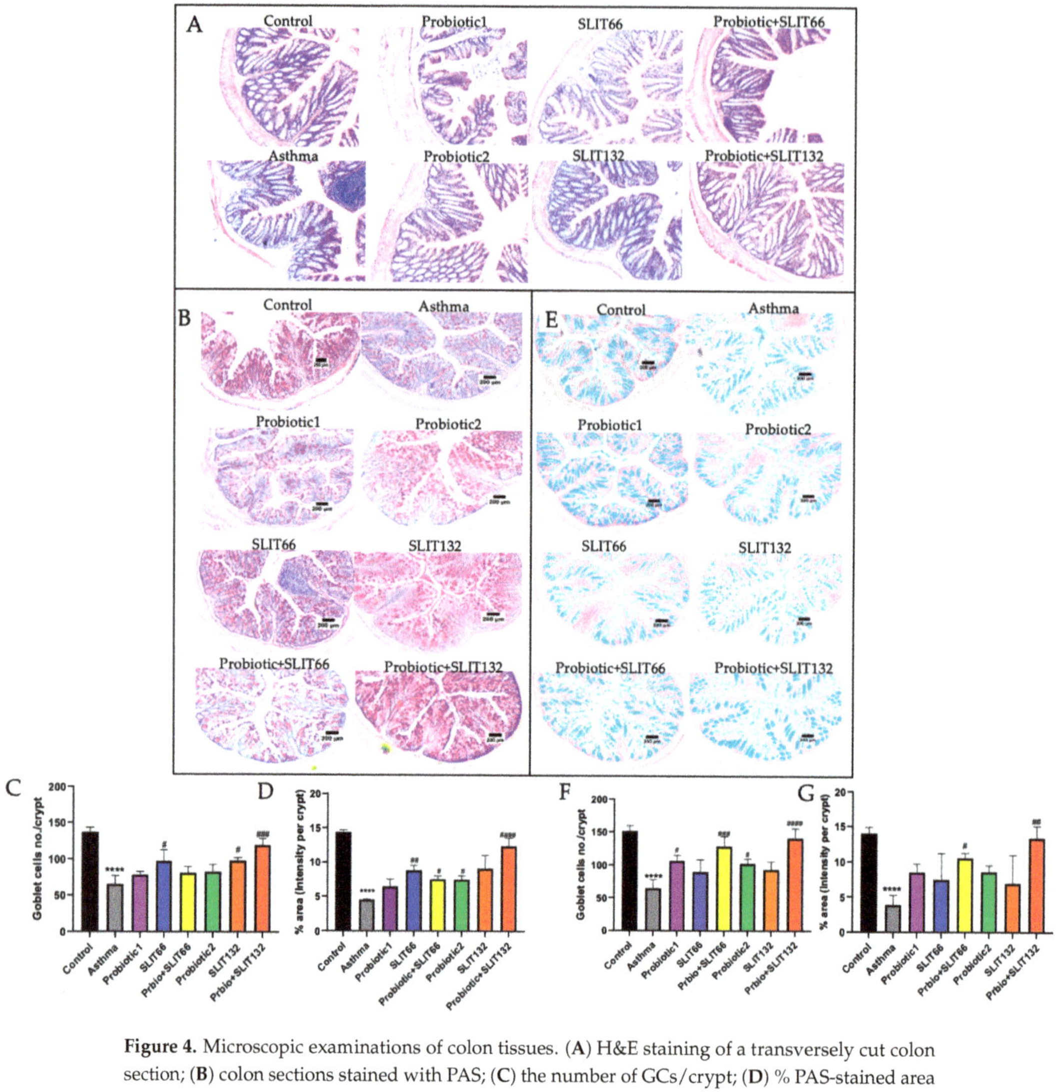

Figure 4. Microscopic examinations of colon tissues. (**A**) H&E staining of a transversely cut colon section; (**B**) colon sections stained with PAS; (**C**) the number of GCs/crypt; (**D**) % PAS-stained area of GCs and mucin; (**E**) colon sections stained with AB staining; (**F**) the number of GCs/crypt in AB-stained areas; and (**G**) % AB-stained areas were assessed in all groups. Magnification: 100×. **** $p < 0.0001$ vs. the control group; # $p < 0.05$, ## $p < 0.01$, ### $p < 0.001$, and #### $p < 0.0001$ vs. the asthma group.

3. Discussion

Our study involved the administration of sublingual allergen therapy, a strategy rooted in prior research showing its potential in modulating T-cell responses and inhibiting eosinophil-mediated inflammation. This method, particularly useful in pediatric populations due to its non-invasive nature, avoids the need for frequent clinical visits or injections [43]. However, the extended treatment typically lasts two to three years—and the gradual increase in dosage can lead to undesirable side effects, potentially reducing patient compliance and carrying concerns about its overall safety [44,45]. Recent advancements have focused on enhancing the efficacy of SLIT while mitigating its side effects. Our investigation aimed to enhance immunity and reduce inflammation through the combined use of probiotics and SLIT, with the expectation that effective regulation can be achieved safely even at low doses and over a short duration.

It is well understood that SLIT follows a dose- and time-dependent relationship, though these aspects remain subjects of ongoing research and discussion [46]. In this study, we implemented two dosage levels: 66 µg (low dose) and 132 µg (relatively higher). Despite the difference, both doses still fall within the low-dose range when compared to previously established SLIT dose standards. The SLIT regimen alone shows poor efficacy in our short-term model; this is consistent with other studies [16]. It is inspiring that the combination therapy exhibited a significant reduction in rubbing counts, indicating a pronounced alleviation of allergy-associated symptoms, which is two-fold lower in dose and 11-fold shorter in duration than other studies that demonstrated beneficial effects [47,48]. This is in agreement with the hypothesis of this study; interestingly, our low-dose SLIT in a short time showed a similar effect and less side function compared to high-dose SLIT in a long time when combined with the probiotics. The efficacy of SLIT may be potentiated with higher doses and prolonged treatment durations, though this can induce a higher incidence of adverse reactions. Moreover, using low doses with longer duration gives conflicting results in some studies. While some showed a good effect [16], others showed a weak one [49].

The significant effects observed in the combined group are based on the restoration of immune balance. This combination treatment strategy led to a marked IgE, eosinophil, and neutrophil level decrease in serum; an increase in anti-inflammatory cytokines like IFN-γ and IL-10; and a reduction in pro-inflammatory cytokines IL-17 and TNF-α. It has better improvement in TNF-α, eosinophils, and IgE than the SLIT group. IgE is the key target for AIT therapy [9–11]; it can serve as a characteristic indicator for evaluating the level of therapies. The lack of a significant reduction in IgE indicates that low-dose, short-term SLIT has limited efficacy in treating asthma. Supporting this, Shima et al. also found that SLIT did not significantly lower IgE but still managed to reduce eosinophilic inflammation [10]. This outcome underscores the potential synergistic role of probiotics in supporting the overall efficacy of SLIT. IL-17 and TNF-α cytokines are essential in neutrophil infiltration within the lungs of asthma patients, and their decline indicates an attenuating of neutrophilic inflammation [50]. Previous studies reported that IL-17 and TNF-α are acting synergistically during the inflammation process [51]. Thus, downregulating these cytokines partially approves combination efficacy. Additionally, the better recovery of eosinophils and neutrophils suggests that the combined group more effectively regulated immune imbalance, thereby achieving better therapeutic outcomes. Moreover, it should be pointed out that the probiotic similarly triggered certain important parameters, i.e., a significant production of IL-10 and decrease in IL-17 levels, and these responses could have helped the promotion of SLIT through pathways mediated by cell signals. We suggest that our probiotic appears consequently to be a probiotic strain that induces, in immature DC, the production of IL-10 concomitant with a low-level induction of IL-17. While the combination therapy did not significantly impact IL-4 levels, it significantly elevated IFN-γ levels, further enhancing the anti-inflammatory effect of the treatment.

Lung inflammation can cause airway epithelial barrier dysfunction and remodeling [52]. It has been known that Th2-secreted cytokines such as IL-4 and IL-5 can release IgE and eosinophil migration to airways (airway eosinophilia), mucus hypersecretion, and GC hyperplasia [53]. In our study, asthma mice displayed inflammatory cell infiltration (both alveolar and peribranchial) as HE- and PAS-stained cells are increased in intensity as shown with a high purple-red color and, with the administration of combination 132, could markedly alleviate inflammation as displayed with the lowest inflammation score compared with other treatment regimens. This complies with other studies' findings [16,17]. This airway barrier injury is most likely related to our immunological findings. Relatedly, we could also analyze colon histopathology to further explore whether asthma has an impact on the intestine, particularly, the colon. Undeniably, intestinal epithelial cells are crucial for maintaining normal intestinal permeability and barrier integrity. Mucins, GC-secreted materials, play a role in maintaining the epithelial barrier [54]. The examination of colon photomicrographs showed a decrease in GCs along with a lower PAS staining intensity in the asthma group compared to the normal control group, implying a lower secretion of neutral mucins. Similar findings have been observed in previous studies where it was seen that asthma induces intestinal injury [55]. While different treatment groups provide variable significant effects in this study, most superior improvements were observed with the combination of SLIT and a probiotic. The combination may lead to an early onset of SLIT efficacy through the additive effects of the probiotic activation of Treg cells in the lung and intestine. However, SCFAs can be a contributor to these effects, which require further exploration as agreed on by other studies [56,57]. In our study, combined 132 group treatment restored the damaged mucosal integrity caused by asthma by replenishing the GC population, implying a favorable modulation of the immune response with the combined treatment.

In summary, we found that the combined treatment of a probiotic with SLIT demonstrated a synergistic effect in reducing inflammation and ameliorating asthma, attenuating the airway and colon barrier primarily in a gut–lung axis-dependent manner and microbiota-dependent modulation. Probiotic treatment alone also showed some level of protection against asthma. The superiority of the SLIT–probiotic combination was most likely clear, potentially because the SLIT mechanism of action is similar to that of a probiotic. However, these results remain contentious, and further research is needed to deeply understand these synergistic effects, including the need for human validation and more profound and comprehensive immunological investigations in mice.

4. Materials and Methods

4.1. Mice, Housing, and Grouping

Six-to-eight-week-old male BALB/c mice (n = 80), weighted 18–20 g, were supplied by Liaoning Changsheng Biotechnology Co., Ltd. (Dalian, China). Mice were cohoused (5/cage) in autoclavable polypropylene cages with free access to chow and water under specific pathogen-free conditions, standard temperature conditions, and humidity with a 12 h light–dark cycle. Mice, who had 7 days of co-acclimatization, were blindly distributed into eight groups (n = 10/group), as described in Table 1.

Table 1. The mice grouping of the study.

Group No.	Group Name	Explanation
Group I	Control	Intranasal (i.n.) 20 µL phosphate-buffered saline (PBS) + 10 µL PBS SLIT
Group II	Asthma	i.n. 25 µg HDM in 20 µL PBS +10 µL PBS SLIT
Group III	Probiotic1	HDM asthma model + 10 µL PBS SLIT + *L. paracasei* (day1–end of model)
Group IV	SLIT66	HDM asthma model+ SLIT 66 µg
Group V	Probiotic + SLIT66	HDM asthma model + (*L. paracasei* + SLIT66 µg combination)
Group VI	Probiotic2	HDM asthma model + 10 µL PBS SLIT + *L. paracasei* (day 5–16)
Group VII	SLIT132	HDM asthma model+ SLIT 132 µg
Group VIII	Probiotic + SLIT132	HDM asthma model + (*L. paracasei* + SLIT132 µg combination)

4.2. Probiotic Culture Conditions

L. paracasei (Department of Pathogen Biology and Microecology, Dalian Medical University) was cultured in sterile Lactobacillus MRS broth (Hopebio, Qingdao, China) at 37 °C for 24–48 h under anaerobic conditions. Cell counts were determined by plating serial dilutions, and the optical density was measured for the subsequent cell number count in the next culture. After being centrifuged for 10 min at 4 °C, 6000× g rpm, the harvested probiotic was washed thrice with PBS and then freshly administered.

4.3. Asthma Model Sensitization and Challenge Protocol

To establish the allergic asthma mouse model, HDM-derived protein Der p powder (*Dermatophagoides (D.) pteronyssinus*, Greer Labs, Lenoir, NC, USA), with a dry weight of

16.7 mg, was first dissolved in 25 mL PBS (Solarbio, Beijing, China) at a final concentration of 6.68 µg/µL. Our asthma model protocol was adopted from a previous one [58] with some modifications. Briefly, mice were given 25 µg HDM extract intranasally on sensitization days 1, 2, and 3 in 20 µL sterile PBS. On days 19–25, mice were challenged with HDM (i.n. 25 µg in 20 µL PBS). PBS (20 µL) was administered in the control group. On day 26, mice were sacrificed (Figure 5).

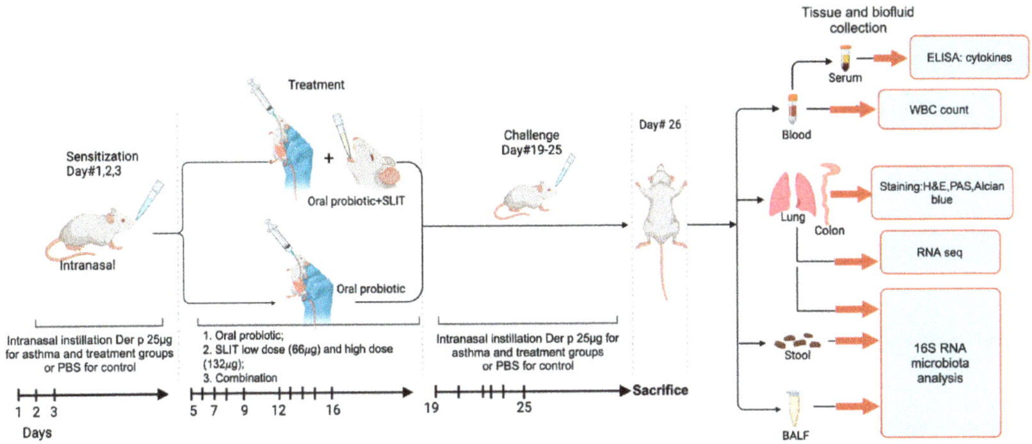

Figure 5. Experimental protocol design of allergic asthma with HDM and *L. paracasei* treatment. Mice were intranasally sensitized to HDM Der p extract (25 µg Der p in 10 µL PBS) for 3 days. SLIT was administered for 5 consecutive days/week for 2 weeks, as either high dose (132 µg/day) or low dose (66 µg/day), followed by 6 days of intranasal challenge exposure (same dose with sensitization). Unlike SLIT HDM-treated groups, control and asthma and probiotic-treated mice received PBS for SLIT.

4.4. SLIT and Probiotic Intervention Protocol

Mice were treated sublingually with either 10 µL PBS alone (control and asthma group), 66 µg HDM extract (SLIT66 alone and Probio + SLIT66 group), or 132 µg HDM extract (SLIT132 alone and Probio + SLIT132 group). Mice received SLIT on day 5 then continued for five days in a row for two weeks with two-day intervals as rest days. In the low-dose group, *L. paracasei* oral intake was performed throughout the experiment days, whereas in the high-dose group, *L. paracasei* was administered only during SLIT days, as depicted in Figure 5. A daily dose of 1.0×10^9 colony-forming units of *L. paracasei* (in 200 µL of PBS) was given intratracheally to each mouse.

4.5. Symptom Sign Evaluation

The number of nasal and facial rubbing induced by HDM stimulation was counted by three observers without prior knowledge of the groups' identity within 15 min immediately after the allergen challenge. The effects of *L. paracasei* and SLIT instillation on the frequency of nasal rubbing after HDM re-exposure at days 19, 21, and 24 were assessed.

4.6. Blood Cytopathological Analysis

The mice were killed on day 26, after which the blood (approximately 0.5–1 mL) was collected from the vena cava vein, placed in a labeled vial containing EDTA, and analyzed for total and differential white blood cell counts. Total cell numbers and numbers of eosinophils and neutrophils were counted for all groups.

4.7. Enzyme-Linked Immunosorbent Assay (ELISA)

Blood was taken from the mice vena cava using a 1 mL syringe. To obtain serum, samples were incubated at room temperature for 1 h, centrifuged at 8000× g at 4 °C for 15 min, and then transferred to new tubes. The IgE concentration and serum cytokines IL-4, TNF-α, IL-17, IFN-γ, and IL-10 were also measured by ELISA (Quanzhou Ruixin Biotechnology Co., Ltd., Quanzhou, China), according to the manufacturer's instructions.

4.8. Tissue Histoprocessing and Staining

After sacrificing the animals, the left lungs and colons of mice were collected and preserved in 4% paraformaldehyde (Seven Biotech, Beijing, China) and sent to a histology lab for paraffin embedding and cutting into 4 μm sections. The sections were rehydrated after deparaffinization and stained with Hematoxylin and Eosin (H&E), Periodic Acid Schiff (PAS), and Alcian Blue (AB) (Solarbio, Beijing, China) as instructed by the kit's protocol to investigate airway and gut pathological and inflammatory processes in the mice. To quantify and evaluate the degree of histopathological inflammation and mucus production, lung and colon sections were examined with a microscope equipped with a camera (McAudi Industrial Group Co., Ltd., Xiamen, China) and images were analyzed with Image J software (version 1.4.3.67). The lung inflammation score was measured as previously described [59]. Briefly, a five-point scoring method was used to determine the inflammatory score: normal = 0, a few cells = 1, one layer of a cell ring = 2, two to four layers of a cell ring = 3, and more than four layers of a cell ring = 4. Using the ImageJ program, the PAS and AB % area stained, as well as the GCs' number and colon crypt, were identified and examined.

4.9. Statistical Analysis

With GraphPad Prism 8 (GraphPad, San Diego, CA, USA), all statistical analyses were carried out using either the one-way analysis of variance (ANOVA) or the t-test (for comparisons between two groups). The findings were presented in the form of the mean ± standard deviation (SD). When p-values were less than 0.05, the results were considered statistically significant.

5. Conclusions

The comprehensive examination of the study purpose, investigating the synergistic impact of combining probiotics with a higher dose of sublingual HDM immunotherapy in an asthma mouse model, yielded notable and promising outcomes. The study findings provide compelling evidence that the combination of probiotics with a high dose of sublingual HDM immunotherapy in an asthma mouse model not only effectively reduces allergic symptoms but also demonstrates immunomodulatory and tissue-protective effects. It is noteworthy that short-term probiotic treatment alone also showed some level of protection against asthma. However, these results remain controversial and need to be confirmed in human studies and more profound and comprehensive immunological investigations in mice. These results suggest a promising avenue for improving therapeutic outcomes while alleviating potential side effects and shortening the duration of treatment.

Author Contributions: Conceptualization, D.A. and W.S.; methodology, D.A.; software, D.A., J.L., X.J., S.R.H.S., A.U. and M.F.Z.A.; formal analysis, D.A.; investigation, W.S.; resources, W.S.; data curation, W.S.; writing—original draft preparation, D.A.; funding acquisition, W.S.; project administration, W.S.; review and editing, W.S. and D.A.; supervision, W.S. All authors have read and agreed to the published version of the manuscript.

Funding: This research was funded by "The National Natural Science Fund Project of China, grant number 81370113".

Institutional Review Board Statement: This study protocol was approved by the Dalian Medical University Animal Ethics Committee (AEE19078).

Informed Consent Statement: Not applicable.

Data Availability Statement: The raw data supporting this study will be made available by the corresponding author upon request.

Conflicts of Interest: The authors declare no conflicts of interest.

References

1. Nunes, C.; Pereira, A.M.; Morais-Almeida, M. Asthma costs and social impact. *Asthma Res. Pract.* **2017**, *3*, 1. [CrossRef] [PubMed]
2. Finotto, S. Resolution of allergic asthma. *Semin. Immunopathol.* **2019**, *41*, 665–674. [CrossRef] [PubMed]
3. Abu Khweek, A.; Kim, E.; Joldrichsen, M.R.; Amer, A.O.; Boyaka, P.N. Insights into Mucosal Innate Immune Responses in House Dust Mite-Mediated Allergic Asthma. *Front. Immunol.* **2020**, *11*, 534501. [CrossRef] [PubMed]
4. Dharmage, S.C.; Perret, J.L.; Custovic, A. Epidemiology of Asthma in Children and Adults. *Front. Pediatr.* **2019**, *7*, 246. [CrossRef]
5. Papi, A.; Blasi, F.; Canonica, G.W.; Morandi, L.; Richeldi, L.; Rossi, A. Treatment strategies for asthma: Reshaping the concept of asthma management. *Allergy Asthma Clin. Immunol.* **2020**, *16*, 75. [CrossRef]
6. Wang, J.; Zhou, Y.; Zhang, H.; Hu, L.; Liu, J.; Wang, L.; Wang, T.; Zhang, H.; Cong, L.; Wang, Q. Pathogenesis of allergic diseases and implications for therapeutic interventions. *Signal Transduct. Target. Ther.* **2023**, *8*, 138. [CrossRef]
7. Robinson, D.; Humbert, M.; Buhl, R.; Cruz, A.A.; Inoue, H.; Korom, S.; Hanania, N.A.; Nair, P. Revisiting Type 2-high and Type 2-low airway inflammation in asthma: Current knowledge and therapeutic implications. *Clin. Exp. Allergy* **2017**, *47*, 161–175. [CrossRef] [PubMed]
8. Luo, W.; Hu, J.; Xu, W.; Dong, J. Distinct spatial and temporal roles for Th1, Th2, and Th17 cells in asthma. *Front. Immunol.* **2022**, *13*, 974066. [CrossRef]
9. Akdis, C.A.; Akdis, M. Mechanisms of allergen-specific immunotherapy. *J. Allergy Clin. Immunol.* **2011**, *127*, 18–27. [CrossRef]
10. Shamji, M.H.; Durham, S.R. Mechanisms of allergen immunotherapy for inhaled allergens and predictive biomarkers. *J. Allergy Clin. Immunol.* **2017**, *140*, 1485–1498. [CrossRef]
11. Shamji, M.H.; Sharif, H.; Layhadi, J.A.; Zhu, R.; Kishore, U.; Renz, H. Diverse immune mechanisms of allergen immunotherapy for allergic rhinitis with and without asthma. *J. Allergy Clin. Immunol.* **2022**, *149*, 791–801. [CrossRef] [PubMed]
12. Rahman, R.S.; Wesemann, D.R. Immunology of allergen immunotherapy. *Immunother. Adv.* **2022**, *2*, ltac022. [CrossRef] [PubMed]
13. Abramson, M.J.; Puy, R.M.; Weiner, J.M. Injection allergen immunotherapy for asthma. *Cochrane Database Syst. Rev.* **2010**, CD001186. [CrossRef] [PubMed]
14. Virchow, J.C.; Backer, V.; Kuna, P.; Prieto, L.; Nolte, H.; Villesen, H.H.; Ljørring, C.; Riis, B.; de Blay, F. Efficacy of a House Dust Mite Sublingual Allergen Immunotherapy Tablet in Adults with Allergic Asthma: A Randomized Clinical Trial. *JAMA* **2016**, *315*, 1715–1725. [CrossRef]
15. Bozek, A.; Galuszka, B.; Gawlik, R.; Misiolek, M.; Scierski, W.; Grzanka, A.; Canonica, G.W. Allergen immunotherapy against house dust mites in patients with local allergic rhinitis and asthma. *J. Asthma* **2022**, *59*, 1850–1858. [CrossRef]
16. Tourdot, S.; Airouche, S.; Berjont, N.; Da Silveira, A.; Mascarell, L.; Jacquet, A.; Caplier, L.; Langelot, M.; Baron-Bodo, V.; Moingeon, P. Evaluation of therapeutic sublingual vaccines in a murine model of chronic house dust mite allergic airway inflammation. *Clin. Exp. Allergy* **2011**, *41*, 1784–1792. [CrossRef]
17. Hagner, S.; Rask, C.; Brimnes, J.; Andersen, P.S.; Raifer, H.; Renz, H.; Garn, H. House Dust Mite-Specific Sublingual Immunotherapy Prevents the Development of Allergic Inflammation in a Mouse Model of Experimental Asthma. *Int. Arch. Allergy Immunol.* **2016**, *170*, 22–34. [CrossRef]
18. Shima, K.; Koya, T.; Tsukioka, K.; Sakagami, T.; Hasegawa, T.; Fukano, C.; Ohashi-Doi, K.; Watanabe, S.; Suzuki, E.; Kikuchi, T. Effects of sublingual immunotherapy in a murine asthma model sensitized by intranasal administration of house dust mite extracts. *Allergol. Int.* **2017**, *66*, 89–96. [CrossRef]
19. Hesse, L.; van Ieperen, N.; Habraken, C.; Petersen, A.H.; Korn, S.; Smilda, T.; Goedewaagen, B.; Ruiters, M.H.; van der Graaf, A.C.; Nawijn, M.C. Subcutaneous immunotherapy with purified Der p1 and 2 suppresses type 2 immunity in a murine asthma model. *Allergy* **2018**, *73*, 862–874. [CrossRef]
20. Kucuksezer, U.C.; Ozdemir, C.; Cevhertas, L.; Ogulur, I.; Akdis, M.; Akdis, C.A. Mechanisms of allergen-specific immunotherapy and allergen tolerance. *Allergol. Int.* **2020**, *69*, 549–560. [CrossRef]
21. Shamji, M.H.; Valenta, R.; Jardetzky, T.; Verhasselt, V.; Durham, S.R.; Würtzen, P.A.; van Neerven, R.J. The role of allergen-specific IgE, IgG and IgA in allergic disease. *Allergy* **2021**, *76*, 3627–3641. [CrossRef] [PubMed]
22. Akdis, M.; Akdis, C.A. Mechanisms of allergen-specific immunotherapy: Multiple suppressor factors at work in immune tolerance to allergens. *J. Allergy Clin. Immunol.* **2014**, *133*, 621–631. [CrossRef] [PubMed]
23. Jutel, M.; Agache, I.; Bonini, S.; Burks, A.W.; Calderon, M.; Canonica, W.; Cox, L.; Demoly, P.; Frew, A.J.; O'Hehir, R.; et al. International Consensus on Allergen Immunotherapy II: Mechanisms, standardization, and pharmacoeconomics. *J. Allergy Clin. Immunol.* **2016**, *137*, 358–368. [CrossRef] [PubMed]
24. Zemelka-Wiacek, M.; Jutel, M. AIT 2023: Current innovation and future outlook. *Allergol. Sel.* **2023**, *7*, 219–228. [CrossRef] [PubMed]
25. Ozdemir, C.; Kucuksezer, U.C.; Akdis, M.; Akdis, C.A. Mechanisms of Aeroallergen Immunotherapy: Subcutaneous Immunotherapy and Sublingual Immunotherapy. *Immunol. Allergy Clin. N. Am.* **2016**, *36*, 71–86. [CrossRef]

26. Głobińska, A.; Boonpiyathad, T.; Satitsuksanoa, P.; Kleuskens, M.; van de Veen, W.; Sokolowska, M.; Akdis, M. Mechanisms of allergen-specific immunotherapy: Diverse mechanisms of immune tolerance to allergens. *Ann. Allergy Asthma Immunol.* **2018**, *121*, 306–312. [CrossRef]
27. Hemarajata, P.; Versalovic, J. Effects of probiotics on gut microbiota: Mechanisms of intestinal immunomodulation and neuro-modulation. *Ther. Adv. Gastroenterol.* **2013**, *6*, 39–51. [CrossRef] [PubMed]
28. Li, L.; Fang, Z.; Liu, X.; Hu, W.; Lu, W.; Lee, Y.K.; Zhao, J.; Zhang, H.; Chen, W. *Lactobacillus reuteri* attenuated allergic inflammation induced by HDM in the mouse and modulated gut microbes. *PLoS ONE* **2020**, *15*, e0231865. [CrossRef]
29. Casaro, M.B.; Thomas, A.M.; Mendes, E.; Fukumori, C.; Ribeiro, W.R.; Oliveira, F.A.; Crisma, A.R.; Murata, G.M.; Bizzarro, B.; Sá-Nunes, A.; et al. A probiotic has differential effects on allergic airway inflammation in A/J and C57BL/6 mice and is correlated with the gut microbiome. *Microbiome* **2021**, *9*, 134. [CrossRef]
30. Ghiamati Yazdi, F.; Zakeri, A.; van Ark, I.; Leusink-Muis, T.; Braber, S.; Soleimanian-Zad, S.; Folkerts, G. Crude Turmeric Extract Improves the Suppressive Effects of *Lactobacillus rhamnosus* GG on Allergic Inflammation in a Murine Model of House Dust Mite-Induced Asthma. *Front. Immunol.* **2020**, *11*, 1092. [CrossRef]
31. Chen, L.H.; Pan, C.H.; Huang, S.Y.; Chan, C.H.; Huang, H.Y. The immunomodulatory effects of long-term supplementation with *Lactobacillus casei* Shirota depend on ovalbumin presentation in BALB/c mice. *Sci. Rep.* **2021**, *11*, 19478. [CrossRef] [PubMed]
32. Cheng, S.H.; Yang, T.Y.; Hsu, C.C.; Wei, Y.H.; Wu, C.C.; Tsai, Y.C. *Lactobacillus paragasseri* BBM171 Ameliorates Allergic Airway Inflammation Induced by Ovalbumin in Mice via Modulating the Th1/Th2 Balance. *Microorganisms* **2022**, *10*, 2041. [CrossRef] [PubMed]
33. Wang, X.; Hui, Y.; Zhao, L.; Hao, Y.; Guo, H.; Ren, F. Oral administration of *Lactobacillus paracasei* L9 attenuates PM2.5-induced enhancement of airway hyperresponsiveness and allergic airway response in murine model of asthma. *PLoS ONE* **2017**, *12*, e0171721. [CrossRef] [PubMed]
34. Xie, A.; Song, J.; Lu, S.; Liu, Y.; Tang, L.; Wen, S. Influence of Diet on the Effect of the Probiotic *Lactobacillus paracasei* in Rats Suffering from Allergic Asthma. *Front. Microbiol.* **2021**, *12*, 737622. [CrossRef]
35. Schenzel, A.; Geiger, A.; Nendel, E.; Yang, Z.; Krammer, S.; Leberle, A.; Brunst, A.K.; Trump, S.; Mittler, S.; Rauh, M.; et al. Fiber rich food suppressed airway inflammation, GATA3 + Th2 cells, and FcεRIα+ eosinophils in asthma. *Front. Nutr.* **2024**, *11*, 1367864. [CrossRef]
36. Huang, M.T.; Chiu, C.J.; Tsai, C.Y.; Lee, Y.R.; Liu, W.L.; Chuang, H.L.; Huang, M.T. Short-chain fatty acids ameliorate allergic airway inflammation via sequential induction of PMN-MDSCs and Treg cells. *J. Allergy Clin. Immunol. Glob.* **2023**, *2*, 100163. [CrossRef]
37. Spacova, I.; Ceuppens, J.L.; Seys, S.F.; Petrova, M.I.; Lebeer, S. Probiotics against airway allergy: Host factors to consider. *Dis. Models Mech.* **2018**, *11*, dmm034314. [CrossRef]
38. Kim, H.J.; Kim, H.Y.; Lee, S.Y.; Seo, J.H.; Lee, E.; Hong, S.J. Clinical efficacy and mechanism of probiotics in allergic diseases. *Korean J. Pediatr.* **2013**, *56*, 369–376. [CrossRef]
39. Kim, B.G.; Kim, J.N.; Jang, A.S.; Shin, M. Combined Effects of *Lactobacillus rhamnosus* and Egg Oral Immunotherapy in a Mouse Model of Egg Allergy. *Allergy Asthma Immunol. Res.* **2020**, *12*, 701–711. [CrossRef]
40. Sim, S.; Park, H.J.; Kim, Y.K.; Choi, Y.; Park, H.S. *Lactobacillus paracasei*-derived extracellular vesicles alleviate neutrophilic asthma by inhibiting the JNK pathway in airway epithelium. *Allergol. Int.* **2024**, *73*, 302–312. [CrossRef]
41. Lin, E.K.; Chang, W.W.; Jhong, J.H.; Tsai, W.H.; Chou, C.H.; Wang, I.J. *Lacticaseibacillus paracasei* GM-080 Ameliorates Allergic Airway Inflammation in Children with Allergic Rhinitis: From an Animal Model to a Double-Blind, Randomized, Placebo-Controlled Trial. *Cells* **2023**, *12*, 768. [CrossRef] [PubMed]
42. Uwaezuoke, S.N.; Ayuk, A.C.; Eze, J.N.; Odimegwu, C.L.; Ndiokwelu, C.O.; Eze, I.C. Postnatal probiotic supplementation can prevent and optimize treatment of childhood asthma and atopic disorders: A systematic review of randomized controlled trials. *Front. Pediatr.* **2022**, *10*, 956141. [CrossRef] [PubMed]
43. Kajiume, T. Sublingual immunotherapy for pediatric patients with mite allergies. *Medicine* **2022**, *101*, e28690. [CrossRef] [PubMed]
44. Pavón-Romero, G.F.; Parra-Vargas, M.I.; Ramírez-Jiménez, F.; Melgoza-Ruiz, E.; Serrano-Pérez, N.H.; Teran, L.M. Allergen Immunotherapy: Current and Future Trends. *Cells* **2022**, *11*, 212. [CrossRef] [PubMed]
45. Fortescue, R.; Kew, K.M.; Leung, M.S.T. Sublingual immunotherapy for asthma. *Cochrane Database Syst. Rev.* **2020**, *9*, CD011293. [CrossRef]
46. Van der Borght, K.; Brimnes, J.; Haspeslagh, E.; Brand, S.; Neyt, K.; Gupta, S.; Knudsen, N.P.H.; Hammad, H.; Andersen, P.S.; Lambrecht, B.N. Sublingual allergen immunotherapy prevents house dust mite inhalant type 2 immunity through dendritic cell-mediated induction of Foxp3+ regulatory T cells. *Mucosal Immunol.* **2024**, *17*, 618–632. [CrossRef]
47. Hesse, L.; Nawijn, M.C. Subcutaneous and Sublingual Immunotherapy in a Mouse Model of Allergic Asthma. *Methods Mol. Biol.* **2017**, *1559*, 137–168. [CrossRef]
48. Hesse, L.; Petersen, A.H.; Nawijn, M.C. Methods for Experimental Allergen Immunotherapy: Subcutaneous and Sublingual Desensitization in Mouse Models of Allergic Asthma. *Methods Mol. Biol.* **2021**, *2223*, 295–335. [CrossRef]
49. Razafindratsita, A.; Saint-Lu, N.; Mascarell, L.; Berjont, N.; Bardon, T.; Betbeder, D.; Van Overtvelt, L.; Moingeon, P. Improvement of sublingual immunotherapy efficacy with a mucoadhesive allergen formulation. *J. Allergy Clin. Immunol.* **2007**, *120*, 278–285. [CrossRef]

50. Wang, Y.H.; Wills-Karp, M. The potential role of interleukin-17 in severe asthma. *Curr. Allergy Asthma Rep.* **2011**, *11*, 388–394. [CrossRef]
51. Li, X.; Ye, C.; Mulati, M.; Sun, L.; Qian, F. Ellipticine blocks synergistic effects of IL-17A and TNF-α in epithelial cells and alleviates severe acute pancreatitis-associated acute lung injury. *Biochem. Pharmacol.* **2020**, *177*, 113992. [CrossRef] [PubMed]
52. Royce, S.G.; Cheng, V.; Samuel, C.S.; Tang, M.L. The regulation of fibrosis in airway remodeling in asthma. *Mol. Cell. Endocrinol.* **2012**, *351*, 167–175. [CrossRef] [PubMed]
53. Walsh, E.R.; August, A. Eosinophils and allergic airway disease: There is more to the story. *Trends Immunol.* **2010**, *31*, 39–44. [CrossRef] [PubMed]
54. Gieryńska, M.; Szulc-Dąbrowska, L.; Struzik, J.; Mielcarska, M.B.; Gregorczyk-Zboroch, K.P. Integrity of the Intestinal Barrier: The Involvement of Epithelial Cells and Microbiota-A Mutual Relationship. *Animals* **2022**, *12*, 145. [CrossRef] [PubMed]
55. Nascimento, C.M.; Casaro, M.C.; Perez, E.R.; Ribeiro, W.R.; Mayer, M.P.A.; Ishikawa, K.H.; Lino-Dos-Santos-Franco, A.; Pereira, J.N.B.; Ferreira, C.M. Experimental allergic airway inflammation impacts gut homeostasis in mice. *Heliyon* **2023**, *9*, e16429. [CrossRef]
56. Liu, X.F.; Shao, J.H.; Liao, Y.T.; Wang, L.N.; Jia, Y.; Dong, P.J.; Liu, Z.Z.; He, D.D.; Li, C.; Zhang, X. Regulation of short-chain fatty acids in the immune system. *Front. Immunol.* **2023**, *14*, 1186892. [CrossRef]
57. Zhou, C.J.; Xie, B.L.; Han, H.Y.; Wang, Y.; Wang, Y.H.; Hong, J.Y.; Wei, Y.X.; Liu, Z.G.; Feng, Y.; Yang, G.; et al. Short-Chain Fatty Acids Promote Immunotherapy by Modulating Immune Regulatory Property in B Cells. *J. Immunol. Res.* **2021**, *2021*, 2684361. [CrossRef]
58. Yang, J.; van 't Veer, C.; Roelofs, J.; van Heijst, J.; de Vos, A.F.; McCrae, K.R.; Revenko, A.S.; Crosby, J.; van der Poll, T. Kininogen deficiency or depletion reduces enhanced pause independent of pulmonary inflammation in a house dust mite-induced murine asthma model. *Am. J. Physiol.-Lung Cell. Mol. Physiol.* **2019**, *316*, L187–L196. [CrossRef]
59. Massoud, A.H.; Charbonnier, L.M.; Lopez, D.; Pellegrini, M.; Phipatanakul, W.; Chatila, T.A. An asthma-associated IL4R variant exacerbates airway inflammation by promoting conversion of regulatory T cells to TH17-like cells. *Nat. Med.* **2016**, *22*, 1013–1022. [CrossRef]

pharmaceuticals

MDPI

Article

β-Tocotrienol Decreases PDGF-BB-Induced Proliferation and Migration of Human Airway Smooth Muscle Cells by Inhibiting RhoA and Reducing ROS Production

Aditya Sri Listyoko *, Ryota Okazaki, Tomoya Harada, Miki Takata, Masato Morita, Hiroki Ishikawa, Yoshihiro Funaki and Akira Yamasaki *

Division of Respiratory Medicine and Rheumatology, Department of Multidisciplinary Internal Medicine, Faculty of Medicine, Tottori University, Yonago 683-8504, Japan; okazaki0222@tottori-u.ac.jp (R.O.); tomo.h.308@tottori-u.ac.jp (T.H.); mikiyamamu@tottori-u.ac.jp (M.T.); drmasato@tottori-u.ac.jp (M.M.); h.ishikawa1990@tottori-u.ac.jp (H.I.); yfunaki@tottori-u.ac.jp (Y.F.)

* Correspondence: adityalistyoko@ub.ac.id (A.S.L.); yamasaki@tottori-u.ac.jp (A.Y.)

Abstract: Background: Tocotrienols exhibit antioxidant and anti-inflammatory activities. RhoA, a small GTPase protein, plays a crucial role in regulating contractility in airway smooth muscle (ASM). Previous studies have demonstrated that γ-tocotrienols reduce ASM proliferation and migration by inhibiting the activation of RhoA. In this present study, we investigate the effect of another vitamin E isoform, β-tocotrienols, on human ASM cell proliferation and migration stimulated by platelet-derived growth factor-BB (PDGF-BB). Methods: Human ASM cells were pre-treated with β-tocotrienol prior to being stimulated with PDGF-BB to induce ASM cell proliferation and migration. The proliferation and migration of PDGF-BB-induced human ASM cells were assessed using colorimetric and transwell migration assays. The intracellular ROS assay kit was employed to quantify reactive oxygen species (ROS) in human ASM cells. Additionally, we explored the effect of β-tocotrienols on the signaling pathways involved in PDGF-BB-induced ASM proliferation and migration. Results: β-tocotrienol inhibited PDGF-BB-induced ASM cell proliferation and migration by reducing RhoA activation and ROS production. However, in this present study, β-tocotrienol did not affect the signaling pathways associated with cyclin D1, phosphorylated Akt1, and ERK1/2. Conclusions: In conclusion, the inhibition of RhoA activation and ROS production by β-tocotrienol, resulting in the reduction in human ASM proliferation and migration, suggests its potential as a treatment for asthma airway remodeling.

Keywords: airway remodeling; ASM; asthma; Rho-A; ROS; tocotrienol; vitamin E

1. Introduction

Asthma typically presents as a heterogeneous disease, often marked by chronic inflammation of the airways [1]. Persistent chronic inflammation in asthma may lead to structural alterations known as airway remodeling [2,3]. Airway remodeling in asthma encompasses a spectrum of structural alterations, including changes such as epithelial alterations including epithelial–mesenchymal transition [4], sub-epithelial fibrosis including a fibroblast-to-myofibroblast transition and deposition of extracellular matrix [5,6], alterations in airway smooth muscle (ASM) [7,8], and remodeling of the airway vasculature [9]. Airway remodeling may be associated with poor asthma outcomes, potentially leading to increased airway hyperresponsiveness and decreased lung function [10–12].

Numerous studies have explored the association between vitamins and asthma, suggesting the potential benefits of supplementary vitamin intake in asthma management to improve outcomes, particularly for individuals deficient in vitamin levels [13–16]. The biological role of vitamin E metabolites has garnered considerable attention, however, exploration of the role of vitamin E metabolites in respiratory diseases remains notably limited. Eight isoforms of vitamin E have been discovered to date, including α, β, γ, and δ-tocotrienol and α, β, γ, and δ-tocopherol [17,18]. Several studies have noted no significant difference in antioxidant capacity between tocopherol and tocotrienol [19,20], emphasizing the importance of considering experimental conditions for accurate comparisons. However, other studies have highlighted the higher potential antioxidant activity in α-tocotrienol compared to α-tocopherol [21] and the potential benefits specifically associated with tocotrienols including antiangiogenic [22], anticancer [23,24], cerebral, and cardioprotective effects [25,26], a potential therapeutic effect on diabetes and hyperlipidemia [27–29], and anti-inflammatory effects [30,31].

In the context of lung disease, despite limited studies, tocotrienols have been observed to provide benefits. For instance, protective effects of γ-tocotrienol against emphysema and lung function were observed in a chronic obstructive pulmonary disease mouse model [32]. Another study observed that tocotrienol has the potential to ameliorate pulmonary fibrosis through mechanisms involving the transforming growth factor-β1 (TGF-β1)/Smad, phosphatidylinositol 3′-kinase/Akt (PI3K/Akt), and translocations of nuclear factor-kappa B (NF-κB) signaling pathways [33]. In the context of asthma, particularly airway remodeling, tocotrienols may offer benefits. Our previous study revealed that γ-tocotrienols could potentially influence airway remodeling by inhibiting RhoA activation in platelet-derived growth factor-BB (PDGF-BB)-induced ASM cell proliferation and migration [34]. Another study determined that γ-tocotrienols hold potential benefits in modulating airway remodeling by inhibiting RhoA activation in TGF-β-stimulated ASM cells [35].

Several studies have compared the antioxidant effects of tocotrienols with inconsistent results. One study, employing peroxide and thiobarbituric acid as markers, assessed similar levels of antioxidant capacity between β-tocopherol and β-tocotrienol, while α-tocotrienol and α-tocopherol were less potent. Moreover, γ-tocotrienol, δ-tocopherol, and δ-tocotrienol exhibited slightly higher potency than either β-tocopherol or β-tocotrienol [36]. Another study observed that administration of a tocotrienol-rich fraction (TRF), containing α-tocotrienol, β-tocotrienol, δ-tocotrienol, γ-tocotrienol, and α-tocopherol, exhibited similar effects on antioxidant levels compared to α-tocopherol alone [37]. Regarding effectiveness as an anticancer treatment, β-tocotrienol showed a notably stronger antiproliferative effect compared to γ-tocotrienols in human breast adenocarcinoma cell lines MDA-MB-231 and MCF7 [38]. Given this, the variability in potency among isoforms of vitamin E can be attributed to several factors. These factors include the source of vitamin E utilized, research methodologies employed, and the intended purpose of administering this isoform, whether as an antioxidant, anticancer agent, or for other potential uses.

Our previous study focused on the use of γ-tocotrienols on ASM cells. However, the effects of various isoforms of tocotrienols as potential therapies for airway remodeling, derived from vitamin E, have not been thoroughly investigated and remain incompletely understood. Furthermore, there have been no studies comparing different isoforms of vitamin E as potential treatments for airway remodeling. In this present study, we investigate the effect of another vitamin E isoform, β-tocotrienols, on human ASM cell proliferation and migration stimulated by platelet-derived growth factor-BB (PDGF-BB). Additionally, we explored the effect of β-tocotrienols on the signaling pathways involved in PDGF-BB-induced ASM proliferation and migration.

2. Results

2.1. *β-Tocotrienols Inhibit PDGF-BB-Induced ASM Cell Proliferation*

Human ASM cells were pre-treated with various concentrations of β-tocotrienols for 1 h before being stimulated with 10 ng/mL PDGF-BB for 48 h to induce ASM cell proliferation. PDGF-BB stimulation increased ASM cell proliferation compared to the non-stimulated (control) group. Pre-treatment with 25 μM β-tocotrienols significantly reduced this effect (Figure 1), indicating that β-tocotrienols have an inhibitory effect on PDGF-BB-induced ASM cell proliferation.

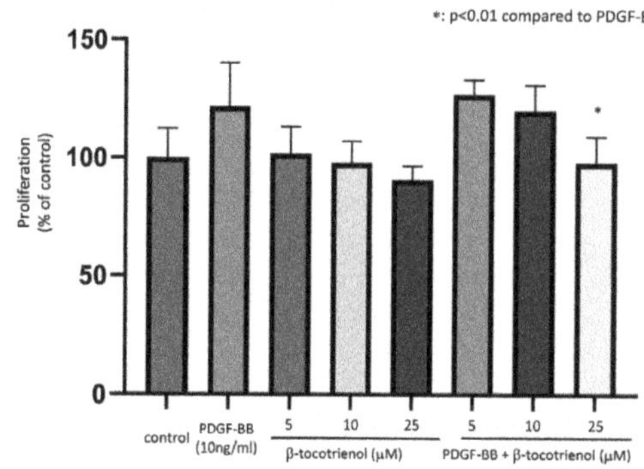

Figure 1. Effect of β-tocotrienols on ASM cell proliferation. Human ASM cells were cultured with 10 ng/mL PDGF-BB, 5–25 μM β-tocotrienols, or pre-treated with 5–25 μM β-tocotrienols before 10 ng/mL PDGF-BB stimulation. The proliferation of ASM cells was measured using the Cell Counting Kit (CCK-8). The results are presented as a percentage of the non-stimulated (control) group and expressed as the mean ± standard deviation (SD) of at least three independent experiments (*: $p < 0.01$ compared to PDGF-BB stimulation alone).

2.2. *β-Tocotrienols Inhibit PDGF-BB-Induced ASM Cell Migration*

Human ASM cells were pre-treated with various concentrations of β-tocotrienols for 1 h before being stimulated with 10 ng/mL PDGF-BB for 5 h to induce ASM cell migration. The migration of ASM cells increased in the PDGF-BB group compared to the non-stimulated (control) group. Pre-treatment with 50 μM β-tocotrienols significantly reduced this effect (Figure 2), indicating the inhibitory effect of β-tocotrienols on PDGF-BB-induced ASM cell migration.

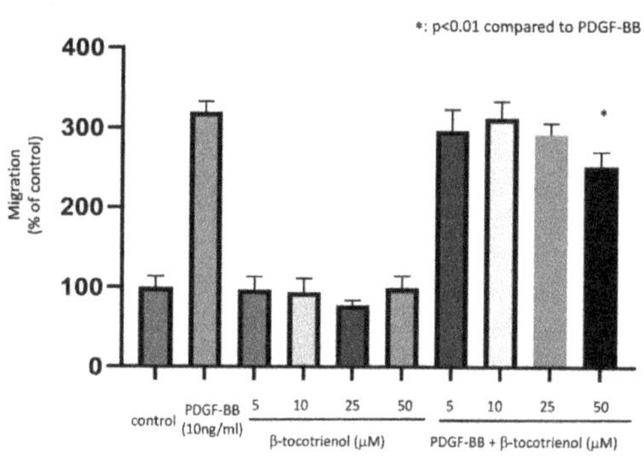

Figure 2. Effect of β-tocotrienols on ASM cell migration. Human ASM cells were cultured with 10 ng/mL PDGF-BB, 5–50 μM β-tocotrienols, or pre-treated with 5–50 μM β-tocotrienols before 10 ng/mL PDGF-BB stimulation. The migration of ASM cells was evaluated using a transwell chamber. The results are presented as a percentage of the non-stimulated (control) group and expressed as the mean ± standard deviation (SD) of at least three independent experiments (*: $p < 0.01$ compared to PDGF-BB stimulation alone).

2.3. *β-Tocotrienols Reduce Intracellular ROS Production*

The generation of oxygen species is essential for the mitogen stimulation of ASM, initiating signal transduction pathways that lead to cell proliferation [39]. In this current study, we assessed the impact of β-tocotrienols on reactive oxygen species (ROS) production. The ROS production decreased after stimulation with β tocotrienols compared to the non-stimulated (control) group, although the result did not reach statistical significance. Following the stimulation with PDGF-BB, ROS production increased, and pre-treatment with β-tocotrienols ameliorated this effect (Figure 3), indicating the inhibitory effect of β-tocotrienols on ROS production.

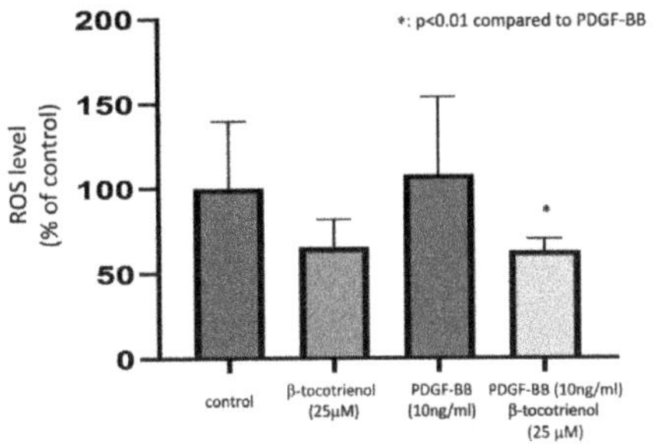

Figure 3. Effect of β-tocotrienols on ROS production. Human ASM cells were cultured with 10 ng/mL PDGF-BB, 25 μM β-tocotrienols, or pre-treated with 25 μM β-tocotrienols before 10 ng/mL PDGF-BB stimulation. The level of ROS in ASM cells was quantified after stimulation with 10 ng/mL PDGF-BB using the Oxiselect intracellular ROS assay kit. The results are presented as a percentage of the non-stimulated (control) group and expressed as the mean ± standard deviation (SD) of at least three independent experiments (*: $p < 0.01$ compared to PDGF-BB stimulation alone).

2.4. The Effect of β-Tocotrienols on Cyclin D1 Levels

Cyclin D1 serves as a crucial regulator of the cell cycle, including that of ASM cells [40–42]. The previous study observed that γ-tocotrienol reduced PDGF-BB-induced cyclin D1 expression [34]. The cyclin D1 level exhibited an upregulation after stimulation with PDGF-BB for 6 h. However, pre-treatment with β-tocotrienols did not reduce this effect (Figure 4), indicating that cyclin D1 may not be associated with the effect of β-tocotrienols on inhibiting PDGF-BB-induced ASM cell proliferation and migration.

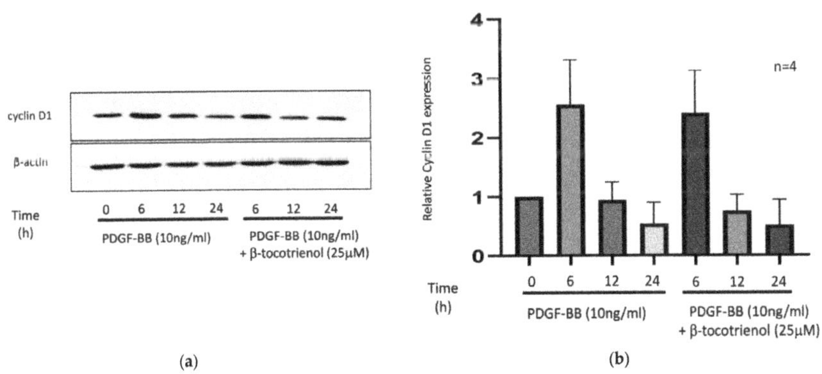

Figure 4. Effect of β-tocotrienols on cyclin D1 expression: (**a**) human ASM cells were cultured with 10 ng/mL PDGF-BB or pre-treated with 25 μM β-tocotrienols before 10 ng/mL PDGF-BB stimulation. Western blot was used to evaluate the expression of cyclin D1. (**b**) The graphic represents densitometry calculations of relative protein expression/β-actin. The results are presented as the mean ± standard deviation (SD) of at least three independent experiments.

2.5. The Effect of β-Tocotrienols on Akt1 and ERK1/2 Signaling Pathways

The previous study observed that the proliferation and migration inhibition effect of γ-tocotrienol on ASM cells was not associated with the Akt1 and ERK1/2 signaling pathways [34]. In this present study, we assessed the effect of β-tocotrienols on the Akt1 and ERK1/2 signaling pathways associated with PDGF-BB-induced proliferation and migration. Phosphorylation of Akt1 and extracellular signal-regulated kinase1/2 (ERK1/2) increased following PDGF-BB stimulation. Pre-treatment with β-tocotrienols did not inhibit this effect (Figure 5), indicating that phosphorylation of Akt1 and ERK1/2 may not be associated with the effect of β-tocotrienols on ASM cell proliferation and migration.

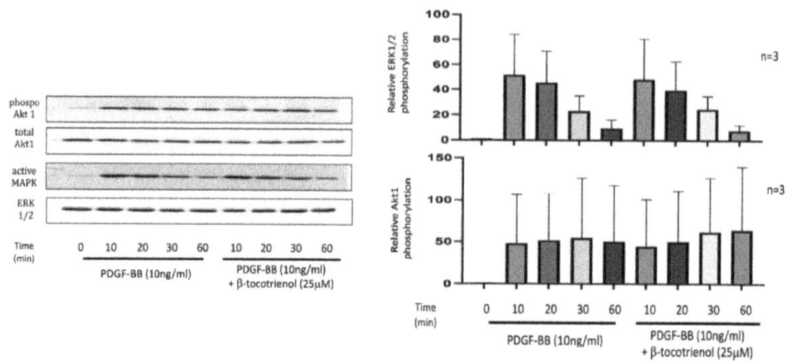

(a) (b)

Figure 5. Effect of β-tocotrienols on Akt1 and ERK1/2 phosphorylation: (**a**) Human ASM cells were cultured with 10 ng/mL PDGF-BB or pre-treated with 25 μM β-tocotrienols before 10 ng/mL PDGF-BB stimulation. Western blot was used to evaluate the expression of Akt1 and ERK1/2. (**b**) The graphic represents densitometry calculations of phosphorylated protein targets to total protein. The results are presented as the mean ± standard deviation (SD) of at least three independent experiments.

2.6. β-Tocotrienols Inhibit PDGF-BB-Induced ASM Cell Proliferation and Migration via RhoA Inactivation

The Rho family serves as a crucial regulator of various cell functions, including migration, adhesion, proliferation, and differentiation [43–45]. The previous study observed that γ-tocotrienol inhibited PDGF-BB-induced RhoA activation [34]. In this current study, we observed that activation of RhoA increased following PDGF-BB stimulation, and pre-treatment with β-tocotrienols reduced this effect (Figure 6), indicating that the inhibition effect of β-tocotrienols on ASM cell proliferation and migration is associated with the RhoA pathway.

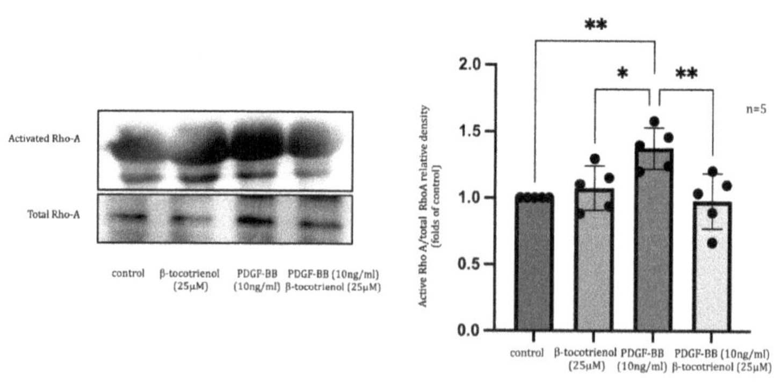

(a) (b)

Figure 6. Effect of β-tocotrienols on RhoA activity: (**a**) human ASM cells were cultured with 10 ng/mL PDGF-BB or pre-treated with 25 μM β-tocotrienols before 10 ng/mL PDGF-BB stimulation. Rho activity was evaluated using a Rho pull-down assay, and the expression was determined with Western blot analysis. (**b**) The graphic represents densitometry calculations of active RhoA to total RhoA. The data are presented as the mean ± standard deviation (SD) of at least three independent experiments. (*: $p < 0.05$, **: $p < 0.01$, compared to PDGF-BB stimulation).

3. Discussion

In this current study, we observed that the proliferation and migration of PDGF-BB-induced ASM cells were effectively inhibited by β-tocotrienol (Figure 7). These recent findings with β-tocotrienol are consistent with our previous study, where γ-tocotrienol inhibited PDGF-BB-induced ASM cell proliferation and migration [34]. Given that ASM proliferation and migration are key contributors to airway remodeling, playing a pivotal role in both promoting and mediating the remodeling process [46,47], these results support the hypothesis that tocotrienols, both of β-tocotrienol and γ-tocotrienol, may hold potential as a treatment for airway remodeling in asthmatic patients.

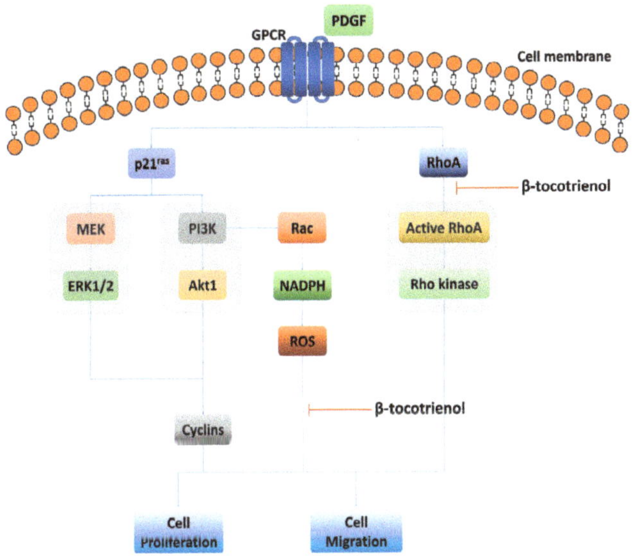

Figure 7. Schematic representation of the effects of β-tocotrienol on inhibiting ASM proliferation and migration. β-tocotrienol directly inhibits ROS production and induces RhoA inactivation. However, β-tocotrienol may not inhibit the Akt1, ERK, and cyclin signaling pathways. Platelet-derived growth factor-BB (PDGF-BB), G protein-coupled receptor (GPCR), extracellular signal-regulated kinase (ERK), phosphatidylinositol 3′-kinase (PI3K), reactive oxygen species (ROS), and nicotinamide adenine dinucleotide phosphate (NADPH).

The mechanism underlying ASM proliferation, migration, growth, and remodeling has been the subject of various studies and literature reviews [7,48–52]. Our findings underscore the importance of targeting the Rho pathway, particularly with tocotrienols, as both β-tocotrienol and γ-tocotrienol inhibit RhoA activation related to ASM proliferation and migration, suggesting that the Rho pathway is an important pathway inhibited by vitamin E isoforms to prevent ASM remodeling [34]. This is supported by several studies and reviews indicating that the Rho/ROCK pathway is a critical regulator of airway remodeling, influencing the regulation, proliferation, and contraction of ASM cells [48,53–55]. The Rho family of GTPases is a group of small signaling G proteins, forming a subfamily within the Ras superfamily and comprising six isoforms (A, B, C, D, E, and G). RhoA has been extensively studied and demonstrates both GDP and GTP binding activities. When stimulated by G protein-coupled receptor (GPCR) agonists, the inactive GDP-bound RhoA can convert into its active state, GTP-bound RhoA [56]. Interestingly, the administration of a selective Rho kinase inhibitor attenuates airway inflammation, eosinophilia, and airway hyperresponsiveness [57–59]. Another study observed that the administration of a selective Rho-A/Rho kinase inhibitor resulted in a significant reduction in inflammatory cell count, decreased mucous secretion, and lowered expression of MUC5AC. These effects were associated with the downregulation of interleukin-17 (IL-17), IL-4, and IL-13 levels, as well as a decline in the expression and phosphorylation of NFκB and signal transducer and activator of transcription 6 (STAT6) [60], indicating the potential therapeutic targeting of the Rho/Rho kinase downstream pathway in asthma.

In this present study, β-tocotrienol did not inhibit the phosphorylation of cyclin D1, Akt1, and ERK 1/2 in PDGF-BB-induced ASM cell proliferation and migration, suggesting that these pathways might not be associated with the inhibitory effect of β-tocotrienol on ASM cell proliferation and migration. Our previous study observed that although γ-tocotrienol also did not affect the Akt1 and ERK 1/2 signaling pathways, cyclin D1 was associated with the inhibition of ASM proliferation and migration. This suggests that various isoforms of vitamin E may have different mechanisms associated with the inhibition of ASM remodeling. ASM proliferation involves crosstalk between inflammatory mediators, contractile agonists, and growth factors released during inflammation. This condition triggers ASM proliferation through activation of the MAPKs, PI3K/AKT, and JAK2/STAT3 signaling pathways. The migration of ASM cells is also a multifaceted process, with several signaling molecules, such as FAK, PI3K, PTEN, ERK, p38, Src, Rho kinase, c-Abl, and Wnt/β-catenin, identified as contributors to the regulation of ASM cell migration [52]. Exploring both upstream and downstream ASM proliferation and migration signaling pathways may provide clear insight into the precise mechanism by which tocotrienol inhibits ASM proliferation and migration.

The reduction in ROS production by β-tocotrienol was observed in this current study. This result is in line with our previous study, which observed a decrease in ROS levels in the γ-tocotrienol pre-treatment group compared to the PDGF-BB group. Several studies have observed the influence of oxygen species generation in ASM proliferation [39,61,62], highlighting the importance of targeting ROS in airway remodeling. The precise mechanism of the antioxidant activity of β-tocotrienol is not fully understood, and further studies are needed to elucidate this aspect. However, several potential mechanisms can be considered, including the enhancement of antioxidant enzymes including glutathione peroxidase activity, scavenging of free radicals, and inhibition of lipid peroxidation [63,64]. The comparative antioxidant strength of β-tocotrienol to other isoforms of vitamin E remains unclear. Nevertheless, tocotrienols, in general, have been suggested to exhibit more potent antioxidant activity than tocopherol [63–66].

In this study, we did not assess the anti-inflammatory effects of β-tocotrienol, and further investigations are required to understand the precise mechanism of β-tocotrienol as an anti-inflammatory agent. β-tocotrienol has the potential to exert a therapeutic effect on airway remodeling by diminishing ASM proliferation and migration. Furthermore, it may possess anti-inflammatory properties, thereby contributing to the amelioration of airway remodeling in asthma. The anti-inflammatory effects of tocotrienol have been observed in several studies. For instance, the reduction in several pro-inflammatory cytokines, including tumor necrosis factor-α (TNF-α), IL-4, and IL-8, through the inhibition of inducible NO synthase (iNOS) and COX-2 expression, was observed after administration of a tocotrienol-rich fraction [31]. Another study observed a reduction in mRNA and protein expressions of TNF-α, IL-1β, IL-6, and iNOS via inhibition of the nuclear translocations of NF-κB and activator protein-1 (AP-1) after treatments with δ-tocotrienol [30], suggesting that tocotrienol has potent anti-inflammatory properties that may be beneficial in airway inflammation and remodeling.

In this study, we did not assess the comparative effects between β-tocotrienol and γ-tocotrienol or with other isoforms of vitamin E. Comparative studies between vitamin E isoforms are limited to antioxidant comparisons between tocotrienol and tocopherol isoforms [36,37], or comparisons in the antiproliferative effects in cancer cells [38]. For instance, comparisons between β-tocotrienol and γ-tocotrienol demonstrated a notably stronger anti-proliferative effect in β-tocotrienol in human breast adenocarcinoma cell lines MDA-MB-231 and MCF7 [38]. This study may offer insight that β-tocotrienol has a more potent cytotoxic effect compared to γ-tocotrienol, suggesting that using β-tocotrienol instead of γ-tocotrienol to target normal cells should be considered for this effect. In this study, we did not conduct viability or apoptotic tests in normal human ASM cells. However, our findings indicated that the administration of 5–25 μM β-tocotrienols alone did not significantly decrease ASM cell proliferation and compared to the non-stimulated group. This suggests that at this dose, β-tocotrienols do not exert a cytotoxic effect on human ASM cell lines.

Clinical studies on Vitamin E administration in asthma have not yet yielded conclusive results to date. Asthmatic patients have been shown to exhibit lower dietary vitamin E levels [67], with severe asthma patients exhibiting lower vitamin E levels compared to those with mild asthma [13]. Additionally, a different study observed that supplemental vitamin E during pregnancy could prevent asthmatic diseases [68]. In the context of clinical studies involving vitamin E isoform, γ-tocopherol administration significantly decreased induced sputum neutrophils compared to the placebo [69], indicating the potential benefit of the vitamin E isoform in reducing neutrophilic airway inflammation. However, one study found that vitamin E supplementation did not affect asthma control in mild to moderate adult asthma subjects [70].

Further investigations are warranted to elucidate the potential benefits of vitamin E and its isoforms for the clinical management of asthma and airway remodeling. Assessing the effects of anti-inflammatory-related vitamin E isoforms should be a priority. Evaluating other signaling molecules or pathways that may indirectly influence ASM remodeling may provide clear insight into the precise mechanism by which tocotrienol inhibits ASM proliferation and migration. Evaluating the effects of other vitamin E isoforms, such as α- or δ-tocotrienol, is also important. Assessing the effects of vitamin E isoforms on other cells, such as airway epithelial cells, may offer benefits as airway remodeling involves not only ASM cells. While the in vitro findings are promising, future studies should validate the efficacy of vitamin E isoform in relevant animal models of asthma to ascertain their therapeutic potential in vivo, including investigating the long-term effects of tocotrienols on ASM remodeling in animal models of asthma or exploring synergistic effects with existing asthma medications, which would enrich the discussion and stimulate further scientific inquiry.

4. Materials and Methods

4.1. Human ASM Cells and Culture Conditions

Immortalized human ASM cells, achieved through stable expression of human telomerase reverse transcriptase (hTERT), were used in this present experiment. These cells were generously provided by Dr. Andrew J. Halayko from the University of Manitoba. The cells were cultured in Dulbecco's Modified Eagle's Medium (DMEM) supplemented with 10% Fetal Bovine Serum (FBS), 100 μg/mL penicillin, and 100 μg/mL streptomycin then incubated at 37 °C in a humidified 5% CO_2 atmosphere until they reached 70–80% confluence. Each experiment utilized a minimum of three distinct cell lines.

4.2. Reagents

β-tocotrienols, the monoclonal antibody against RhoA, PDGF-BB were purchased from Cayman Chemical (Ann Arbor, MI, USA), Santa Cruz Biotechnology (Dallas, TX, USA), and Wako (Osaka, Japan), respectively. In our previous study, it was observed that PDGF-BB at a concentration of 10 ng/mL induced ASM proliferation and migration. A dosage of 5–50 μM of γ-tocotrienol was used to assess the inhibitory effect on PDGF-BB-induced ASM proliferation and migration, and this effect was effectively reduced by the administration of 25 μM γ-tocotrienol [34]. Therefore, this dosage was selected for use in the current experiment.

4.3. Cell Proliferation Assay

Human ASM cells were seeded in 96-well plates at a density of 5.0×10^3 cells/well in DMEM supplemented with 0.3% bovine serum albumin (BSA) and allowed to adhere for 24 h. Subsequently, the cells were treated with 5–25 μM β-tocotrienols for one hour, followed by incubation with 10 ng/mL PDGF-BB for 48 h. The Cell Counting Kit (CCK-8) (Dojindo, Kumamoto, Japan) was used to measure the proliferation of cells. A Sunrise microplate analyzer (TECAN, Mannedorf, Switzerland) was used to measure the results at 450 nm with a reference wavelength of 600 nm.

4.4. Cell Migration Assay

Cell migration was evaluated using a transwell chamber (Costar, Corning Incorporated, Corning, NY, USA). Human ASM cells were cultured in 100-mm dishes until nearly confluent, then maintained in a serum-free medium for 24 h. Following trypsinization, cells were resuspended in DMEM containing 0.3% BSA. After a one-hour treatment with 5–50 μM β-tocotrienols, 100 μL (5.0×10^4 cells/well) of the suspension was added to the upper wells of the chamber, while 5 ng/mL PDGF-BB with 5–50 μM β-tocotrienols was placed in the bottom of the chambers. Following five hours of incubation, the cells were stained using Diff-Quick (Sysmex, Kobe, Japan) and then fixed with 10% formalin. Swabbing was employed to eliminate non-migrating cells from the top of the chambers. Migrated cells were counted manually in 10 randomly selected fields, and the average cell count per field was compared to that of the non-stimulated group.

4.5. Preparation of Cell Lysate and Western Blotting

Cells were rinsed with ice-cold phosphate-buffered saline (PBS) and subsequently lysed using a lysate buffer consisting of 500 μL 1× lysis buffer and 5 μL 100 mM PMSF. Equal amounts of protein were then subjected to electrophoresis and transferred onto polyvinylidene difluoride (PVDF) membranes (Amersham Hybond-P, GE Healthcare Lifescience, Buckinghamshire, UK). The membranes were incubated with primary rabbit antibodies: cyclin D1 (1:2000; Cell Signaling Technology); anti-rabbit phosphorylated and non-phosphorylated Akt1 (1:1000; Cell Signaling Technology, Danvers, MA, USA); polyclonal rabbit anti-phosphorylated or total antibodies for ERK1/2 (1:5000; Promega, Madison, WI, USA), followed by a second antibody incubation for 1 h at room temperature with horseradish peroxidase-conjugated anti-rabbit IgG (1:5000; GE Healthcare Lifescience). The bands were then visualized on an ImageQuant LAS 4000 mini (GE Healthcare Lifescience) using ECL reagent (GE Healthcare Lifescience) and densitometry quantified using TotalLab Quant software version 7.0 (Newcastle, UK).

4.6. Active Rho Detection Assay

Rho activity was measured according to the manufacturer's instructions using an Active Rho detection kit (Cell Signaling Technology, Danvers, MA, USA). Human ASM cells were cultured in 100-mm dishes until they reached 60–70% confluence, followed by 24 h of maintenance in Ham's F-12 (serum-free medium). The cells were then preincubated for one hour with 25 μM β-tocotrienols before being stimulated with 10 ng/mL PDGF-BB for five minutes. Subsequently, the cells were lysed in the lysis buffer (20 mM HEPES, 10 mM EGTA, 40 mM β-glycerophosphate, 1% Triton-X-100, 20 mM $MgCl_2$, 2 mM Na_3VO_4, 1 mM DTT, 10 μg/mL leupeptin, 10 μg/mL aprotinin, 1 mM PMSF, 100 mM NaCl). To the cell lysate, 400 μg GST-Rhotekin-RBD was added and gently rocked for 1 h at 4 °C. Samples were run through gel electrophoresis and subsequently transferred onto PVDF membranes (Immobilon-P, Millipore, Billerica, MA, USA). Following this, the membranes were blocked with 5% non-fat dry milk in Tris-buffered saline (20 mM Tris, 150 mM NaCl, pH 7.6) containing 0.1% Tween 20 (TBS-T) for 1 h at room temperature. Then, the membranes were incubated overnight at 4 °C with 0.1% TBS-T containing primary mouse monoclonal IgG for RhoA (1:1000; Santa Cruz Biotechnology). After being washed with TBS-T, the membranes were incubated with a secondary antibody for 1 h at room temperature, using horseradish peroxidase-conjugated anti-mouse IgG antibody (1:3000). The bands were then visualized on an ImageQuant LAS 4000 mini (GE Healthcare Lifescience) using ECL reagent (GE Healthcare Lifescience) and densitometry quantified using TotalLab Quant software (Newcastle, UK).

4.7. Intracellular Reactive Oxygen Species Quantification

The level of ROS in ASM cells was measured utilizing the Oxiselect intracellular ROS assay kit (Cell Biolabs, San Diego, CA, USA) according to the manufacturer's guidelines. The assay utilizes the cell-permeable fluorogenic probe 2′,7′-Dichlorodihydrofluorescin diacetate (DCFH-DA). Cellular esterases deacetylate DCFH-DA to the non-fluorescent 2′,7′-Dichlorodihydrofluorescin (DCFH), which is then rapidly oxidized to the highly fluorescent 2′,7′-Dichlorohihydrofluorescin (DCF) by ROS. In this investigation, serum-starved ASM cells were treated with 0.1 mM DCFH-DA for 1 h at 37 °C. Subsequently, human ASM cells were stimulated with PDGF-BB in the presence or absence of a 1-h pre-treatment with 25 μM β-tocotrienols. The intracellular ROS level was determined through fluorescence intensity, and quantification was carried out using a fluorescence plate reader (Infinite 500, TECAN).

4.8. Statistical Analysis

The data are presented as mean ± standard deviation (SD). Statistical differences between groups were analyzed using ANOVA. A subsequent multiple comparison test between pairs of groups was performed, with statistical significance defined as $p < 0.05$.

5. Conclusions

In conclusion, β-tocotrienols have demonstrated efficacy in reducing ASM cell proliferation and migration. We have also elucidated the key components of the downstream signaling cascade associated with the effects of β-tocotrienols on ASM cell proliferation and migration. This involves the inhibition of ROS production and RhoA inactivation. These findings suggest that β-tocotrienols may hold potential as a treatment for airway remodeling, which could benefit individuals with asthma. Further investigations are warranted to fully understand the potential of β-tocotrienols in addressing airway remodeling, especially through laboratory and clinical studies.

Author Contributions: Investigation: A.S.L., R.O., T.H., M.T., M.M., H.I., Y.F. and A.Y.; writing-original draft preparation: A.S.L.; review and editing: A.S.L., R.O., T.H., M.T., M.M., H.I., Y.F. and A.Y.; conceptualization: R.O., T.H. and A.Y.; supervision: A.Y. All authors have read and agreed to the published version of the manuscript.

Funding: This work was supported by JPPS KAKENI II 24500976.

Institutional Review Board Statement: Not applicable.

Informed Consent Statement: Not applicable.

Data Availability Statement: Data is contained within the article.

Acknowledgments: We express our gratitude to Andrew J. Halayko from the University of Manitoba for generously providing immortalized human ASM cells.

Conflicts of Interest: The authors declare no conflicts of interest.

References

1. GINA. From the Global Strategy for Asthma Management and Prevention, Global Initiative for Asthma (GINA). 2023. Available online: https://ginasthma.org/gina-reports/ (accessed on 8 February 2024).
2. Vignola, A.M.; Mirabella, F.; Costanzo, G.; Di Giorgi, R.; Gjomarkaj, M.; Bellia, V.; Bonsignore, G. Airway Remodeling in Asthma. *Chest* **2003**, *123* (Suppl. S3), 417S–422S. [CrossRef] [PubMed]
3. Hough, K.P.; Curtiss, M.L.; Blain, T.J.; Liu, R.-M.; Trevor, J.; Deshane, J.S.; Thannickal, V.J. Airway Remodeling in Asthma. *Front. Med.* **2020**, *7*, 191. Available online: https://www.frontiersin.org/articles/10.3389/fmed.2020.00191 (accessed on 8 February 2024). [CrossRef]
4. Sun, Z.; Ji, N.; Ma, Q.; Zhu, R.; Chen, Z.; Wang, Z.; Qian, Y.; Wu, C.; Hu, F.; Huang, M.; et al. Epithelial-Mesenchymal Transition in Asthma Airway Remodeling Is Regulated by the IL-33/CD146 Axis. *Front. Immunol.* **2020**, *11*, 1598. [CrossRef] [PubMed]

5. Michalik, M.; Wójcik-Pszczoła, K.; Paw, M.; Wnuk, D.; Koczurkiewicz, P.; Sanak, M.; Pękala, E.; Madeja, Z. Fibroblast-to-myofibroblast transition in bronchial asthma. *Cell. Mol. Life Sci.* **2018**, *75*, 3943–3961. [CrossRef]
6. Yu, Y.; Sakai, H.; Misawa, M.; Chiba, Y. Matrix Metalloproteinases-9 (MMPs-9) and -12 Are Upregulated in the Airways of Mice with Chronic Airway Inflammation and Remodeling. *ISRN Pulmonol.* **2012**, *2012*, 840489. [CrossRef]
7. Salter, B.; Pray, C.; Radford, K.; Martin, J.G.; Nair, P. Regulation of human airway smooth muscle cell migration and relevance to asthma. *Respir. Res.* **2017**, *18*, 156. [CrossRef]
8. Redhu, N.S.; Shan, L.; Movassagh, H.; Gounni, A.S. Thymic Stromal Lymphopoietin Induces Migration in Human Airway Smooth Muscle Cells. *Sci. Rep.* **2013**, *3*, 2301. [CrossRef]
9. McDonald, D.M. Angiogenesis and Remodeling of Airway Vasculature in Chronic Inflammation. *Am. J. Respir. Crit. Care Med.* **2001**, *164*, S39–S45. [CrossRef]
10. Gabehart, K.E.; Royce, S.G.; Maselli, D.J.; Miyasato, S.K.; Davis, E.C.; Tang, M.L.K.; Jourdan Le Saux, C. Airway hyperresponsiveness is associated with airway remodeling but not inflammation in aging Cav1$^{-/-}$mice. *Respir. Res.* **2013**, *14*, 110. [CrossRef] [PubMed]
11. Pepe, C.; Foley, S.; Shannon, J.; Lemiere, C.; Olivenstein, R.; Ernst, P.; Ludwig, M.S.; Martin, J.G.; Hamid, Q. Differences in airway remodeling between subjects with severe and moderate asthma. *J. Allergy Clin. Immunol.* **2005**, *116*, 544–549. [CrossRef]
12. Ward, C.; Johns, D.P.; Bish, R.O.S.; Pais, M.; Reid, D.W.; Ingram, C.; Feltis, B.; Walters, E.H. Reduced Airway Distensibility, Fixed Airflow Limitation, and Airway Wall Remodeling in Asthma. *Am. J. Respir. Crit. Care Med.* **2001**, *164*, 1718–1721. [CrossRef]
13. Allen, S.; Britton, J.R.; Leonardi-Bee, J.A. Association between antioxidant vitamins and asthma outcome measures: Systematic review and meta-analysis. *Thorax* **2009**, *64*, 610–619. [CrossRef]
14. Jolliffe, D.A.; Greenberg, L.; Hooper, R.L.; Griffiths, C.J.; Camargo, C.A., Jr.; Kerley, C.P.; Jensen, M.E.; Mauger, D.; Stelmach, I.; Urashima, M.; et al. Vitamin D supplementation to prevent asthma exacerbations: A systematic review and meta-analysis of individual participant data. *Lancet Respir. Med.* **2017**, *5*, 881–890. [CrossRef]
15. Wang, M.; Liu, M.; Wang, C.; Xiao, Y.; An, T.; Zou, M.; Cheng, G. Association between vitamin D status and asthma control: A meta-analysis of randomized trials. *Respir. Med.* **2019**, *150*, 85–94. [CrossRef]
16. Nurmatov, U.; Devereux, G.; Sheikh, A. Nutrients and foods for the primary prevention of asthma and allergy: Systematic review and meta-analysis. *J. Allergy Clin. Immunol.* **2011**, *127*, 724–733.e30. [CrossRef]
17. Zhao, Y.; Lee, M.-J.; Cheung, C.; Ju, J.-H.; Chen, Y.-K.; Liu, B.; Hu, L.-Q.; Yang, C.S. Analysis of Multiple Metabolites of Tocopherols and Tocotrienols in Mice and Humans. *J. Agric. Food Chem.* **2010**, *58*, 4844–4852. [CrossRef]
18. Jiang, Q. Metabolism of natural forms of vitamin E and biological actions of vitamin E metabolites. *Free Radic. Biol. Med.* **2022**, *179*, 375–387. [CrossRef]
19. Müller, L.; Theile, K.; Böhm, V. In vitro antioxidant activity of tocopherols and tocotrienols and comparison of vitamin E concentration and lipophilic antioxidant capacity in human plasma. *Mol. Nutr. Food Res.* **2010**, *54*, 731–742. [CrossRef]
20. Yoshida, Y.; Niki, E.; Noguchi, N. Comparative study on the action of tocopherols and tocotrienols as antioxidant: Chemical and physical effects. *Chem. Phys. Lipids* **2003**, *123*, 63–75. [CrossRef]
21. Suzuki, Y.J.; Tsuchiya, M.; Wassall, S.R.; Choo, Y.M.; Govil, G.; Kagan, V.E.; Packer, L. Structural and dynamic membrane properties of .alpha.-tocopherol and .alpha.-tocotrienol: Implication to the molecular mechanism of their antioxidant potency. *Biochemistry* **1993**, *32*, 10692–10699. [CrossRef]
22. Inokuchi, H.; Hirokane, H.; Tsuzuki, T.; Nakagawa, K.; Igarashi, M.; Miyazawa, T. Anti-angiogenic Activity of Tocotrienol. *Biosci. Biotechnol. Biochem.* **2003**, *67*, 1623–1627. [CrossRef]
23. Pang, K.-L.; Mai, C.-W.; Chin, K.-Y. Molecular Mechanism of Tocotrienol-Mediated Anticancer Properties: A Systematic Review of the Involvement of Endoplasmic Reticulum Stress and Unfolded Protein Response. *Nutrients* **2023**, *15*, 1854. [CrossRef]
24. Samant, G.V.; Wali, V.B.; Sylvester, P.W. Anti-proliferative effects of γ-tocotrienol on mammary tumour cells are associated with suppression of cell cycle progression. *Cell Prolif.* **2010**, *43*, 77–83. [CrossRef]
25. Ramli, F.F.; Ali, A.; Ibrahim, N. Protective Effects of Tocotrienols in Cerebral and Myocardial Ischemia-Reperfusion Injury: A Systematic Review. *Appl. Sci.* **2021**, *11*, 7994. [CrossRef]
26. Lekli, I.; Ray, D.; Mukherjee, S.; Gurusamy, N.; Ahsan, M.K.; Juhasz, B.; Bak, I.; Tosaki, A.; Gherghiceanu, M.; Popescu, L.M.; et al. Co-ordinated autophagy with resveratrol and γ-tocotrienol confers synergetic cardioprotection. *J. Cell. Mol. Med.* **2010**, *14*, 2506–2518. [CrossRef]
27. Baliarsingh, S.; Beg, Z.H.; Ahmad, J. The therapeutic impacts of tocotrienols in type 2 diabetic patients with hyperlipidemia. *Atherosclerosis* **2005**, *182*, 367–374. [CrossRef]
28. Mahjabeen, W.; Khan, D.A.; Mirza, S.A.; Pervez, M.A. Effects of delta-tocotrienol supplementation on Glycemic Control, oxidative stress, inflammatory biomarkers and miRNA expression in type 2 diabetes mellitus: A randomized control trial. *Phyther. Res.* **2021**, *35*, 3968–3976. [CrossRef]
29. Daud, Z.A.M.; Tubie, B.; Sheyman, M.; Osia, R.; Adams, J.; Tubie, S.; Khosla, P. Vitamin E tocotrienol supplementation improves lipid profiles in chronic hemodialysis patients. *Vasc. Health Risk Manag.* **2013**, *9*, 747–761. [CrossRef]
30. Shen, J.; Yang, T.; Xu, Y.; Luo, Y.; Zhong, X.; Shi, L.; Hu, T.; Guo, T.; Nie, Y.; Luo, F.; et al. δ-Tocotrienol, Isolated from Rice Bran, Exerts an Anti-Inflammatory Effect via MAPKs and PPARs Signaling Pathways in Lipopolysaccharide-Stimulated Macrophages. *Int. J. Mol. Sci.* **2018**, *19*, 3022. [CrossRef]

31. Wu, S.-J.; Liu, P.-L.; Ng, L.-T. Tocotrienol-rich fraction of palm oil exhibits anti-inflammatory property by suppressing the expression of inflammatory mediators in human monocytic cells. *Mol. Nutr. Food Res.* **2008**, *52*, 921–929. [CrossRef]
32. Peh, H.Y.; Tan, W.S.D.; Chan, T.K.; Pow, C.W.; Foster, P.S.; Wong, W.S.F. Vitamin E isoform γ-tocotrienol protects against emphysema in cigarette smoke-induced COPD. *Free Radic. Biol. Med.* **2017**, *110*, 332–344. [CrossRef]
33. Lu, Y.; Zhang, Y.; Xu, D.; Wang, Y.; Pan, D.; Wang, P.; Xia, J.; Yin, S.; Liao, W.; Wang, S.; et al. Tocotrienol-Rich Fractions Offer Potential to Suppress Pulmonary Fibrosis Progression. *Int. J. Mol. Sci.* **2022**, *23*, 14331. [CrossRef]
34. Harada, T.; Yamasaki, A.; Chikumi, H.; Hashimoto, K.; Okazaki, R.; Takata, M.; Fukushima, T.; Watanabe, M.; Kurai, J.; Halayko, A.J.; et al. γ-Tocotrienol reduces human airway smooth muscle cell proliferation and migration. *Pulm. Pharmacol. Ther.* **2015**, *32*, 45–52. [CrossRef]
35. Fukushima, T.; Yamasaki, A.; Harada, T.; Chikumi, H.; Watanabe, M.; Okazaki, R.; Takata, M.; Hasegawa, Y.; Kurai, J.; Yanai, M.; et al. γ-Tocotrienol Inhibits TGF-β1-Induced Contractile Phenotype Expression of Human Airway Smooth Muscle Cells. *Yonago Acta Med.* **2017**, *60*, 16–23.
36. Ko, S.-N.; Kim, C.-J.; Kim, C.-T.; Kim, Y.; Kim, I.-H. Effects of tocopherols and tocotrienols on the inhibition of autoxidation of conjugated linoleic acid. *Eur. J. Lipid Sci. Technol.* **2010**, *112*, 496–501. [CrossRef]
37. Nor Azman, N.; Goon, J.; Abdul Ghani, S.; Hamid, Z.; Wan Ngah, W. Comparing Palm Oil, Tocotrienol-Rich Fraction and α-Tocopherol Supplementation on the Antioxidant Levels of Older Adults. *Antioxidants* **2018**, *7*, 74. [CrossRef]
38. Idriss, M.; Hodroj, M.H.; Fakhoury, R.; Rizk, S. Beta-Tocotrienol Exhibits More Cytotoxic Effects than Gamma-Tocotrienol on Breast Cancer Cells by Promoting Apoptosis via a P53-Independent PI3-Kinase Dependent Pathway. *Biomolecules* **2020**, *10*, 577. [CrossRef]
39. Brar, S.S.; Kennedy, T.P.; Whorton, A.R.; Murphy, T.M.; Chitano, P.; Hoidal, J.R. Requirement for Reactive Oxygen Species in Serum-induced and Platelet-derived Growth Factor-induced Growth of Airway Smooth Muscle*. *J. Biol. Chem.* **1999**, *274*, 20017–20026. [CrossRef]
40. Qiao, L.; Xu, Y.; Liu, X.; Xie, J.; Wang, J.; Du, C.; Zhang, J.; Ni, W.; Chen, S. Role of protein kinase C α and cyclin D1 in the proliferation of airway smooth muscle in asthmatic rats. *Chin. Med. J.* **2008**, *121*, 2070–2076. [CrossRef] [PubMed]
41. Page, K.; Li, J.; Wang, Y.; Kartha, S.; Pestell, R.G.; Hershenson, M.B. Regulation of Cyclin D1 Expression and DNA Synthesis by Phosphatidylinositol 3-Kinase in Airway Smooth Muscle Cells. *Am. J. Respir. Cell Mol. Biol.* **2000**, *23*, 436–443. [CrossRef] [PubMed]
42. Yang, K.; Hitomi, M.; Stacey, D.W. Variations in cyclin D1 levels through the cell cycle determine the proliferative fate of a cell. *Cell Div.* **2006**, *1*, 32. [CrossRef]
43. Guan, X.; Guan, X.; Dong, C.; Jiao, Z. Rho GTPases and related signaling complexes in cell migration and invasion. *Exp. Cell Res.* **2020**, *388*, 111824. [CrossRef]
44. Evers, E.E.; Zondag, G.C.M.; Malliri, A.; Price, L.S.; ten Klooster, J.-P.; van der Kammen, R.A.; Collard, J.G. Rho family proteins in cell adhesion and cell migration. *Eur. J. Cancer* **2000**, *36*, 1269–1274. [CrossRef]
45. Sadok, A.; Marshall, C.J. Rho GTPases. *Small GTPases* **2014**, *5*, e983878. [CrossRef]
46. Black, J.L.; Roth, M.; Lee, J.; Carlin, S.; Johnson, P.R.A. Mechanisms of Airway Remodeling. *Am. J. Respir. Crit. Care Med.* **2001**, *164*, S63–S66. [CrossRef]
47. Madison, J.M. Migration of Airway Smooth Muscle Cells. *Am. J. Respir. Cell Mol. Biol.* **2003**, *29*, 8–11. [CrossRef]
48. Yang, Q.; Shi, W. Rho/ROCK-MYOCD in regulating airway smooth muscle growth and remodeling. *Am. J. Physiol. Cell. Mol. Physiol.* **2021**, *321*, L1–L5. [CrossRef]
49. Lv, C.; Huang, Y.; Yan, R.; Gao, Y. Vascular endothelial growth factor induces the migration of human airway smooth muscle cells by activating the RhoA/ROCK pathway. *BMC Pulm. Med.* **2023**, *23*, 505. [CrossRef]
50. Liu, L.; Zhai, C.; Pan, Y.; Zhu, Y.; Shi, W.; Wang, J.; Yan, X.; Su, X.; Song, Y.; Gao, L.; et al. Sphingosine-1-phosphate induces airway smooth muscle cell proliferation, migration, and contraction by modulating Hippo signaling effector YAP. *Am. J. Physiol. Cell. Mol. Physiol.* **2018**, *315*, L609–L621. [CrossRef]
51. Li, N.; Cai, R.; Niu, Y.; Shen, B.; Xu, J.; Cheng, Y. Inhibition of angiotensin II-induced contraction of human airway smooth muscle cells by angiotensin-(1-7) via downregulation of the RhoA/ROCK2 signaling pathway. *Int. J. Mol. Med.* **2012**, *30*, 811–818. [CrossRef]
52. Yap, H.M.; Israf, D.A.; Harith, H.H.; Tham, C.L.; Sulaiman, M.R. Crosstalk Between Signaling Pathways Involved in the Regulation of Airway Smooth Muscle Cell Hyperplasia. *Front. Pharmacol.* **2019**, *10*, 1148. [CrossRef]
53. Raqeeb, A.; Jiao, Y.; Syyong, H.T.; Paré, P.D.; Seow, C.Y. Regulatable stiffness in relaxed airway smooth muscle: A target for asthma treatment? *J. Appl. Physiol.* **2011**, *112*, 337–346. [CrossRef]
54. Chiba, Y.; Misawa, M. The role of RhoA-mediated Ca^{2+} sensitization of bronchial smooth muscle contraction in airway hyperresponsiveness. *J. Smooth Muscle Res.* **2004**, *40*, 155–167. [CrossRef]
55. Wei, B.; Shang, Y.X.; Li, M.; Jiang, J.; Zhang, H. Cytoskeleton changes of airway smooth muscle cells in juvenile rats with airway remodeling in asthma and the RhoA/ROCK signaling pathway mechanism. *Genet. Mol. Res.* **2014**, *13*, 559–569. [CrossRef]
56. Zhang, Y.; Saradna, A.; Ratan, R.; Ke, X.; Tu, W.; Do, D.C.; Hu, C.; Gao, P. RhoA/Rho-kinases in asthma: From pathogenesis to therapeutic targets. *Clin. Transl. Immunol.* **2020**, *9*, e1134. [CrossRef]

57. Schaafsma, D.; Bos, I.S.T.; Zuidhof, A.B.; Zaagsma, J.; Meurs, H. The inhaled Rho kinase inhibitor Y-27632 protects against allergen-induced acute bronchoconstriction, airway hyperresponsiveness, and inflammation. *Am. J. Physiol. Cell. Mol. Physiol.* **2008**, *295*, L214–L219. [CrossRef]
58. Henry, P.J.; Mann, T.S.; Goldie, R.G. A Rho kinase inhibitor, Y-27632 inhibits pulmonary eosinophilia, bronchoconstriction and airways hyperresponsiveness in allergic mice. *Pulm. Pharmacol. Ther.* **2005**, *18*, 67–74. [CrossRef]
59. Chiba, Y.; Matsusue, K.; Misawa, M. RhoA, a Possible Target for Treatment of Airway Hyperresponsiveness in Bronchial Asthma. *J. Pharmacol. Sci.* **2010**, *114*, 239–247. [CrossRef]
60. Xie, T.; Luo, G.Y.; Zhang, Y.; Wang, X.; Wang, X.Y.; Wu, M.; Li, G.P. Rho-kinase inhibitor fasudil reduces allergic airway inflammation and mucus hypersecretion by regulating STAT6 and NFκB. *Clin. Exp. Allergy* **2015**, *45*, 1812–1822. [CrossRef]
61. Pandya, H.C.; Snetkov, V.A.; Twort, C.H.C.; Ward, J.P.T.; Hirst, S.J. Oxygen regulates mitogen-stimulated proliferation of fetal human airway smooth muscle cells. *Am. J. Physiol. Cell. Mol. Physiol.* **2002**, *283*, L1220–L1230. [CrossRef]
62. Svensson Holm, A.-C.B.; Bengtsson, T.; Grenegård, M.; Lindström, E.G. Platelets stimulate airway smooth muscle cell proliferation through mechanisms involving 5-lipoxygenase and reactive oxygen species. *Platelets* **2008**, *19*, 528–536. [CrossRef]
63. Maniam, S.; Mohamed, N.; Shuid, A.N.; Soelaiman, I.N. Palm Tocotrienol Exerted Better Antioxidant Activities in Bone than α-Tocopherol. *Basic Clin. Pharmacol. Toxicol.* **2008**, *103*, 55–60. [CrossRef]
64. Rossi, M.; Alamprese, C.; Ratti, S. Tocopherols and tocotrienols as free radical-scavengers in refined vegetable oils and their stability during deep-fat frying. *Food Chem.* **2007**, *102*, 812–817. [CrossRef]
65. Packer, L.; Weber, S.U.; Rimbach, G. Molecular Aspects of α-Tocotrienol Antioxidant Action and Cell Signalling. *J. Nutr.* **2001**, *131*, 369S–373S. [CrossRef]
66. Serbinova, E.; Kagan, V.; Han, D.; Packer, L. Free radical recycling and intramembrane mobility in the antioxidant properties of alpha-tocopherol and alpha-tocotrienol. *Free Radic. Biol. Med.* **1991**, *10*, 263–275. [CrossRef]
67. de Luis, D.A.; Armentia, A.; Aller, R.; Asensio, A.; Sedano, E.; Izaola, O.; Cuellar, L. Dietary intake in patients with asthma: A case control study. *Nutrition* **2005**, *21*, 320–324. [CrossRef]
68. Wu, H.; Zhang, C.; Wang, Y.; Li, Y. Does vitamin E prevent asthma or wheeze in children: A systematic review and meta-analysis. *Paediatr. Respir. Rev.* **2018**, *27*, 60–68. [CrossRef]
69. Hernandez, M.L.; Wagner, J.G.; Kala, A.; Mills, K.; Wells, H.B.; Alexis, N.E.; Lay, J.C.; Jiang, Q.; Zhang, H.; Zhou, H.; et al. Vitamin E, γ-tocopherol, reduces airway neutrophil recruitment after inhaled endotoxin challenge in rats and in healthy volunteers. *Free Radic. Biol. Med.* **2013**, *60*, 56–62. [CrossRef]
70. Pearson, P.J.K.; Lewis, S.A.; Britton, J.; Fogarty, A. Vitamin E supplements in asthma: A parallel group randomised placebo controlled trial. *Thorax* **2004**, *59*, 652–656. [CrossRef]

pharmaceuticals

MDPI

Systematic Review

Evidence Gaps in Clinical Trials of Pharmacologic Treatment for H1-Antihistamine-Refractory Chronic Spontaneous Urticaria: A Systematic Review and Future Perspectives

Surapon Nochaiwong [1,2,*], Mati Chuamanochan [2,3], Chidchanok Ruengorn [1,2] and Kednapa Thavorn [2,4,5,*]

1 Department of Pharmaceutical Care, Faculty of Pharmacy, Chiang Mai University, Chiang Mai 50200, Thailand
2 Pharmacoepidemiology and Statistics Research Center (PESRC), Chiang Mai University, Chiang Mai 50200, Thailand
3 Division of Dermatology, Department of Internal Medicine, Faculty of Medicine, Chiang Mai University, Chiang Mai 50200, Thailand
4 Ottawa Hospital Research Institute, Ottawa Hospital, Ottawa, ON K1H 8L6, Canada
5 School of Epidemiology and Public Health, Faculty of Medicine, University of Ottawa, Ottawa, ON K1G 5Z3, Canada
* Correspondence: surapon.nochaiwong@cmu.ac.th (S.N.); kthavorn@ohri.ca (K.T.); Tel.: +66-53-944-342 (S.N.); +66-613-7378899 (ext. 72330) (K.T.)

Abstract: No data addressing issues concerning disparities in participant and trial characteristics and trial outcome reporting have been established in clinical trials for H1-antihistamine-refractory chronic spontaneous urticaria (CSU). To better harmonize and compare the different treatment interventions, we systematically evaluated the overall landscape of pharmacological treatments for H1-antihistamine-refractory CSU clinical trials published between 2000 and 2021. This systematic review included 23 randomized clinical trials involving 2480 participants from 22 countries. We found significant increases in the number of globally published and newly tested drugs, especially biologic drugs. Regarding relatively small trials, we found that people living with H1-antihistamine-refractory CSU who were identified as members of minority groups (non-white population), populations of regions other than North America/Europe, and populations of low- to lower/upper-middle-income countries are underrepresented. Most trials were designed to evaluate treatment efficacy and safety profiles; however, less than half of the included trials reported the patient's perspective in terms of patient-reported outcomes. Disparities in outcome reporting, including clinimetric tools for assessing treatment response and outcome sets, were observed. To close the evidence gap in H1-antihistamine refractory CSU trials, strategies for improving trial and participant enrollment and standardizing core outcome sets for trial reporting are needed.

Keywords: biologic agents; chronic spontaneous urticaria; clinical trials; core outcomes sets; evidence gaps; H1-antihistamine-refractory; minority groups

1. Introduction

Chronic spontaneous urticaria (CSU) is characterized by wheals and itching lasting for more than six weeks, with or without angioedema and with no identifiable trigger [1]. This condition affects patients of all ages and has an estimated global prevalence of 4.4%, which has been increasing over time [2]. Despite the widespread use of licensed doses and up-dosing (i.e., two- to four-fold higher than approved doses) of H1-antihistamines, less than half of patients with CSU responded adequately to this first-line therapy [1,3]. Furthermore, CSU can severely impact health-related quality of life (HRQOL), reduce physical and social interactions, affect work or school performance, and negatively affect mental health and psychosocial issues, particularly refractory cases [1,4].

Over the past decade, therapy for people living with CSU, mainly those unresponsive to licensed doses and up-dosing of H1-antihistamines, has evolved rapidly [5–7]. Currently, randomized trials of novel therapies to offer pharmacological treatment options for the management of H1-antihistamine-refractory CSU are ongoing [1,5]. These promising pharmacological therapies possess biological, immunosuppressive, and other pharmacological qualities. Recent evidence has suggested that biologic agents such as ligelizumab (72 or 240 mg) and omalizumab (300 or 600 mg) appear to be effective treatments (moderate to large beneficial effect) and were closely associated with improved HRQOL in people living with H1-antihistamine-refractory CSU [8,9].

To date, there is a need to improve disparities in the diversity of participant enrollment based on equity and representativeness to close the gap in dermatologic trials [10]. According to the United States Food and Drug Administration (FDA), in 2014, an action plan was recognized and developed to support and encourage diversity in randomized clinical trials so that more concise information regarding the representativeness of participants in trials can be published [11]. Theoretically, effective treatments may limit generalizability or effectiveness for all populations when diverse populations are lacking or underrepresented in clinical trials [12]. Recently, a standardized set of outcomes to capture and assess treatment intervention effectiveness and safety profiles has been brought to the scientific community's attention.

To our knowledge, no data addressing issues concerning disparities in participant and trial characteristics and trial outcome reporting have been established in clinical trials for H1-antihistamine-refractory CSU. To better harmonize and compare the different treatment interventions, we performed a systematic review to assess the evidence gap, consistency in outcome reporting, and representation across global pharmacological treatment clinical trials involving people living with H1-antihistamine-refractory CSU.

2. Methods

2.1. Protocol and Literature Search

The pre-specified protocol and living systematic review update was registered on the International Prospective Register of Systematic Reviews (PROSPERO, CRD42020196592). However, the pre-specified protocol was amended to focus on randomized clinical trials owing to the limited availability of relevant data on comparative effectiveness observational studies. Therefore, we decided not to include non-randomized studies in the present study. This systematic review followed the Preferred Reporting Items for Systematic Reviews and Meta-Analyses 2020 statement [13]. Due to the nature of the systematic review and meta-analysis, ethical approval was not required.

Regarding the pre-specified protocol, with the help of an experienced medical librarian, we searched seven electronic databases including Medline, Embase, PubMed, Cochrane Library, Web of Science, Scopus, and CINAHL. We also searched grey literature on Google Scholar, clinical trial registers, and preprints reports. We constructed the search strategy based on the combinations of main keywords or medical subject headings regarding CSU (e.g., "Chronic spontaneous urticaria" OR "Chronic idiopathic urticaria" OR "Refractory urticaria" OR "Hives"). Moreover, search terms in relation to types of interventions were browsed according to the individual drugs or their pharmacological classes (e.g., "Anti-immunoglobulin E" OR "Monoclonal antibody" OR "Bruton tyrosine kinase inhibitor" OR "CRTH2 antagonist" OR "IL-1 inhibitor" OR "anti-tumor necrosis factor alpha" OR "Immunosuppressive Agent" OR "Calcineurin inhibitor").

A comprehensive literature search was performed from the inception of each database until 19 April 2021, with no language restrictions. Potential trials were also supplemented by searching the reference lists of included studies, previous systematic reviews, and major international scientific conference meetings (dermatology, allergy, and immunology congress). The search strategy details for each database are available in Supplementary Tables S1 and S2.

2.2. Article Screening

Two investigators (SN and MC) independently screened the eligible titles and abstracts of articles identified by the systematic search. Subsequently, potentially relevant full-text articles were reviewed against the study inclusion/exclusion criteria for the final set of included studies. Potential non-English-language eligible studies were translated before the full-text appraisal. Any disagreement was resolved through team discussion.

The inclusion and exclusion criteria details were described previously (Supplementary Table S3) [8,9]. In brief, we included randomized clinical trials (parallel and cross-over trials) that (i) involved adolescents or adults (12 years or older) who were diagnosed with CSU refractory to H1-antihistamines (standard dose or up-dosing) and (ii) used validated measurement tools for urticaria treatment response assessment with a follow-up period of two weeks onward. For companion trials with overlapping participants and study periods, relevant information was assembled from the study that provided the most detailed information.

However, we excluded clinical trials that investigated body weight-based or immunoglobulin E level-based dosing of omalizumab, as early studies among patients with CSU showed no benefit of this approach [14]. Moreover, trials that used terfenadine up-dosed or combined with other treatments were excluded from this review because this treatment is no longer available in current practice. All placebos across the included trials were defined as standard doses or an up-dosing of H1-antihistamines in conjunction with rescue medications.

2.3. Data Extraction

After screening articles against the inclusion and exclusion criteria, data were collected via full-text abstraction of the included clinical trials. Two investigators (SN and MC) independently extracted pre-specified information using a standardized approach. Pre-specified data extraction was managed via a Microsoft Excel spreadsheet (data extraction details are described in Table 1). The categorization of race and ethnicity was based on the National Institutes of Health—United States Office of Budget and Management, Revisions to the Standards for the Classification of Federal Data on Race and Ethnicity, 2020 [15]. Based on participant-level characteristics, we classified trials that indicated any race other than white as a trial involving a non-white population. To establish the underrepresentation of race and ethnicity across the included clinical trials, the cutoff value (<20%) that reflects the United States census was employed [10]. Discrepancies and uncertainties were resolved through discussion until a consensus was reached. Two investigators (CR and KT) independently cross-checked the final dataset.

2.4. Risk-of-Bias Assessment

Two investigators (SN and MC) independently and critically appraised the methodological quality of each included trial using the Cochrane revised tool for risk of bias assessment (RoB 2) [16]. Cochrane RoB 2 consists of six bias domains, including the randomization process, deviations from intended interventions, missing outcome data, measurement of the outcome, and selection of the reported result. The overall risk of bias of the included trials was then classified as low, some concerns, or high risk of bias [16].

Table 1. Pre-specified data extraction.

Domain	Detail
Participant characteristics	• Number of participants enrolled • Mean or median age of study participants and age inclusion criteria • Reported proportion of females • Race or ethnicity reporting based on National Institutes of Health—United States Office of Budget and Management, 2020 • Definition of H1-antihistamine-refractory CSU: refractory to (i) licensed-dose antihistamines, (ii) up-dosing antihistamines (two- to four-fold the licensed-dose), (iii) mixed/not specified • Duration of CSU • Pharmacologic intervention class: biologic drugs, immunosuppressive drugs, and others
Trial characteristics	• Year of publication • Trial setting: monocentric vs. multicenter • Trial location: North America/Europe, others, and international • Trial design: parallel-group vs crossover design • Control group in trial: placebo-controlled vs. active-controlled trial • Trial blinding: open-label, single-blind, double-blind, triple-blind, or quadruple-blind • Number of arms in trial • Study treatment period in week • Funding: industry sponsorship, partial industry sponsorship, academic/government, none, or not reported • Overall risk of bias based on the Cochrane revised tool for risk-of-bias assessment (RoB2): low, some concerns, or high-risk of bias
Outcomes of interest	• Measurement tools and definition of outcomes • Treatment efficacy: urticaria symptom, pruritus severity, and hive severity • Safety profiles: all-cause study dropout, incidence of adverse events, incidence of serious adverse events • Patient-reported outcomes: HRQOL (i.e., dermatology-specific, chronic urticaria-specific, angioedema-specific, or generic measure), impact on sleep, treatment satisfaction, or others mental health and psychosocial issues

Abbreviations: CSU, chronic spontaneous urticaria; HRQOL, health-related quality of life.

2.5. Statistical Analysis

Descriptive statistics were used and are expressed as frequency and percentage, mean ± standard deviation, or median with a range (min–max), as appropriate. To explore the disparities and evaluate the evidence gap across continents and the capacity to conduct clinical trials, the included trials were classified as high-income or lower/upper-middle-income country trials based on the World Bank 2021 income grouping. Statistical significance of differences in the evidence gap in terms of participant and trial characteristics and outcomes of interest across the included trials according to the World Bank income grouping was determined using Fisher's exact tests. Two-tailed tests with p-values < 0.05 were considered statistically significant. All analyses were performed using Stata 14.0 (StataCorp LLC).

3. Results and Discussion

3.1. Overview of Included Trials for H1-Antihistamine-Refractory CSU

Based on a systematic search approach, 20,796 records were identified. After deduplication and screening based on title and abstract, we identified 492 articles for full-text review. Of these, 23 randomized clinical trials (21 parallel-group [14,17–36] and two crossover [37,38] trials) fulfilled the study inclusion and exclusion criteria, and were included in this systematic review (Figure 1).

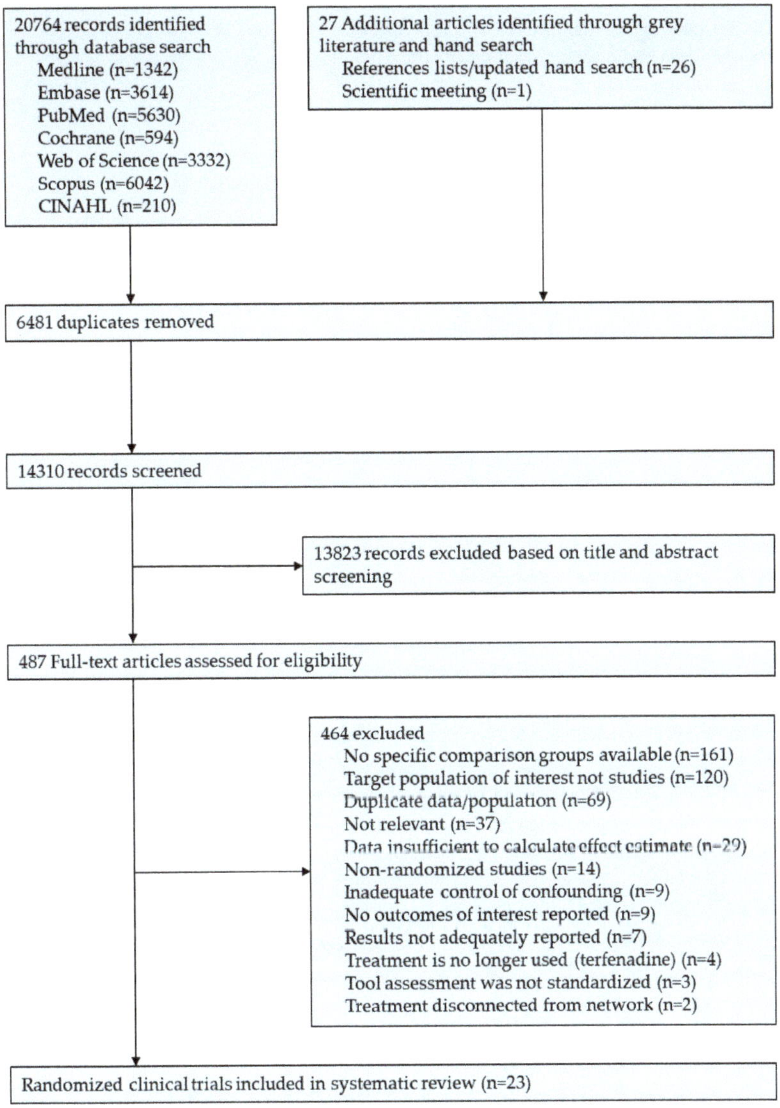

Figure 1. Preferred Reporting Items for Systematic Reviews and Meta-Analyses (PRISMA) flow diagram of trials included in the systematic review.

3.2. Participant and Trial Characteristics

The participant and trial characteristics of all the included trials are illustrated in Table 2. The included trials comprised 2480 participants (range, 20–340 participants per trial) from 22 different countries, with a treatment duration of 12.0 ± 7.1 (range, 3.0–24.0) weeks. The reported mean age was 41.2 ± 3.4 years (range, 32.2–45.7; mainly adult participants) and the reported proportion of women was 64.8% (range, 6.2–86.7%). However, 10 (43.5%) trials did not report race or ethnicity. More than one-half of the included trials (13 trials, 56.5%) were conducted in participants who were unresponsive to licensed doses of H1-antihistamine. Regarding trial characteristics, 15 (65.2%) of the included trials were multicenter trials, 21 (91.3%) were placebo-controlled trials, 20 (87.0%) used a double-blind trial design, 18 (78.3%) were two-arm trials, and 13 (56.5%) received industry sponsorship. Of the 23 included trials, 13 (56.5%) had a low risk of bias, 10 (43.5%) had some concerns, and no studies had a high risk of bias.

Table 2. Characteristics of included trials.

Participant and Trial Characteristics	Number of Trials (%)			*p*-Value
	Overall (*n* = 23)	High-Income Countries (*n* = 18) †	Lower/Upper-Middle-Income Countries (*n* = 5) †	
Total enrollment, participants; median (range, min–max)	2480; 75 (20–340)	2251; 83 (20–340)	229; 35 (29–80)	0.279
<50 participants	10 (43.5)	7 (38.9)	3 (60.0)	0.563
50–100 participant	8 (34.8)	6 (33.3)	2 (40.0)	
>100 participants	5 (21.7)	5 (27.8)	0 (0.0)	
Reported mean age in year, grand mean ± S.D.; Median (range, min–max); missing data for one trial (4.3%)	41.2 ± 3.4; 42.5 (32.2–45.7)	41.3 ± 1.8; 42.7 (38.7–45.7)	36.2 ± 4.7; 34.9 (32.2–42.8)	<0.001
Age inclusion				
Only adults included	16 (69.6)	12 (66.7)	4 (80.0)	1.000
Mixed children and adolescents/adults included	7 (30.4)	6 (33.3)	1 (20.0)	
Reported % female, grand mean ± S.D.; Median (range, min– max); missing data for one trial (4.3%)	64.8 ± 19.2; 69.6 (6.2–86.7)	63.9 ± 20.6; 70.6 (6.2–86.7)	68.5 ± 12.4; 65.0 (58.6–85.4)	0.677
Race/ethnicity reporting				
>80% white representation	9 (39.1)	9 (50.0)	0 (0.0)	0.108
≥20% non-white representation	4 (17.4)	3 (16.7)	1 (20.0)	
Neither race nor ethnicity reported	10 (43.5)	6 (33.3)	4 (80.0)	
Type of refractory CSU				
Refractory to licensed-dose antihistamines	9 (39.1)	9 (50.0)	0 (0.0)	0.108
Refractory to up-dosing antihistamines (two- to four-fold the licensed-dose)	10 (43.5)	6 (33.3)	4 (80.0)	
Mixed/not specified	4 (17.4)	3 (16.7)	1 (20.0)	
Duration of CSU in year, grand mean ± S.D.; Median (range, min–max); missing data for six trials (26.1%)	5.0 ± 2.8; 5.1 (0.5–11.5)	5.9 ± 2.4; 5.9 (2.4–11.5)	2.4 ± 2.4; 1.7 (0.5–5.9)	0.029
Pharmacologic intervention class of studies: Specific intervention (no. of trials) ‡				
Biologic drugs: Canakinumab (1), Ligelizumab (1), Omalizumab (10), Quilizumab (1)	12 (52.2)	11 (61.1)	1 (20.0)	0.214
Immunosuppressive drugs: Azathioprine (1), Cyclosporine (4), Methotrexate (2)	5 (21.7)	3 (16.7)	2 (40.0)	
Others: AZD1981—CRTh2 antagonist (1), Dapsone (1), Hydroxychloroquine (1), Miltefosine (1), Montelukast (1), Zafirlukast (1)	6 (26.1)	4 (22.2)	2 (40.0)	
Year of publication				
Before 2015	10 (43.5)	8 (44.4)	2 (40.0)	1.000
2015–2021	13 (56.5)	10 (55.6)	3 (60.0)	
Trial setting				
Monocentric	8 (34.8)	4 (22.2)	4 (80.0)	0.033
Multicenter	15 (65.2)	14 (77.8)	1 (20.0)	
Trial location: Country (no. of trials)				
North America/Europe: France (1), Germany (3), Italy (1), Switzerland (2), Türkiye (1), United Kingdom (1), United States (3)	12 (52.2)	11 (61.1)	1 (20.0)	0.001
Others: Colombia (1), India (2), Thailand (1)	4 (17.4)	0 (0.0)	4 (80.0)	
International (includes Australia, Canada, Denmark, France, Germany, Greece, Italy, Japan, Korea, New Zealand, Poland, Russian Federation, Singapore, Spain, Taiwan, Türkiye, United Kingdom, United States)	7 (30.4)	7 (38.9)	0 (0.0)	

Table 2. *Cont.*

Participant and Trial Characteristics	Number of Trials (%) Overall (*n* = 23)	High-Income Countries (*n* = 18) †	Lower/Upper-Middle-Income Countries (*n* = 5) †	*p*-Value
Trial Design				
Parallel-group	21 (91.3)	17 (94.4)	4 (80.0)	0.395
Crossover	2 (8.7)	1 (5.6)	1 (20.0)	
Control group in trial				
Placebo-controlled trial	21 (91.3)	18 (100.0)	3 (60.0)	0.040
Active-controlled trial	2 (8.7)	0 (0.0)	2 (40.0)	
Trial Blinding				
Open-label/single-blind	3 (13.0)	0 (0.0)	3 (60.0)	0.006
Double-blind	20 (87.0)	10 (100.0)	2 (40.0)	
Arms in trial				
2	18 (78.3)	13 (72.2)	5 (100.0)	0.545
≥3	5 (21.7)	5 (27.8)	0 (0.0)	
Study treatment duration in week, grand mean ± S.D.; Median (range, min–max)	12.0 ± 7.1; 12.0 (3.0–24.0)	12.2 ± 7.9; 12.0 (3.0–24.0)	11.6 ± 3.6; 12.0 (6.0–16.0)	0.910
<8 weeks	8 (34.8)	7 (38.9)	1 (20.0)	0.371
8–12 weeks	7 (30.4)	4 (22.2)	3 (60.0)	
>12 weeks	8 (34.8)	7 (38.9)	1 (20.0)	
Funding				
Industry sponsorship	13 (56.5)	13 (72.2)	0 (0.0)	0.001
Partial industry sponsorship	3 (13.0)	3 (16.7)	0 (0.0)	
Academic/government	4 (17.4)	2 (11.1)	2 (40.0)	
None	1 (4.4)	0 (0.0)	1 (20.0)	
Not reported	2 (8.7)	0 (0.0)	2 (40.0)	
Overall risk of bias				
Low	13 (56.5)	12 (66.7)	1 (20.0)	0.127
Some concern	10 (43.5)	6 (33.3)	4 (80.0)	

† On the basis of primary site economy. ‡ Interventions were counted independently, as many trials included multiple interventions. Abbreviations: CSU, chronic spontaneous urticaria; S.D., standard deviation.

Twelve (52.2%) of the included trials were conducted in North America or Europe, seven (30.4%) in international trial locations, and four (17.4%) in other locations. Based on the global distribution of pharmacological treatments for H1-antihistamine-refractory CSU, the top two countries that conducted trials were Germany (nine trials) and the United States (eight trials).

The included trials were published between the years 2000 and 2021. The type of pharmacological intervention was identified as biologic drugs in 12 (52.2%) trials, immunosuppressive drugs in five (21.7%), and others in six (26.1%), which investigated 18 different pharmacological interventions or dosages and one placebo (usual care treatment). Notably, in 2015 and 2021, the number of biological drugs used dramatically increased by 300% and 800%, respectively; the number in 2005 was zero (Figure 2). Meanwhile, the number of non-biological drugs investigated in clinical trials annually revealed little change over time.

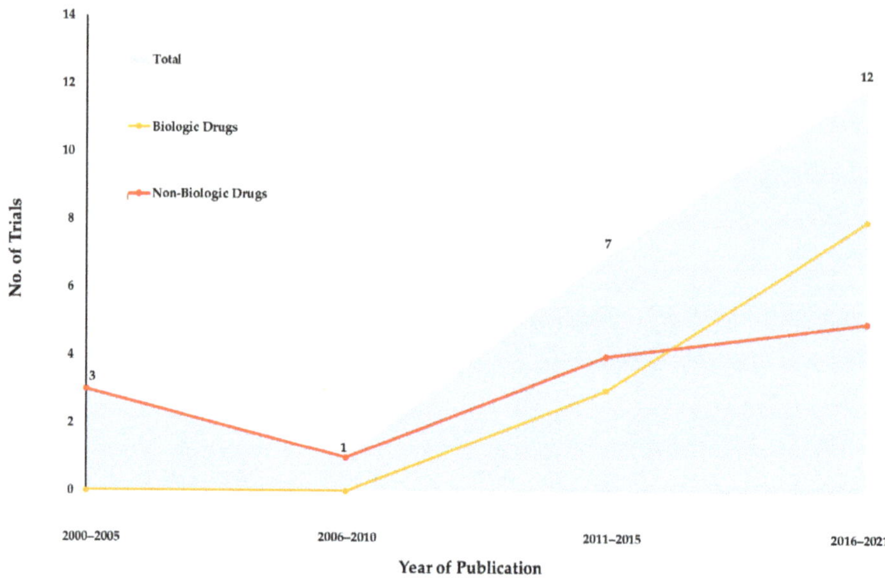

Figure 2. Time trend in the publication of pharmacologic treatments for H1-antihistamine-refractory chronic spontaneous urticaria trials.

3.3. Trial Outcome Reporting

The outcomes of interest were categorized into three groups: (i) treatment efficacy, (ii) safety profiles, and (iii) patient-reported outcomes (Table 3). Regarding treatment efficacy, 16 (69.6%) trials reported treatment response for urticaria symptoms using the urticaria activity score over 7 days (UAS7). Meanwhile, 13 (56.5%) and 12 (52.2%) trials reported the component of urticaria symptoms—pruritus and hives severity, respectively. Regarding safety profiles, the unacceptability of treatment (all-cause study dropout), incidence of adverse events, and serious adverse events were the most reported outcome theme (≥80% of the included trials). However, less than half of the included trials recognized patient-reported outcomes. Based on validated tools, patient-reported outcomes included a measure of HRQOL (dermatology-specific, chronic urticaria-specific, angioedema-specific, and generic measures), impact on sleep, and general well-being. Regarding treatment-level comparisons, all possible individual pharmacological nodes for each outcome of interest are illustrated in Figure 3.

3.4. Evidence Gap across Included Trials

No clinical trials are available in African and low-income countries. Meanwhile, limited clinical trials have been conducted in regions other than America and Europe. Based on the World Bank income grouping, 18 (78.3%) of the included trials were conducted in high-income countries and five (21.7%) in lower/upper-middle-income countries. The distribution of participants and trial characteristics (Table 2), including age ($p < 0.001$), duration of CSU ($p = 0.029$), trial setting ($p = 0.033$), trial location and continent ($p = 0.001$), the control group in a trial ($p = 0.040$), trial blinding ($p = 0.006$), and funding ($p = 0.001$), demonstrated a statistically significant association with the country income groups (high-income vs. lower/upper-middle-income countries). Moreover, trials in high-income countries were more likely to use a well-established tool—UAS7—and report on the component of urticaria symptoms (severity of pruritus and hives) compared with trials conducted in lower/upper-middle-income countries (all $p < 0.050$, Table 3). However, disparities in reported results, particularly patient-reported outcomes in the core outcome set and measurement tools, were observed across the included trials.

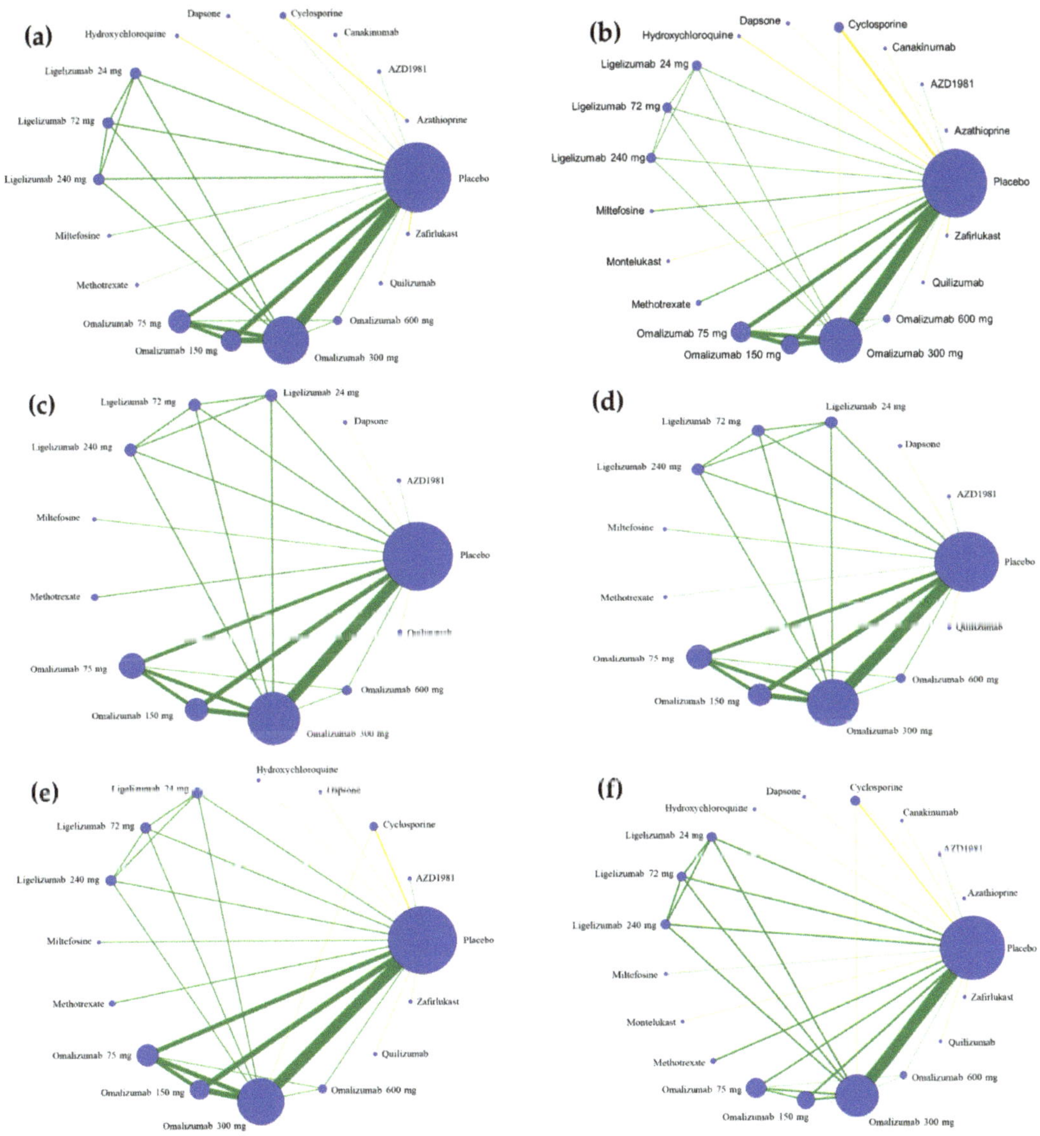

Figure 3. Geometry networks for pharmacologic treatment-level comparisons. (**a**) urticaria symptoms; (**b**), unacceptability of treatment (all-cause study dropout); (**c**) pruritus severity; (**d**) hive severity; (**e**) adverse event; (**f**), serious adverse event. Nodes denote pharmacological treatments and lines denote trials of the corresponding treatment comparison. The size of a node is proportional to the number of trials that included the corresponding treatment. The thickness of the lines corresponds to the number of trials performing each comparison (green and yellow lines represent studies with a low risk of bias and some concerns, respectively, according to the overall risk-of-bias assessment).

Table 3. Outcome categorization and frequency of outcome reporting.

Outcomes	Number of Trials (%)			*p*-Value
	Overall (*n* = 23)	**High-Income Countries (*n* = 18) †**	**Lower/Upper-Middle-Income Countries (*n* = 5) †**	
Treatment Efficacy (Specific Assessment Tool): Urticaria symptom				
UAS7 (scale, 0–42)	16 (69.6)	15 (83.3)	1 (20.0)	0.017
Daily UAS (scale, 0–3),	1 (4.4)	0 (0.0)	1 (20.0)	
USS (scale, 0–93),	1 (4.4)	0 (0.0)	1 (20.0)	
VAS (scale, 0–100)	1 (4.4)	1 (5.6)	0 (0.0)	
Not reported	4 (17.4)	2 (11.1)	2 (40.0)	
Treatment Efficacy (Specific Assessment Tool): Pruritus severity				
UAS7-subscale itch (scale, 0–21)	13 (56.5)	13 (72.2)	0 (0.0)	0.007
Daily UAS-subscale itch (scale, 0–3)	1 (4.4)	0 (0.0)	1 (20.0)	
VAS (scale, 0–100)	1 (4.4)	1 (5.6)	0 (0.0)	
Not reported	8 (34.8)	4 (22.2)	4 (80.0)	
Treatment Efficacy (Specific Assessment Tool): Hive severity				
UAS7-subscale hive/wheal (scale, 0–21)	12 (52.2)	12 (66.7)	0 (0.0)	0.006
Daily UAS-subscale hive/wheal (scale, 0–3)	1 (4.4)	0 (0.0)	1 (20.0)	
Not reported	10 (43.5)	6 (33.3)	4 (80.0)	
Safety Profile				
Unacceptability of treatment (all-cause study dropout)	22 (95.6)	18 (100.0)	4 (80.0)	0.217
Occurrence of adverse events reported (participant with ≥1 adverse events)	20 (87.0)	17 (94.4)	3 (60.0)	0.107
Occurrence of serious adverse events reported (participant with ≥1 serious adverse events)	23 (100.0)	18 (100.0)	5 (100.0)	1.000
Patients-Reported Outcomes (Specific Assessment Tools) ‡				
HRQOL: dermatology—specific measure (DLQI)	10 (43.5)	8 (44.4)	2 (40.0)	1.000
HRQOL: chronic urticaria—specific measure (CU-Q2oL)	4 (17.4)	4 (22.2)	0 (0.0)	0.539
HRQOL: angioedema—specific measure (AE-QoL)	1 (4.4)	1 (5.6)	0 (0.0)	1.000
HRQOL—generic measure (MOSS-SF12)	1 (4.4)	1 (5.6)	0 (0.0)	1.000
Impact on sleep (UPDD-weekly sleep, VAS [scale, 0–100])	1 (4.4)	1 (5.6)	0 (0.0)	1.000
General well-being (WHO-5 well-being index)	5 (21.7)	5 (27.8)	0 (0.0)	0.545

† On the basis of primary site economy. ‡ Patient-reported outcomes were counted independently, as many trials included multiple interventions. Abbreviations: AE-QoL, angioedema-quality of life; CU-Q2oL, chronic urticaria-quality of life; DLQI, Dermatology Life Quality Index; HRQOL, health-related quality of life; MOSS-SF12, Medical Outcomes Study Survey—Short Form 12 Item; UAS, urticaria activity score; UAS7, urticaria activity score over 7 days; UPDD, urticaria patient daily diary; USS, urticaria severity score; VAS, visual analog scale; WHO, World Health Organization.

3.5. Summary of the Findings

This systematic review highlighted a global evidence gap and provided important information regarding pharmacological treatments for H1-antihistamine-refractory CSU clinical trials. Significant global increases in published clinical trials and new investigational medicinal products, especially biologic drugs, demonstrate the progress made between 2000 and 2021. However, we hypothesized that people living with H1-antihistamine-refractory CSU who are members of minority groups (non-white population), part of regions other than North America/Europe (i.e., Africa, Asia, and South America), and live in low- to lower/upper-middle-income countries would be underrepresented in CSU clinical trials.

Currently, licensed biologic therapy—omalizumab (anti-immunoglobulin E)—has become the frontline treatment and revolutionized the management of H1-antihistamine-refractory CSU [1]. Subsequently, overall increases were observed in the number of H1-antihistamine-refractory CSU drugs investigated. Based on promising mechanisms, there has been a rapid surge of clinical trials among new biologics drugs that reduce mast cell activation by blocking activating pathways and engaging inhibitory receptors or mast cell members [5–7].

3.6. Comparison with Other Studies

The poor representation of minority groups in this study is consistent with previous systematic reviews [10]. Chen et al. (2022) [39] examined the diversity of participants in dermatologic clinical trials in the United States published conducted between 2010 and 2020 and found that clinical trials that included at least 20% non-white participants were noticeably few. Of note, 10 (43.5%) of the trials included in this study did not report on race or ethnicity. One possible explanation for the poor enrollment of racial/ethnic minority groups in clinical trials is that existing national or international policies for promoting patient engagement in randomized clinical trials are not effective. Currently, the United States FDA has implemented an action plan to support and encourage diversity in randomized clinical trials conducted by the industry to improve and publish transparent data regarding race or ethnicity [11]. However, these FDA regulations focus on investigating new drugs and are not implemented in all industry-sponsored and non-industry-sponsored clinical trials.

Regarding infrastructure and economic indices for clinical trials, only five (21.7%) of 23 trials were conducted in lower/upper-middle-income countries between 2000 and 2021. Moreover, the included trials were generally small-scale, with a median sample size of 75 (range, 20–340) participants and a median study treatment duration of 12 (range, 3–24) weeks. Remarkably, our study illustrated a statistically significantly different in the age of participants, duration of CSU, trial setting, trial location and continent, the control group in a trial, trial blinding, and funding between high-income and lower/upper-middle-income countries. Unfortunately, we found no clinical trials in African regions or low-income countries, suggesting that the pharmaceutical industry and clinical research organizations need to set policies and harmonize trial designs to increase participants' demographic and geographical diversity.

Regarding outcome reporting, most included trials were designed to evaluate urticaria treatment responses and safety profiles. However, disparities in the clinimetric tools for assessing treatment responses have been observed. More than one-half of the included trials (16 trials, 69.6%) used UAS7—a validated tool suggested by the 2021 joint update guideline recommendations from the European Academy of Allergology and Clinical Immunology, Global Allergy and Asthma European Network, European Dermatology Forum, and the Asia Pacific Association of Allergy, Asthma and Clinical Immunology [1]; other trials used other clinimetric tools, including daily UAS, urticaria severity score (USS), or visual analog scale (VAS, scale 0–100). Beyond treatment efficacy and safety profiles, less than half of the included trials reported patients' perspectives regarding patient-reported outcomes. Most trials assessed HRQOL, but lacked information regarding other aspects of patient-reported outcomes, such as sleep problems, symptom burden, psychosocial and mental health problems, and work or school impairment. Although the Cochrane Skin—Core Outcome Set Initiative has been developed as a core outcome set for several skin conditions, there is a lack of specific outcome sets for patients with CSU [40]. To better compare across-trial results, we recommend that standardized reporting in core outcome sets for people living with CSU (including efficacy, safety events, and patient-reported outcomes) be developed and applied to make trial evidence more useful [41].

3.7. Strengths and Limitations

To the best of our knowledge, this is the first systematic review to elucidate the disparities and evidence gaps across pharmacologic treatment clinical trials for H1-antihistamine-refractory CSU. However, our systematic review has some limitations. First, age was reported in various ways—by category, mean, range, and percentage older than 12 years, with the exclusion age criteria (i.e., 65, 70, or 75 years)—resulting in difficulty in addressing age disparities. Second, we could not assess representativeness based on sexual identity and orientation because of the lack of information on these issues. Third, 10 (43.5%) trials did not report race or ethnicity; therefore, we had to deduce racial makeup based on the country or judge that neither race nor ethnicity was reported owing to insufficient data. Lastly, we only assessed published H1-antihistamine-refractory CSU randomized clinical trials that used validated measurement tools for outcomes assessment. As a result, we lack information on ongoing studies based on clinical trial registries, non-randomized studies, and post-marketing trials, as well as other aspects of dermatology trials.

3.8. Implications for Conducting Clinical Trials, Future Research, and Conclusion

Establishing disparities and evidence gaps in H1-antihistamine-refractory CSU clinical trials is the first step toward developing a system for conducting clinical trials that involve an increasingly diverse population. Given that the clinical trials included in this systematic review were generally small, we postulate that our findings are informative for the pharmaceutical industry, researchers, patients, and policymakers to promote medical innovation in CSU. Collectively, we advocate the inclusion of diverse populations in CSU trials globally. Different study site selections in industry-sponsored clinical trials based on multinational studies are required to improve diversity in participant enrollment and drug development for diverse populations. Besides population availability and timely recruitment, patient enrollment based on heterogonous inclusion of age, sex, and race or ethnicity should be employed in the protocol generation phase. Ultimately, to conduct clinical trials, experience is not required; the pharmaceutical industry and clinical research organizations should collaborate with inexperienced trial sites, particularly in low- or lower/upper-middle-income countries, if they have access to the relevant patient population.

To facilitate and encourage the formation of a highly motivating environment for pharmaceutical innovation, it is essential for future research and development strategies to create equitable access to new investigational medical products and the efficiency of pharmaceutical research in high- and lower/upper-middle-income countries. Furthermore, apart from international collaborative clinical trials, the approaches being considered at present will need head-to-head trials with high methodological quality and harmonized trial design and outcomes to help inform subsequent international guidelines for managing people living with CSU.

4. Conclusions

In this systematic review, the number of randomized clinical trials for the pharmacologic treatment of H1-antihistamine-refractory CSU increased between 2000 and 2021, particularly in biologic drug intervention trials. However, relatively small trial sizes, underrepresentation of minority groups (non-white populations, populations of regions other than North America/Europe, and low- to lower/upper-middle-income countries), and disparities in outcome reporting were observed across H1-antihistamine-refractory CSU clinical trials. To close the evidence gap in H1-antihistamine-refractory CSU clinical trials, strategies for improving clinical trials and participant enrollment and standardizing core outcome sets for trial reporting are needed.

Supplementary Materials: The following supporting information can be downloaded at: https://www.mdpi.com/article/10.3390/ph15101246/s1, Table S1: Systematic review search strategy; Table S2: Grey literature search; Table S3: The PICOTS: study inclusion/exclusion criteria.

Author Contributions: Conceptualization, S.N. and C.R.; methodology, S.N., M.C., C.R. and K.T.; software; S.N. and C.R.; validation, C.R. and K.T.; formal analysis, S.N. and C.R.; investigation, all authors; re-sources, S.N. and M.C.; data curation, S.N. and M.C.; writing—original draft preparation, S.N.; writing—review and editing, M.C., C.R. and K.T.; visualization, S.N. and M.C., supervision, S.N. and K.T.; project administration, S.N. and M.C.; funding acquisition, S.N. All authors have read and agreed to the published version of the manuscript.

Funding: This research was supported by a grant from the Pharmacoepidemiology and Statistics Research Center (PESRC) through Chiang Mai University.

Institutional Review Board Statement: Not applicable.

Informed Consent Statement: Not applicable.

Data Availability Statement: Not applicable.

Acknowledgments: The authors thank the research assistances and all staff of Pharmacoepidemiology and Statistics Research Center (PESRC), Chiang Mai, Thailand.

Conflicts of Interest: The authors declare no conflict of interest.

References

1. Zuberbier, T.; Abdul Latiff, A.H.; Abuzakouk, M.; Aquilina, S.; Asero, R.; Baker, D.; Ballmer-Weber, B.; Bangert, C.; Ben-Shoshan, M.; Bernstein, J.A.; et al. The international EAACI/GA^{2}LEN/EuroGuiDerm/APAAACI guideline for the definition, classification, diagnosis, and management of urticaria. *Allergy* **2022**, *77*, 734–766. [CrossRef] [PubMed]
2. Fricke, J.; Ávila, G.; Keller, T.; Weller, K.; Lau, S.; Maurer, M.; Zuberbier, T.; Keil, T. Prevalence of chronic urticaria in children and adults across the globe: Systematic review with meta-analysis. *Allergy* **2020**, *75*, 423–432. [CrossRef] [PubMed]
3. Maurer, M.; Weller, K.; Bindslev-Jensen, C.; Giménez-Arnau, A.; Bousquet, P.J.; Bousquet, J.; Canonica, G.W.; Church, M.K.; Godse, K.V.; Grattan, C.E.; et al. Unmet clinical needs in chronic spontaneous urticaria. A GA^{2}LEN task force report. *Allergy* **2011**, *66*, 317–330. [CrossRef] [PubMed]
4. Gonçalo, M.; Gimenéz-Arnau, A.; Al-Ahmad, M.; Ben-Shoshan, M.; Bernstein, J.A.; Ensina, L.F.; Fomina, D.; Galvàn, C.A.; Godse, K.; Grattan, C.; et al. The global burden of chronic urticaria for the patient and society. *Br. J. Dermatol.* **2021**, *184*, 226–236. [CrossRef]
5. Maurer, M.; Khan, D.A.; Elieh Ali Komi, D.; Kaplan, A.P. Biologics for the Use in Chronic Spontaneous Urticaria: When and Which. *J. Allergy Clin. Immunol. Pract.* **2021**, *9*, 1067–1078. [CrossRef]
6. Metz, M.; Sussman, G.; Gagnon, R.; Staubach, P.; Tanus, T.; Yang, W.H.; Lim, J.J.; Clarke, H.J.; Galanter, J.; Chinn, L.W.; et al. Fenebrutinib in H(1) antihistamine-refractory chronic spontaneous urticaria: A randomized phase 2 trial. *Nat. Med.* **2021**, *27*, 1961–1969. [CrossRef]
7. Altrichter, S.; Staubach, P.; Pasha, M.; Singh, B.; Chang, A.T.; Bernstein, J.A.; Rasmussen, H.S.; Siebenhaar, F.; Maurer, M. An open-label, proof-of-concept study of lirentelimab for antihistamine-resistant chronic spontaneous and inducible urticaria. *J. Allergy Clin. Immunol. Pract.* **2022**, *149*, 1683–1690.e1687. [CrossRef]
8. Nochaiwong, S.; Chuamanochan, M.; Ruengorn, C.; Awiphan, R.; Tovanabutra, N.; Chiewchanvit, S. Evaluation of Pharmacologic Treatments for H1 Antihistamine-Refractory Chronic Spontaneous Urticaria: A Systematic Review and Network Meta-analysis. *JAMA Dermatol.* **2021**, *157*, 1316–1327. [CrossRef]
9. Nochaiwong, S.; Chuamanochan, M.; Ruengorn, C.; Awiphan, R.; Tovanabutra, N.; Chiewchanvit, S.; Hutton, B.; Thavorn, K. Impact of Pharmacological Treatments for Chronic Spontaneous Urticaria with an Inadequate Response to H1-Antihistamines on Health-Related Quality of Life: A Systematic Review and Network Meta-Analysis. *J. Allergy Clin. Immunol. Pract.* **2022**, *10*, 297–308. [CrossRef]
10. Charrow, A.; Xia, F.D.; Joyce, C.; Mostaghimi, A. Diversity in Dermatology Clinical Trials: A Systematic Review. *JAMA Dermatol.* **2017**, *153*, 193–198. [CrossRef]
11. Diversifying clinical trials. *Nat. Med.* **2018**, *24*, 1779. [CrossRef] [PubMed]
12. Ramamoorthy, A.; Pacanowski, M.A.; Bull, J.; Zhang, L. Racial/ethnic differences in drug disposition and response: Review of recently approved drugs. *Clin. Pharmacol. Ther.* **2015**, *97*, 263–273. [CrossRef] [PubMed]
13. Page, M.J.; McKenzie, J.E.; Bossuyt, P.M.; Boutron, I.; Hoffmann, T.C.; Mulrow, C.D.; Shamseer, L.; Tetzlaff, J.M.; Akl, E.A.; Brennan, S.E.; et al. The PRISMA 2020 statement: An updated guideline for reporting systematic reviews. *BMJ* **2021**, *372*, n71. [CrossRef]
14. Saini, S.; Rosen, K.E.; Hsieh, H.J.; Wong, D.A.; Conner, E.; Kaplan, A.; Spector, S.; Maurer, M. A randomized, placebo-controlled, dose-ranging study of single-dose omalizumab in patients with H1-antihistamine-refractory chronic idiopathic urticaria. *J. Allergy Clin. Immunol.* **2011**, *128*, 567–573.e561. [CrossRef]
15. National Institutes of Health; US Office of Budget and Management. Revisions to the Standards for the Classifications of Federal Data on Race and Ethnicity. Available online: https://orwh.od.nih.gov/toolkit/other-relevant-federal-policies/OMB-standards (accessed on 15 July 2022).
16. Sterne, J.A.C.; Savović, J.; Page, M.J.; Elbers, R.G.; Blencowe, N.S.; Boutron, I.; Cates, C.J.; Cheng, H.Y.; Corbett, M.S.; Eldridge, S.M.; et al. RoB 2: A revised tool for assessing risk of bias in randomised trials. *BMJ* **2019**, *366*, l4898. [CrossRef] [PubMed]
17. Maul, J.T.; Distler, M.; Kolios, A.; Maul, L.V.; Guillet, C.; Graf, N.; Imhof, L.; Lang, C.; Navarini, A.A.; Schmid-Grendelmeier, P. Canakinumab Lacks Efficacy in Treating Adult Patients with Moderate to Severe Chronic Spontaneous Urticaria in a Phase II Randomized Double-Blind Placebo-Controlled Single-Center Study. *J. Allergy Clin. Immunol. Pract.* **2021**, *9*, 463–468.e463. [CrossRef]

18. Leducq, S.; Samimi, M.; Bernier, C.; Soria, A.; Amsler, E.; Staumont-Sallé, D.; Gabison, G.; Chosidow, O.; Bénéton, N.; Bara, C.; et al. Efficacy and safety of methotrexate versus placebo as add-on therapy to H1 antihistamines for patients with difficult-to-treat chronic spontaneous urticaria: A randomized, controlled trial. *J. Am. Acad. Dermatol.* **2020**, *82*, 240–243. [CrossRef] [PubMed]
19. Pathania, Y.S.; Bishnoi, A.; Parsad, D.; Kumar, A.; Kumaran, M.S. Comparing azathioprine with cyclosporine in the treatment of antihistamine refractory chronic spontaneous urticaria: A randomized prospective active-controlled non-inferiority study. *World Allergy Organ. J.* **2019**, *12*, 100033. [CrossRef]
20. Oliver, E.T.; Chichester, K.; Devine, K.; Sterba, P.M.; Wegner, C.; Vonakis, B.M.; Saini, S.S. Effects of an Oral CRTh2 Antagonist (AZD1981) on Eosinophil Activity and Symptoms in Chronic Spontaneous Urticaria. *Int. Arch. Allergy Immunol.* **2019**, *179*, 21–30. [CrossRef]
21. Maurer, M.; Giménez-Arnau, A.M.; Sussman, G.; Metz, M.; Baker, D.R.; Bauer, A.; Bernstein, J.A.; Brehler, R.; Chu, C.Y.; Chung, W.H.; et al. Ligelizumab for Chronic Spontaneous Urticaria. *N. Engl. J. Med.* **2019**, *381*, 1321–1332. [CrossRef]
22. Sánchez, J.; Zakzuk, J.; Cardona, R. Evaluation of a Guidelines-Based Approach to the Treatment of Chronic Spontaneous Urticaria. *J. Allergy Clin. Immunol. Pract.* **2018**, *6*, 177–182.e171. [CrossRef] [PubMed]
23. Jörg, L.; Pecaric-Petkovic, T.; Reichenbach, S.; Coslovsky, M.; Stalder, O.; Pichler, W.; Hausmann, O. Double-blind placebo-controlled trial of the effect of omalizumab on basophils in chronic urticaria patients. *Clin. Exp. Allergy* **2018**, *48*, 196–204. [CrossRef] [PubMed]
24. Metz, M.; Staubach, P.; Bauer, A.; Brehler, R.; Gericke, J.; Kangas, M.; Ashton-Chess, J.; Jarvis, P.; Georgiou, P.; Canvin, J.; et al. Clinical efficacy of omalizumab in chronic spontaneous urticaria is associated with a reduction of FcεRI-positive cells in the skin. *Theranostics* **2017**, *7*, 1266–1276. [CrossRef] [PubMed]
25. Hide, M.; Park, H.S.; Igarashi, A.; Ye, Y.M.; Kim, T.B.; Yagami, A.; Roh, J.; Lee, J.H.; Chinuki, Y.; Youn, S.W.; et al. Efficacy and safety of omalizumab in Japanese and Korean patients with refractory chronic spontaneous urticaria. *J. Dermatol. Sci.* **2017**, *87*, 70–78. [CrossRef]
26. Boonpiyathad, T.; Sangasapaviliya, A. Hydroxychloroquine in the treatment of anti-histamine refractory chronic spontaneous urticaria, randomized single-blinded placebo-controlled trial and an open label comparison study. *Eur. Ann. Allergy Clin. Immunol.* **2017**, *49*, 220–224. [CrossRef]
27. Staubach, P.; Metz, M.; Chapman-Rothe, N.; Sieder, C.; Bräutigam, M.; Canvin, J.; Maurer, M. Effect of omalizumab on angioedema in H1 -antihistamine-resistant chronic spontaneous urticaria patients: Results from X-ACT, a randomized controlled trial. *Allergy* **2016**, *71*, 1135–1144. [CrossRef]
28. Harris, J.M.; Cabanski, C.R.; Scheerens, H.; Samineni, D.; Bradley, M.S.; Cochran, C.; Staubach, P.; Metz, M.; Sussman, G.; Maurer, M. A randomized trial of quilizumab in adults with refractory chronic spontaneous urticaria. *J. Allergy Clin. Immunol.* **2016**, *138*, 1730–1732. [CrossRef]
29. Saini, S.S.; Bindslev-Jensen, C.; Maurer, M.; Grob, J.J.; Bülbül Baskan, E.; Bradley, M.S.; Canvin, J.; Rahmaoui, A.; Georgiou, P.; Alpan, O.; et al. Efficacy and safety of omalizumab in patients with chronic idiopathic/spontaneous urticaria who remain symptomatic on H1 antihistamines: A randomized, placebo-controlled study. *J. Investig. Dermatol.* **2015**, *135*, 67–75. [CrossRef]
30. Sharma, V.K.; Singh, S.; Ramam, M.; Kumawat, M.; Kumar, R. A randomized placebo-controlled double-blind pilot study of methotrexate in the treatment of H1 antihistamine-resistant chronic spontaneous urticaria. *Indian J. Dermatol. Venereol. Leprol.* **2014**, *80*, 122–128. [CrossRef]
31. Maurer, M.; Rosén, K.; Hsieh, H.J.; Saini, S.; Grattan, C.; Gimenéz-Arnau, A.; Agarwal, S.; Doyle, R.; Canvin, J.; Kaplan, A.; et al. Omalizumab for the treatment of chronic idiopathic or spontaneous urticaria. *N. Engl. J. Med.* **2013**, *368*, 924–935. [CrossRef]
32. Magerl, M.; Rother, M.; Bieber, T.; Biedermann, T.; Brasch, J.; Dominicus, R.; Hunzelmann, N.; Jakob, T.; Mahler, V.; Popp, G.; et al. Randomized, double-blind, placebo-controlled study of safety and efficacy of miltefosine in antihistamine-resistant chronic spontaneous urticaria. *J. Eur. Acad. Dermatol. Venereol.* **2013**, *27*, e363–e369. [CrossRef] [PubMed]
33. Kaplan, A.; Ledford, D.; Ashby, M.; Canvin, J.; Zazzali, J.L.; Conner, E.; Veith, J.; Kamath, N.; Staubach, P.; Jakob, T.; et al. Omalizumab in patients with symptomatic chronic idiopathic/spontaneous urticaria despite standard combination therapy. *J. Allergy Clin. Immunol.* **2013**, *132*, 101–109. [CrossRef] [PubMed]
34. Vena, G.A.; Cassano, N.; Colombo, D.; Peruzzi, E.; Pigatto, P. Cyclosporine in chronic idiopathic urticaria: A double-blind, randomized, placebo-controlled trial. *J. Am. Acad. Dermatol.* **2006**, *55*, 705–709. [CrossRef] [PubMed]
35. Bagenstose, S.E.; Levin, L.; Bernstein, J.A. The addition of zafirlukast to cetirizine improves the treatment of chronic urticaria in patients with positive autologous serum skin test results. *J. Allergy Clin. Immunol.* **2004**, *113*, 134–140. [CrossRef] [PubMed]
36. Grattan, C.E.; O'Donnell, B.F.; Francis, D.M.; Niimi, N.; Barlow, R.J.; Seed, P.T.; Kobza Black, A.; Greaves, M.W. Randomized double-blind study of cyclosporin in chronic 'idiopathic' urticaria. *Br. J. Dermatol.* **2000**, *143*, 365–372. [CrossRef] [PubMed]
37. Morgan, M.; Cooke, A.; Rogers, L.; Adams-Huet, B.; Khan, D.A. Double-blind placebo-controlled trial of dapsone in antihistamine refractory chronic idiopathic urticaria. *J. Allergy Clin. Immunol. Pract.* **2014**, *2*, 601–606. [CrossRef] [PubMed]
38. Erbagci, Z. The leukotriene receptor antagonist montelukast in the treatment of chronic idiopathic urticaria: A single-blind, placebo-controlled, crossover clinical study. *J. Allergy Clin. Immunol.* **2002**, *110*, 484–488. [CrossRef]
39. Chen, V.; Akhtar, S.; Zheng, C.; Kumaresan, V.; Nouri, K. Assessment of Changes in Diversity in Dermatology Clinical Trials Between 2010–2015 and 2015–2020: A Systematic Review. *JAMA Dermatol.* **2022**, *158*, 288–292. [CrossRef]

40. CHORD COUSIN Collaboration. The Cochrane Skin-Core Outcome Set Initiative (CS-COUSIN). Available online: http://cs-cousin.org/ (accessed on 17 July 2022).
41. Dodd, S.; Clarke, M.; Becker, L.; Mavergames, C.; Fish, R.; Williamson, P.R. A taxonomy has been developed for outcomes in medical research to help improve knowledge discovery. *J. Clin. Epidemiol.* **2018**, *96*, 84–92. [CrossRef]

MDPI AG
Grosspeteranlage 5
4052 Basel
Switzerland
Tel.: +41 61 683 77 34

Pharmaceuticals Editorial Office
E-mail: pharmaceuticals@mdpi.com
www.mdpi.com/journal/pharmaceuticals

www.ingramcontent.com/pod-product-compliance
Lightning Source LLC
Chambersburg PA
CBHW062037220926
51850CB00010B/2578